Lecture Notes on
Clinical Medicine

KU-465-823

Lecture Notes on Clinical Medicine

DAVID RUBENSTEIN
M.A. M.D. F.R.C.P. (Lond.)
Physician, Addenbrooke's Hospital,
Cambridge

DAVID WAYNE
M.A. B.M. F.R.C.P. (Lond. & Edin.)
Physician, James Paget
District General Hospital,
Gorleston, Great Yarmouth

FOURTH EDITION

OXFORD

BLACKWELL SCIENTIFIC PUBLICATIONS

LONDON EDINBURGH BOSTON

MELBOURNE PARIS BERLIN VIENNA

©1976, 1980, 1985, 1991 by
Blackwell Scientific Publications
Editorial Offices:
Osney Mead, Oxford OX2 0EL
25 John Street, London WC1N 2BL
23 Ainslie Place, Edinburgh EH3 6AJ
3 Cambridge Center, Cambridge,
  Massachusetts 02142, USA
54 University Street, Carlton
  Victoria 3053, Australia

Other Editorial Offices:
Arnette SA
2, rue Casimir-Delavigne
75006 Paris
France

Blackwell Wissenschaft
Meinekestrasse 4
D–1000 Berlin 15
Germany

Blackwell MZV
Feldgasse 13
A–1238 Wein
Austria

All rights reserved. No part of this publication
may be reproduced, stored in a retrieval system,
or transmitted, in any form or by any means,
electronic, mechanical, photocopying, recording or otherwise without the prior permission of
the copyright owner

First published 1976
Reprinted 1977, 1978, 1979
Second edition 1980
Reprinted 1981, 1982, 1983, 1984
Third edition 1985
Reprinted 1986, 1987, 1990
Portuguese translation 1981
Spanish translation 1984
German translation 1986
Fourth edition 1991
Four Dragons edition 1991

Set by Times Graphics Ltd, Singapore
Printed and bound in Great Britain
by Hartnolls Ltd, Bodmin, Cornwall

DISTRIBUTORS

Marston Book Services Ltd
PO Box 87
Oxford OX2 0DT
(Orders: Tel. 0865 791155
        Fax: 0865 791927
        Telex: 837515)

USA
  Mosby–Year Book, Inc.
  11830 Westline Industrial Drive
  St Louis, Missouri 63146
  (Orders: Tel: (800) 633–6699)

Canada
  Mosby–Year Book, Inc.
  5240 Finch Avenue East
  Scarborough, Ontario
  (Orders: Tel: (416) 298–1588)

Australia
  Blackwell Scientific Publications
  (Australia) Pty Ltd
  54 University Street
  Carlton, Victoria 3053
  (Orders: Tel: (03) 347–0300)

British Library
Cataloguing in Publication Data

Rubenstein, David 1939–
  Lecture notes on clinical medicine.—4th. ed.
  1. Man. Diseases
  I. Title II. Wayne, David
  616
ISBN 0–632–02780–0 (BSP)
ISBN 0–632–03073–9 (Four Dragons)

Contents

Cardiovascular system, 62

Arterial pulse: volume and character. Neck veins: raised jugular venous pressure. Heart: difficult systolic murmurs, continuous murmurs, heart failure. Hypertension. Myocardial infarction. Cardiac arrest. Cardiac arrhythmias. Electrocardiograms: interpretation, electrocardiographic deflections, special patterns, sample electrocardiograms, notes, mean frontal QRS axis. Echocardiography: mitral valve disease, aortic valve disease, cardiomyopathy. Cardiac pressure studies. Cardiac radionucleide studies

Haematology, 91

Anaemia. Blood count: notes. Skin haemorrhage. Coagulation defects: notes. Lymphadenopathy

Diabetes, 102

Management: diet, drugs, assessment of diabetic control, insulin resistance, symptoms of poor control. Examination. Screening in diabetes. Diabetes and pregnancy. Diabetes and illness. Diabetes and surgery. Diabetes and driving

Skin, 109

History. Examination

PART 2: ESSENTIAL BACKGROUND INFORMATION

Neurology, 113

Headache. Unilateral facial pain: migraine, cluster headaches, neuralgias, temporal arteritis, atypical facial pain, unilateral pain. Cerebrovascular disease: 'strokes', transient ischaemic attacks, lateral medullary syndrome, extracerebral haemorrhage. Brain death. Epilepsy. Narcolepsy. Multiple sclerosis. Motor neurone disease. Parkinson's disease and extrapyramidal disorders: Parkinson's disease, hepatolenticular degeneration, chorea. Cerebral tumours: symptoms and signs, acoustic neuroma, benign intracranial hypertension. Peripheral neuropathy. Brachial neuralgia. Mononeuritis multiplex. Hereditary ataxias: Friedreich's ataxia, cerebellar degenerations, hereditary spastic paraplegia. Meningitis: meningococcal meningitis, pneumococcal meningitis, *Haemophilus influenzae* meningitis, acute bacterial meningitis of unknown cause, tuberculous meningitis. Intracranial abscess. Acute postinfective polyneuropathy. Poliomyelitis. Syphilis of the nervous system.
Disorders of spinal cord: syringomyelia, syringobulbia, subacute combined degeneration of the cord, peroneal muscular atrophy, cord compression, cervical spondylosis. Disorders of muscles: mixed connective tissue disease, polymyositis and allied disorders, myasthenia gravis, myotonia, muscular dystrophies.
Psychiatry: depression, mania, anxiety, hysteria, acute confusional states, dementia, schizophrenia

Connective tissue and rheumatic diseases, 161

Systemic lupus erythematosus. Polyarteritis nodosa. Dermatomyositis. Polymyositis. Scleroderma (systemic sclerosis). Mixed connective tissue disease. Polymyalgia rheumatica. Temporal arteritis (giant cell arteritis, cranial arteritis). Organ-specific autoimmune disease. Rheumatoid arthritis. Diseases resembling rheumatoid arthritis: Still's disease, Sjögren's syndrome, Felty's syndrome, psoriatic arthritis. Ankylosing spondylitis (sacroiliitis). Reiter's syndrome. Acute generalised arthritis: Still's disease—juvenile form. Acute rheumatic fever. Postinfectious arthralgia. Osteoarthritis

Endocrine disease, 179

Thyroid: non-toxic goitre, thyrotoxicosis (hyperthyroidism), hypothyroidism, autoimmune thyroiditis, acute thyroiditis, thyroid cancer. Pituitary: hypopituitarism (Simmond's disease), acromegaly, diabetes insipidus, prolactinoma. Adrenal: adrenal glands, Cushing's syndrome, Conn's syndrome (primary hyperaldosteronism), adrenogenital syndrome, adrenal insufficiency (Addison's disease), phaeochromocytoma, multiple endocrine adenomatosis (MEA syndrome). Shortness of stature

Metabolic disease, 198

Diabetes mellitus: diabetic coma, diabetes in surgery and in pregnancy. Carcinoid syndrome. Porphyria. Hyperlipidaemia: classification of particles, classification of diseases. Metabolic bone disease: osteoporosis, osteomalacia and rickets, uraemic bone disease (renal osteodystrophy), Paget's diease. Endocrine bone disease: osteogenesis imperfecta, hyperparathyroidism, hypoparathyroidism. Hypercalcaemia. Gout and hyperuricaemia. Nutrition: obesity, malnutrition, anorexia nervosa

Renal disease, 229

Proteinuria. Nephrotic syndrome. Haematuria. Acute renal failure (acute uraemia). Chronic renal failure (chronic uraemia). Glomerulonephritis: acute streptococcal glomerulonephritis (acute nephritic syndrome). Urinary tract infection. Chronic interstitial nephritis. Polycystic kidney disease. Hepatorenal syndrome. Haemolytic uraemic syndrome (diffuse intravascular coagulation). Fluids and electrolytes: salt and water depletion, water excess, hypokalaemia, hyperkalaemia, metabolic acidosis, hyperaldosteronism, hypercalcaemia, hypocalcaemia, hypomagnesaemia

Liver disease, 249

Acute hepatitis: acute viral hepatitis. Chronic hepatitis: chronic persistent hepatitis, chronic lobular hepatitis, chronic active hepatitis. Alcoholic hepatitis. Cirrhosis: hepatocellular failure (chronic), portal hypertension, management of ascites in cirrhosis, Budd–Chiari syndrome. Rare cirrhoses: idiopathic haemochromatosis (bronzed diabetes), hepatolenticular degeneration (Wilson's disease). Drug jaundice: hypersensitivity reactions, direct hepatotoxicity, haemolytic jaundice

Gastroenterology, 260

Gastric and duodenal ulceration. Endocrine tumours of the gut: apudomas, Zollinger–Ellison syndrome, other endocrine tumours of the gut. Gastrointestinal haemorrhage: upper gut, lower gut. Reflux oesophagitis. Ulcerative colitis. Crohn's disease (regional enteritis). Steatorrhoea and malabsorption: gluten-sensitive enteropathy (coeliac disease), other causes of malabsorption. Diverticular disease. Irritable bowel syndrome (irritable colon; spastic colon; nervous colon; mucous colitis). Ischaemic colitis. Pancreas: carcinoma, acute pancreatitis, chronic pancreatitis. Gall bladder: acute cholecystitis, chronic cholecystitis, gallstones

Respiratory disease, 282

Chronic bronchitis and emphysema. Bronchiectasis. Cystic fibrosis. Asthma: severe asthma. Respiratory failure: acute on chronic respiratory failure. Acute anaphylaxis. Pneumonia: bronchopneumonia, lobar pneumonia, other bacterial pneumonias, recurrent bacterial pneumonia, viral pneumonia, mycoplasma pneumonia, opportunistic infection of the lungs, aspiration pneumonia, lung abscess. Carcinoma of the bronchus. Bronchial adenoma. Sarcoidosis. Tuberculosis: primary tuberculosis, post-primary tuberculosis. Occupational lung diseases: dust diseases; asthma, extrinsic allergic alveolitis, irritant gases. Pulmonary embolism. Pneumothorax. Hyperventilation syndrome. Fibrosing alveolitis (diffuse interstitial pulmonary fibrosis). Adult respiratory distress syndrome (ARDs, shock lung)

Cardiovascular disease, 308

Ischaemic heart disease: factors associated with coronary athero-sclerosis: angina, myocardial infarction. Heart failure. Hypertension. Valvular heart disease: mitral stenosis, mitral regurgitation, aortic stenosis, aortic regurgitation, tricuspid regurgitation, pulmonary stenosis, atrial myxoma. Congenital heart disease: working classifica-tion, artial septal defect, patent ductus arteriosus, ventricular septal defect, Fallot's tetralogy, pulmonary stenosis, coarctation of the aorta, Eisenmenger's syndrome. Infective endocarditis: acute, subacute, 'culture-negative endocarditis'. Acute pericarditis. Constrictive pericarditis. Syphilitic aortitis and carditis. Cardiomyopathy: hypertrophic cardiomyopathy, dilated (congestive) cardiomyopathy, restrictive cardiomyopathy. Peripheral arterial disease: intermittent claudication, acute obstruction, ischaemic foot, Raynaud's phenomenon

Dermatology, 344

Primary skin disorders: psoriasis, lichen planus, pityriasis rosea, dermatitis and eczema, acne vulgaris, rosacea. Fungus infections: candidiasis (monilia, thrush), pityriasis versicolor, ringworm (tinea), treatment of dermatophytes in general. Drug eruptions: urticarial reactions, purpura, other disorders. Skin manifestations of systemic disease: erythema nodosum, Lyme disease (erythema chronicum migrans), haemolytic streptococcal infection, malignancy, xanthomatosis, other rare manifestations. Mucosal ulceration: Behçet's disease. Bullous lesions: dermatitis herpetiformis, pemphigus vulgaris, pemphigoid, erythema multiforme, skin pigmentation

Haematology, 355

Anaemia: classification, iron deficiency anaemia, B_{12} and folic acid deficiency, pernicious anaemia, haemolytic anaemia, paroxysmal nocturnal haemoglobinuria, marrow aplasia. Leukaemias: acute lymphatic leukaemia, chronic lymphatic leukaemia, acute myeloid leukaemia, chronic myeloid leukaemia. Multiple myelomatosis. Hodgkin's disease. Non-Hodgkin's lymphoma. Infectious mononucleosis. Postviral syndrome

Drug overdoses, 368

Clinical presentation, management

Imported diseases and infections, 373

Imported diseases. Malaria. Typhoid. Dysentery: bacillary dysentery, amoebic dysentery. Giardiasis. Pyrexia of unknown origin. Other imported pathogens: nematodes, schistosomes. Septicaemia (bacteriaemia): post-operative bacteriaemia. Infections in the immunocompromised. AIDS (acquired immune deficiency syndrome).

Recommended reading, 387

Journals
General texts
Specialist texts

SI units conversion table, 390

Index, 391

Preface to the fourth edition

It is now 6 years since the third edition was published. We have revised the book extensively but have kept the basic structure unchanged. Where fields have changed markedly, we have covered them in more detail. As in previous editions, we have asked colleagues to read through the revised chapters.

Readers:
Renal disease—John Bradley
Respiratory disease—David Ellis
Infections—Mark Farrington
Connective tissue and rheumatic diseases—Peter Forster
Dermatology—Tina Green
Endocrinology—Philip Heyburn
Metabolism—Philip Heyburn
Gastroenterology—Stuart Hishon
Liver disease—Stuart Hishon
Cardiovascular disease—Kim Priestley
Neurology—A. K. Vishnau
Haematology—Jennifer Wimperis

We are much indebted to them for their patience and expertise. If you find errors—for which we must be responsible—please write and tell us. Our thanks are due to those readers who have written to us in the past. Again, the late Sir Edward Wayne read the text and made many valuable suggestions.

We have made every effort to ensure that the advice and information contained in this book is accurate at the date of going to press. Dosage recommendations change frequently so please check doses in the current edition of the *British National Formulary* before prescribing.

David Rubenstein
David Wayne

Preface to the first edition

This book is intended primarily for the junior hospital doctor in the period between qualification and the examination for Membership of the Royal Colleges of Physicians. We think that it will also be helpful to final year medical students and to clinicians reading for higher specialist qualifications in surgery and anaesthetics.

The hospital doctor must not only acquire a large amount of factual information but also use it effectively in the clinical situation. The experienced physician has acquired some clinical perspective through practice: we hope that this book imparts some of this to the relatively inexperienced. The format and contents are designed for the examination candidate but the same approach to problems should help the hospital doctor in his everyday work.

The book as a whole is not suitable as a first reader for the undergraduate because it assumes much basic knowledge and considerable detailed information has had to be omitted. It is not intended to be a complete textbook of medicine and the information it contains must be supplemented by further reading. The contents are intended only as lecture notes and the margins of the pages are intentionally large so that the reader may easily add additional material of his own.

The book is divided into two parts: *the clinical approach* and *essential background information*. In the first part we have considered the situation which a candidate meets in the clinical part of an examination or a physician in the clinic. This part of the book thus resembles a manual on techniques of physical examination, though it is more specifically intended to help the candidate carry out an examiner's request to perform a specific examination. It has been our experience in listening to candidates' performances in examinations and hearing the examiner's subsequent assessment, that it is the failure of a candidate to examine cases systematically and his failure to behave as if he were used to doing this every day of his clinical life that leads to adverse comments.

In the second part of the book a summary of basic clinical facts is given in the conventional way. We have included most common diseases but not all, and we have tried to emphasise points which are understressed in many textbooks. Accounts are given of many conditions which are relatively rare. It is necessary for the clinician to know about these and to be on the lookout for them both in the clinic and in examinations. Supplementary reading is essential to understand their basic pathology but the information we give is probably all that need be remembered by the non-specialist reader and will provide adequate working knowledge in a clinical situation. It should not be forgotten that some rare diseases are of great importance in practice because they are treatable or preventable, e.g. infective endocarditis, hepatolenticular degeneration, attacks of acute porphyria. Some conditions are important to examination candidates because patients are ambulant and appear commonly in examinations, e.g. neurosyphilis, syringomyelia, atrial and ventricular septal defects.

We have not attempted to cover the whole of medicine but by cross-referencing between the two sections of the book and giving information in summary form we have completely omitted few subjects. Some highly special-ised fields such as the treatment of leukaemia were thought unsuitable for inclusion.

A short account of psychiatry is given in the section on neurology since many patients with mental illness attend general clinics and it is hoped that readers may be warned of gaps in their knowledge of this important field. The section on dermatology is incomplete but should serve for quick revision of common skin disorders.

Wherever possible we have tried to indicate the relative frequency with which various conditions are likely to be seen in hospital practice in this country and have selected those clinical features which in our view are most commonly seen and where possible have listed them in order of importance. The frequency with which a disease is encountered by any individual physician will depend upon its prevalence in the district from which his cases are drawn and also on his known special interests. Nevertheless rare conditions are rarely seen; at least in the clinic. Examinations, however, are a 'special case'.

We have used many generally accepted abbreviations, e.g. ECG, ESR, and have included them in the index instead of suppling a glossary.

Despite our best efforts, some errors of fact may have been included. As with every book and authority, question and check everything—and please write to us if you wish.

We should like to thank all those who helped us with producing this book and in particular. Sir Edward Wayne and Sir Graham Bull who have kindly allowed us to benefit from their extensive experience both in medicine and in examining for the Colleges of Physicians.

David Rubenstein
David Wayne
November 1975

Part 1
The clinical approach

Nervous system

The candidate is usually asked to examine a specific area, e.g. *'Examine the cranial nerves', 'Examine the lower limbs', 'Examine the arms'* or *'Examine the eyes'*. By far the commonest neurological disorders suitable for a clinical examination are multiple sclerosis and the results of cerebrovascular disease. Diabetes is a common disorder which fairly frequently gives rise to neurological manifestations. Carcinomatous neuropathy should always be considered when the signs are difficult to synthesise. Parkinsonism is relatively common. Motor neurone disease (MND), myopathies, myasthenia gravis and the neurological manifestations of vitamin B_{12} deficiency are all rare in practice but more frequently seen in examinations. Neurosyphilis is becoming progressively rarer—the patient will belong to the prepenicillin era, i.e. be over 50 years old.

In terms of examination technique the practising physician must examine case after case, both normal and abnormal, until he has developed a system which is rapid, accurate and second nature to him. An appearance of professionalism in your neurological examination may encourage the examiner to take a less unfavourable view of minor errors than he might if you appear hesitant, clumsy or imprecise. Analysis of clinical signs is improved if you can remember some anatomical diagrams (pages 5, 6, 117, 118 and 122)

CRANIAL NERVES
'Examine the cranial nerves'
Many abnormalities of the cranial nerves are the results of chronic disease and patients with them are commonly seen in examinations.

The commonest disorders in examinations are multiple sclerosis (optic atrophy, nystagmus [often ataxic], cerebellar dysarthria), stroke, and Bell's palsy. The manifestation of cerebral tumour, aneurysm, syphilis, dystrophia myotonica and myasthenia gravis are seen much less frequently. It is useful to memorise diagrams of cross-sections of the brain-stem and one of the floor of the fourth ventricle (page 6) since these may greatly improve analysis of a cranial nerve lesion. Do not spend long on the first or second cranial nerves unless there is good reason to suspect an abnormality. If the optic fundus is abnormal, the examiner is likely to ask you to look at it specifically. Eye movements must be carefully examined. Do not confuse ptosis (third nerve or sympathetic) with paresis of the orbicularis oculi (seventh nerve). Make sure you can explain clearly and concisely the difference between an upper and lower motor neurone (UMN and LMN) lesion of the seventh nerve. The corneal reflex is an essential part of the complete examination of the cranial nerves.

The following approach is recommended:

Smell

'*Has there been any recent change in your sense of smell?*' If so, test formally with fresh 'smell bottles' (e.g. freshly ground coffee or instant coffee granules). Colds and sinusitis are the most likely cause.

Eyes

Observe, and test when necessary, for:
- *visual acuity* either quickly with literature from the bedside locker, or formally with Snellen's charts
- *ptosis*

Third nerve lesion (complete or partial ptosis).

Sympathetic lesion (partial ptosis) as part of Horner's syndrome. Muscle weakness of myasthenia gravis (and rarely, dystrophia myotonica, facio-scapulo-humeral dystrophy, congenital and in tabo-paresis).

NB   Ptosis is not due to a seventh nerve lesion.
- *pupillary responses* (page 9)
- *visual fields* to confrontation (second nerve) (page 5)
- *external ocular movements* (third, fourth and sixth nerves) (pages 7 and 8) and *nystagmus* (page 11)
- *the fundi* (second nerve)(page 30)

Face (seventh nerve)

- '*Screw up your eyes very tightly.*' Compare how deeply the eyelashes are buried on the two sides. Unilateral weakness is invariably due to a lower motor neurone lesion
- '*Grin.*' Compare the nasolabial grooves

Mouth

- '*Clench your teeth*' (fifth nerve, motor). Feel the masseters and test the jaw jerk if indicated. The jaw jerk is obtained from placing one finger horizontally across the front of the jaw and tapping the finger with a tendon hammer with the jaw relaxed and the mouth just open. An increased jaw jerk occurs in upper motor neurone lesions of the fifth cranial nerve (pseudobulbar palsy, page 14)
- '*Open your mouth and keep it open*' (fifth nerve, motor: pterygoids). You should not be able to force it closed. With a unilateral lesion, the jaw deviates towards the weaker side (the weak muscle cannot keep it open)
- '*Say aaah*'(ninth and tenth nerves) both mixed, but the ninth is mainly sensory for the pharynx and palate, and the tenth for motor. Normally the uvula and soft palate move upwards and remain central and the posterior pharyngeal wall moves a little. With a unilateral lesion the soft palate is pulled away from the weaker side (there may also be 'curtain movement' of the posterior pharyngeal wall away from the weaker side)
- '*Put your tongue out*' (twelfth nerve). Look for wasting, fasciculation and

whether it protrudes to one side (towards the weaker side since the weaker muscle cannot push it out)

Neck (eleventh nerve)
- 'Lift your head off the pillows' or 'Put your chin on your right (or left) shoulder' while you resist the movement. Look at, and palpate the sternomastoids. 'Shrug your shoulders' while you push them down. Look at and palpate the bulk of trapezius

Ears (eighth nerve)

Test hearing by whispering in each ear and perform Weber and Rinne tests (page 10). You should ask for an auriscope if indicated. The commonest cause of conductive (air conduction) deafness is wax

Facial sensation (fifth nerve)

Test the three divisions on both sides with cotton wool. Check the corneal reflexes (often the first clinical deficit in fifth nerve lesions). Ask the patient if the sensation is equally unpleasant on the two sides.

NB   It is frequently helpful to be able to draw cross-sections of the spinal cord and brain-stem when considering lesions in those areas (figures 1–3).

Field defects

In principle you are comparing the patient's visual fields with your own. When testing his right eye, he should be level with you and look straight into your left eye with his head held at arm's length. 'Keep looking at my eye and tell me when you first see my finger out of the corner of your eye.' Then bring your finger towards the centre of the field of vision from the four main directions (right, left, up, down). It is preferable to use a white-headed hat pin if you have one. The nasal and superior fields are limited by the nose and eyebrow respectively but this is not often of clinical importance. Field defects are described by the side of the visual field which is lost, i.e. temporal field loss

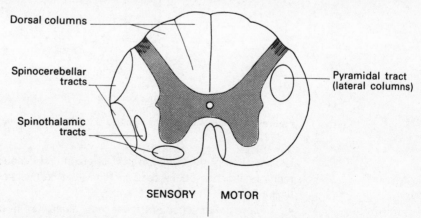

Figure 1.   Cross-section through spinal cord.

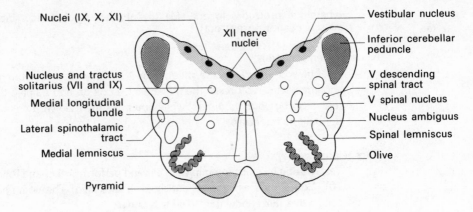

Figure 2.   Cross-section through open medulla.

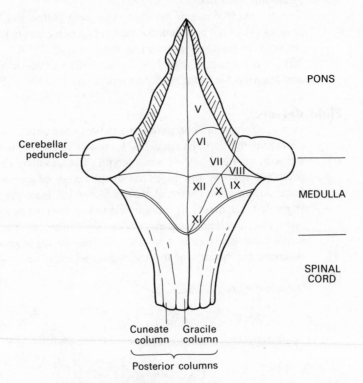

Figure 3.   Floor of the fourth ventricle showing cranial nerve nuclei.

indicates loss of the temporal field of vision and denotes damage to the nasal retina or its connections back to the visual cortex. Perimetry will accurately define defects.

• *Temporal hemianopia* in one eye alone or in both eyes (bitemporal hemianopia) suggests a chiasmal compression usually from a pituitary tumour

- *Homonymous hemianopia,* i.e. loss of nasal field in one eye and temporal field in the other. This may occur with any postchiasmal lesion, commonly following a posterior cerebral vascular lesion (usually with macular sparing). The side of the field loss is opposite to the side of the damaged cortex (i.e. a right-sided cerebral lesion produces a left homonymous hemianopia)
- *Upper quadrantic field loss* suggests a temporal lesion of the opposite cortex or optic radiation. It is homonymous
- *Central scotoma.* Loss of vision in the centre of the visual field is detected by passing a small-diameter white- or red-tipped pin across the front of the eyes which are held looking forward. This occurs in acute retrobulbar neuritis most commonly due to multiple sclerosis
- Test for visual inattention by presenting the stimulus simultaneously to both eyes

Blindness

A history of transient blindness, total or partial (with specific field defects usually in one eye) is not uncommon in migraine. It may also follow arteriography and carotid transient ischaemic attacks.

Sudden blindness also occurs with:
- retinal detachment
- acute glaucoma
- vitreous haemorrhage in diabetes
- temporal arteritis and retinal artery or vein obstruction
- fractures of the skull
- raised intracranial pressure

NB   The light reflex is absent except in cortical blindness.

Senile changes and *glaucoma* account for about two-thirds of blindness in this country. Diabetes is the major non-ocular (systemic) cause (7–10%) due chiefly to vitreous haemorrhage and cataract. Trachoma is a common cause on a world-wide basis. *Hysterical blindness* is uncommon and should never be confidently assumed.

The blindness of *temporal arteritis* is preventable if steroid therapy is started in time.

Eye movements

These are controlled by the third, fourth and sixth nerves and conjugate movement integrated by the medial longitudinal bundle. This connects the above nuclei together and to the cerebellum and the vestibular nuclei.

Squint (Strabismus)

Congenital concomitant squints are present from childhood and are due to a defect of one eye. The angle between the longitudinal axes of the eyes remains constant on testing extraocular movements, and there is no diplopia.

Paralytic squint is acquired and results from paralysis of one or more of the muscles which move the eye, or paralysis from proptosis. On testing external ocular movements, the angle between the eye axes varies and there is diplopia.

The following rules should be borne in mind:

1 Diplopia is maximum when looking in the direction of action of the paralysed muscle.

2 The image further from the midline arises from the 'paralysed' eye. This may be determined by covering up each eye in turn and asking which image has disappeared.

NB It is sometimes easier to test movements in each eye separately.

'Do you see double?'

If so, ask him in which direction it is worst, move your forefinger in that direction and then ask him if the two fingers which he sees are parallel to each other (lateral rectus palsy: sixth nerve) or at an angle (superior oblique palsy: fourth nerve). If he has not noticed diplopia, test the movements formally, right and left, up and down, and note if there is any nystagmus.

Apart from local lesions such as pressure from tumour or aneurysm, isolated external ocular palsies may result from diabetes mellitus (ischaemia), multiple sclerosis, migraine, raised intracranial pressure, mononeuritis multiplex (e.g. polyarteriti), sarcoidosis, syphilis (ischaemia) and meningitis (usually tuberculosis or pneumococcal).

Lateral rectus palsy (sixth nerve)

This produces failure of lateral movement with convergent strabismus. It is the commonest external ocular palsy. The diplopia is maximal on looking to the affected side. The images are parallel and separated horizontally. The outermost image comes from the affected eye and disappears when that eye is covered. The palsy is produced as a false localising sign in raised intracranial pressure or by direct involvement with tumour, aneurysm, or rarely with acoustic neuroma (page 135).

Superior oblique palsy (fourth nerve)

This type is rare. Palsy produces diplopia maximal on downward gaze. The two images are then at an angle to each other when the palsied eye is abducted and one above the other when the eye is adducted. The diplopia is therefore noticed most on reading or descending stairs.

Third nerve palsy

It may not present with diplopia because there may be complete ptosis. When the lid is lifted the eye is seen to be 'down and out' (divergent strabismus) and there is severe (angulated) diplopia. The pupil may be dilated. It occurs with space-occupying lesions, brain-stem vascular lesions (Weber's syndrome) after surgery (e.g. for pituitary lesions) and aneurysm of the posterior communicating artery (painful).

The muscles themselves are involved in myasthenia gravis and in the ophthalmoplegia of thyrotoxicosis (particularly looking up and out).

Pupillary reflexes

The balance between parasympathetic (constrictor) and sympathetic (dilator tone controls pupil size.

Constriction of the pupil in response to light is relayed via the optic nerve, optic tract, lateral geniculate nuclei, the Edinger–Westphal nucleus of the third nerve and the ciliary ganglion. The cortex is not involved.

Constriction of the pupil with accommodation. Convergence originates within the cortex and is relayed to the pupil via the third nerve nuclei. The optic nerve and tract and the lateral geniculate nucleus are not involved.
   Therefore:
• if the direct light reflex is absent and the convergence reflex is present, a local lesion in the brain-stem or ciliary ganglion is implied possibly due to degeneration in the ciliary ganglia, e.g. Argyll Robertson pupil
• if the convergence reflex is absent and the light reflex is present, a lesion of the cerebral cortex is implied, e.g. cortical blindness
   Examination of the pupillary reflexes should be performed in subdued light. The pupil should be positively inspected for irregularity. A torch is flashed twice at each eye (once for direct and once for consensual responses), preferably from the side so that the patient does not focus on it (and hence have an accommodation-convergence reflex).

If the pupil is constricted consider: Horner's syndrome (below); morphine; pilocarpine; pontine haemorrhage; Argyll Robertson pupil (must be irregular and have no light reflex). It also occurs in old age.

If the pupil is dilated consider: mydriatics (e.g. homatropine, tropicamide or cyclopentolate); a third nerve lesion; the Holmes–Adie syndrome (pupils constrict sluggishly to light, e.g. in half an hour in a bright room, and absent tendon reflexes); and congenital (ask the patient). In the unconscious patient a fixed dilated pupil (third nerve lesion) may indicate temporal lobe herniation (from raised intracranial pressure) on the same side, intracranial bleeding, tumour or abscess.

Horner's syndrome

This is rare in practice but common in examinations. The syndrome comprises unilateral:
• ptosis (partial, i.e. sympathetic)
• miosis (constricted pupil) with normal reactions
• anhidrosis (decreased sweating over face)
• enophthalmos (indrawing of orbital contents)
i.e. everything gets smaller or contracts.
The syndrome results from lesions of the sympathetic nerves to the eye, anywhere from the hypothalamus downwards through the sympathetic nucleus of the brain-stem and during their passage through the cervical and upper

thoracic cord, the anterior spinal first thoracic root, the sympathetic chain, stellate ganglion and carotid sympathetic plexus. It is essential to look for evidence of a T1 lesion (page 26) and to palpate the neck and supraclavicular fossae for malignant glands.

Aetiology

Carcinoma of the bronchus (T1, Pancoast tumour).

Cervical node secondary deposits.

Cervical sympathectomy (look for the scar)

Brain-stem vascular disease (lateral medullary syndrome, page 120) and demyelinating disease.

Local neoplasms and trauma in the neck.

Rarely carotid or aortic aneurysms.

Very rarely syringomyelia and intrinsic cervical cord disease (vascular and neoplastic).

Hearing

Roughly assess auditory acuity in each ear in succession, by blocking the sound in the other ear with a restless finger tip, and then whisper at arm's length. Compare the ears. A clockwork watch is a suitable alternative—if available.

Weber test

A vibrating tuning fork is held in the middle of the forehead. In the absence of nerve deafness, the sound is louder in the ear where air conduction is impaired, e.g. wax or otitis media. (This can easily be tested by placing a vibrating tuning fork on one's own forehead and putting a finger in one ear.)

Rinne test

Air conduction is normally better than bone conduction. The vibrating tuning fork is first placed behind the ear on the mastoid process and then rapidly held with its prongs in line with the external meatus. The patient is asked 'Is it louder behind (with the tuning fork on the mastoid) or in front (with the tuning fork in line with the external meatus)?' Normally it is louder in front—this is termed Rinne positive. Negative is abnormal and implies conductive (air) deafness in that ear—usually wax.

Dizziness and giddiness

Dizziness and giddiness are very common neurological presenting features.

The important clinical observation is to determine whether there is true vertigo or not (see below). If this is present, it strongly suggests a disorder of the brain-stem (vascular or demyelinating) or its vestibular connections, e.g. labyrinthitis, Menière's disease (see below). Dizziness or unsteadiness without vertigo, particularly if intermittent, may suggest postural hypotension—which is relatively common in the elderly, in those on over-enthusiastic hypotensive regimes and in those who stand stationary too long particularly in warm weather. It may also suggest a cardiovascular disorder such as a transient cardiac arrhythmia including heart block, or, less commonly, aortic stenosis or emboli e.g. from carotid artery stenosis. Transient dizzy sensations may very rarely be a feature of temporal lobe epilepsy (page 125). Usually no organic cause is found and the complaint may be a marker of emotional distress.

NB   'Something wrong with the brain, think of the heart.'

Vertigo

Vertigo refers to unsteadiness with a subjective sensation of rotation of the patient or of the environment around him. Vertigo results from disease of the inner ear, eighth cranial nerve or its connections in the brain-stem.

Labyrinthine. Menière's disease, acute labyrinthitis.
Eighth nerve. Acoustic neuroma and other posterior fossa tumours, aminoglycosides (streptomycin and gentamicin).
Brain-stem. Neoplasm, vascular disease (vertebrobasilar ischaemia, lateral medullary syndrome), demyelination (multiple sclerosis), migraine, aneurysms, degeneration (syringobulbia).

Menière's disease

The onset is usually in people over 40 years old with progressive deafness and tinnitus usually only in one ear. There are attacks of vertigo, nausea and vomiting. Attacks cease when deafness is complete. Progression may be so slow that this may never occur. Examination shows a defect of eighth nerve conduction and abnormal results to caloric tests of vestibular function. Nystagmus is present during attacks of vertigo.

Treatment

Phenothiazines (e.g. prochlorperazine, thiethylperazine) and some antihistamines (e.g. promethazine) act as sedatives and against nausea during acute episodes. They may reduce the incidence and severity of attacks. Betahistine, a histamine analogue, may specifically help in this condition by reducing endolymph pressure. If very severe, ultrasonic destruction of the labyrinth should be considered, though it results in total deafness on that side.

Nystagmus

Nystagmus may result from any disturbance of either the eighth nerve and its connections in the brain-stem or the cerebellum, and in phenytoin intoxication. Its direction is named after the quick phase (or 'saw-tooth' nystagmus). Nystagmus is usually more pronounced when the patient looks in the direction of the quick phase. Nystagmoid jerks may be produced in normal eyes by errors of examination technique: either holding the object too close to the patient or too far to one side.

Horizontal nystagmus

Vestibular nystagmus occurs following damage to the inner ear, eighth nerve or to its brain-stem connections and is present only in the first few weeks after the damage because central compensation occurs. It is greater on looking *away* from the side of a destructive lesion. It may be caused by acute viral labyrinthitis, acute alcoholism, Menière's disease, middle ear disease and surgery. It is usually associated with vertigo and often with vomitting, deafness and tinnitus. Multiple sclerosis, basilar artery ischaemia, and syringobulbia cause less constitutional upset.

Cerebellar nystagmus usually occurs with lateral lobe lesions: even central (vermis) lesions causing severe truncal ataxia may cause no nystagmus. Since cerebellar disease is frequently bilateral, nystagmus may occur to both sides. If it is unilateral it is greater *towards* the side of the destructive lesion.

Cerebellar lesions occur in multiple sclerosis, hereditary ataxias and vascular disease.

Nystagmus is often seen in patients who have taken high doses (though often within the therapeutic range) of sedative drugs, especially phenytoin and barbiturates.

Ataxic nystagmus. The degree of nystagmus in the abducting eye is greater than in the adducting eye, which may fail to adduct completely. This is virtually pathognomonic of multiple sclerosis and is due to damage to the medial longitudinal bundle.

Vertical nystagmus

The direction of jerks is vertical. Vertical gaze usually makes it more pronounced. It may be produced by sedative drugs (especially phenytoin) but otherwise localises disease to the brain-stem (although brain-stem disorders more commonly produce horizontal nystagmus).

Pendular and rotary nystagmus

Unlike all the above, the phases of the nystagmus are equal in duration. It is secondary to an inability to fix objects and focus with one or both eyes due to partial blindness, e.g. albinism, coal miners.

Facial palsy

In unilateral upper motor neurone lesions (e.g. stroke) movements of the upper face are retained because it is represented on both sides of the cerebral cortex. The flattened forehead and sagging lower eyelid are seen in complete lower motor neurone lesions (e.g. Bell's palsy and middle ear surgery). Taste sensation from the tongue in the chorda tympani leaves the facial nerve in the middle ear, and therefore loss of taste over the anterior two-thirds of the tongue means that a facial nerve paresis must be due to a lesion above this level, e.g. herpes zoster of the geniculate ganglion—the Ramsay Hunt syndrome. Lesions caused by tumours of the parotid gland do not give these signs. Facial palsy is a very late sign of acoustic neuroma. It may occur in an unusually extensive lateral medullary syndrome.

Aetiology of cranial nerve palsies

The causes of single-nerve palsies include cerebral aneurysm, diabetes mellitus, trauma, surgery, cerebral tumour and multiple sclerosis. The various eponymous vascular lesions of the brain-stem need not be separately remembered, but you should be able to discuss the localisation of such lesions with the help of diagrams: they are relatively common causes of cranial nerve palsy. Polyarteritis nodosa, sarcoidosis, meningitis, Lyme disease, syphilis and Wernicke's encephalopathy are less common causes.

Speech disorders

'Would you like to ask this patient some questions?'
It is likely that the patient has a speech disorder, but there may be some degree of dementia (page 158).

Ask name, age, occupation and address.
Test orientation in time (date, season) and place, for dementia.
If indicated, test memory and intellectual capacity.
Test ability to name familiar objects (pen, coins, watch): nominal dysphasia.
Test articulation, e.g. 'baby hippopotamus', 'West Register Street'.
If dysarthria is present, look in the mouth for local lesions and test the lower cranial nerves.

Dysphasia (or aphasia)

A disorder of the symbolic aspects of language, both written and spoken, which usually follows cerebrovascular accidents of the dominant cortex and hence is common. Test by asking patient to name familiar objects, e.g. pen, watch. Failure to name an object spontaneously but with recognition of the correct answer on prompting suggests a motor dysphasia (nominal or expressive dysphasia), classically due to a lesion in the posterior inferior part of the dominant frontal lobe (Broca's area). Sensory dysphasia (receptive dysphasia) describes a specific failure to understand the meaning of words. It is classically localised to the dominant superior temporal lobe (Wernicke's area).

Dysarthria

Inability to articulate properly due to local lesions in the mouth or disorders of the muscles of speech or their connections. There is no disorder of the content of speech.

Paralysis of cranial nerves, e.g. Bell's palsy (seventh), ninth, tenth or twelfth nerves.
Cerebellar disease—'scanning' speech or staccato, seen in multiple sclerosis.
Parkinson's disease: speech is slow, quiet, slurred and monotonous.
Pseudobulbar palsy (spastic dysarthria): monotonous, high pitched 'hot potato' speech (rare).
Progressive bulbar palsy (rare).

General paralysis of the insane (very rare nowadays).
Stutter (usually physiological).

Bulbar and pseudobulbar palsies (table 1)

Both forms are rare. The symptoms of dysarthria, dysphagia and nasal regurgitation result from paralysis of the ninth, tenth and twelfth cranial nerves.

Pseudobulbar (upper motor neurone) palsy is commoner than bulbar palsy and is due to bilateral lesions of the internal capsule, most often the result of cerebrovascular accidents affecting both sides, usually sequentially. It can also occur in multiple sclerosis (page 127). Bulbar (lower motor neurone) palsy is rare because motor neurone disease, and the infective causes (poliomyelitis, Guillain–Barré) are rare.

Table 1. Clinical signs of bulbar and pseudobulbar palsies.

	Pseudobulbar (UMN lesion)	Bulbar (LMN lesion)
Emotions	Labile	Normal
Dysarthria	Donald Duck speech	Nasal
Tongue	Spastic, small for mouth	Flaccid, fasciculating
Jaw jerk	Increased	Normal or absent
Associated findings	Bilateral upper motor neurone lesions of limbs	Sometimes other evidence of MND, e.g. fasciculation in limbs

TESTS OF HIGHER CEREBRAL FUNCTIONS

'Would you like to have a few words with this patient?' or *'Assess the higher cerebral functions'* or *'Assess this patient's personality/mental state/intellectual function.'*

This usually implies dysphasia (page 13), dysarthria (page 13) or dementia (page 158). You should have some all-purpose questions to ask such as 'What is your name?', 'Where do you live?' or 'What is your job?' The answers to these questions may give you some indication of the best lines for further questioning.

Orientation. Orientation in time and space is assessed by asking the patient his name, the date and the place of the interview.

Motivation. Non-dominant lesions may cause loss of motivation.

Personality and mood. Subtle personality changes are best obtained from the relatives' history. Recent personality changes are common in depression with feelings of exhaustion, guilt and self-depreciation and a tendency to cry when asked 'Are you depressed?' (see Depression, page 155).

In dementia, the common personality changes are lack of social awareness, e.g. a previously religious man blaspheming in front of the vicar; lack of love for close and previously loved relatives and lack of interest in dress and appearance. In disseminated sclerosis, patients frequently appear artificially happy despite serious disability. (This is also seen in lesions of the frontal lobes.) Labile emotional expression with alternate laughing and crying for no obvious cause and often without appropriate mood, is a feature of pseudobulbar palsy (see page 14) .

Intellectual function. Intellectual function tests must be related to the patient's previous abilities.

Loss of memory for recent events more than for distant events is a feature of organic cerebral disease and an early feature of dementia. Commonly used tests of intellectual function are:

1 Naming the Monarch, Prime Minister, members of favourite sports teams, famous places and capitals.

2 Serial 7's: the patient is asked to subtract successive 7's from 100.

3 Ability to remember numbers forward and backward. Most can remember 5 or more forward and 4 or more backward.

4 Repetition of complex sentences, e.g. the Babcock sentence: 'The one thing a nation requires to be rich and famous is a large secure supply of wood.'

5 Interpretation of proverbs, e.g. 'People who live in glass houses should not throw stones.'

Dysphasia. The inability to comprehend or express the symbols of speech. In right-handed people and 50% of left-handed people the left hemisphere is dominant in this respect. Before assessing dysphasia it is important to exclude dysarthria from neuromuscular lesions affecting the speech. Depression and parkinsonism may cause slow response but not dysphasia.

Pure expressive dysphasia tends to result from lesions of the frontal lobe (Broca's area, see figure 43, page 117) and a pure receptive dysphasia from lesions of the temporo-parietal lobes (Wernicke's area, see figure 43, page 117).

A form of expressive dysphasia where patients cannot name objects whilst knowing what they are is called 'nominal dysphasia'. (e.g. Ask when holding up a pen, 'What is this?' Pause. 'Is it a watch?' 'No.' 'Is it a key?' 'No.' 'Is it a pen?' 'Yes'.)

Dyslexia (difficulty in reading); dysgraphia (difficulty in writing) and dyscalculia (difficulty in calculating) are usually features of lesions in the posterior parietal lobe.

Agnosia is inability to understand or recognise objects and forms in the presence of normal peripheral sensation. Tactile agnosia is most common and tested by asking the patient to recognise and distinguish objects placed in the hand (astereognosis) or figures drawn on the palm with the eyes closed (dysgraphaesthesia).

Agnosia denotes damage to the contralateral sensory cortex. Inability to recognise objects when viewed (visual agnosia) denotes a lesion of the occipital cortex.

Apraxia is the inability to perform complex and sequential actions to command in the presence of normal coordination, sensation and motor power. It occurs with lesions of the parietal cortices connected by the corpus callosum; e.g. inability to light a match (given the closed box); difficulty dressing ('dressing dyspraxia') and inability to copy designs ('constructional dyspraxia'—most often seen in patients with hepatocellular failure).

ARMS

'Examine this patient's arms (neurologically)'

You may be asked to look at a patient whose neurological syndrome involving the arm is part of a more central lesion such as a stroke or cerebral tumour (perhaps producing 'cortical' sensory or motor loss), a cerebellar lesion, brain-stem involvement or cervical cord disease (e.g. vascular disease, tumour, syringomyelia). Peripheral neuropathies affecting the hands are uncommon (cf. isolated peripheral nerve lesions).

Amongst the commonest neurological lesions of the arms are:

Carpal tunnel syndrome (median nerve palsy).
Ulnar nerve palsy (involved in the ulnar groove at the elbow—usually osteo-arthritis or trauma).
Cervical spondylosis (usually of roots C5 and C6 but occasionally lower).

All three syndromes may present with motor and/or sensory signs and symptoms. A mononeuropathy is usually due to a mechanical cause or old injury and is only rarely due to polyarteritis, diabetes mellitus, sarcoidosis or underlying carcinoma. Leprosy is very rare in Britain.

In an examination the examiner may indicate that neurological examination is required. If not, it is important to ensure that there are no obvious bone, soft tissue or joint abnormalities. Quickly look at the face for parkinsonism or signs of a stroke. (Ask 'Are the arms or joints painful?') Then try to identify the problem more precisely by asking the patient 'Have you any loss of strength in your arms or hands?' and 'Have you had any numbness or tingling in your hands?' If you suspect a specific lesion, demonstrate the complete syndrome. If not, perform a methodical examination. The following scheme is recommended.

Motor system

'Examine the motor system'(page 24)

Look for obvious muscle wasting and test the strength of the appropriate muscle if it is present. If there is wasting of the small hand muscles, note whether it is generalised (ulnar) or thenar (median). Note any fasciculation or tremor (page 28).

Test muscle tone—easiest at the elbow though cogwheel rigidity may be more obvious at the wrist.

Test muscle power in groups (table 2). 'I am going to test the strength of some of your muscles.'

● *Shoulder: C5.* 'Hold both arms out in front of you and close your eyes.' Look for drifting of one arm. This test checks not only weakness of the muscles at the

Table 2. Motor root values (including reflexes).

Joint	Movement	Roots	Muscles	Reflex
Shoulder	Abduction	C4,5,6	Supraspinatus, deltoid	
	External rotation	C4,5,6	Infraspinatus	
	Adduction	C6,7,8	Pectorales	+
Elbow	Flexion	C5,6	Biceps	+
	Extension	C7,8	Triceps	+
	Pronation	C6,7		
	Supination	C5,6	Biceps	+
Wrist	Flexion (palmar): radial	C6,7		
	ulnar	C8		
	Extension (dorsiflexion)	C6,7		
Fingers (long) and thumb	Flexion	C8		+
	Extension	C7		
Fingers (short)	Flexion	T1		
Hips	Flexion	L1,2,3	Iliopsoas	
	Extension	L5	Glutei	
		S1,2		
	Adduction	L2,3,4	Adductors	+
	Abduction	L1,4,5	Glutei and tensor	
		S1	fasciae latae	
Knee	Flexion	L5	Hamstrings	
		S1,2		
	Extension	L3,4	Quadriceps	+
Ankle	Dorsiflexion	L4,5	Anterior tibial	
	Plantar flexion	S1,2	Calf	+
	Eversion	L,5	Peronei	
		S1		
	Inversion	L4	Anterior and	
			posterior tibial	
Toes	Flexion	S1,2		
	Extension	L5		
		S1		
Anus		S2,3,4,5		+
Cremaster		L1,2		+

NB **1** A simple *aide-mémoire* for reflexes and controlling muscle groups is:

Ankle jerk	S1, 2	Biceps jerk	C5, 6
Knee jerk	L3, 4	Triceps jerk	C7, 8

2 All muscles on the 'back' of the upper limb (triceps, wrist extensors and finger extensors) are innervated by C7.

3 T1 innervates the small muscles of the hand.

shoulder but also for loss of position sense (when there is no evidence of weakness) and for lesions of the cerebral cortex (when the patient will not be aware of the drift, sometimes even when his eyes are open). You should also notice any winging of the scapula (nerve to seratus anterior, C5,6,7).

- *Elbow flexion: C5,6: biceps.* 'Bend your elbow up; don't let me straighten it.'
- *Elbow extension: C7: triceps.* 'Now straighten your elbows and push me away.'
- *Wrist and finger extension: C7.* 'Keep your wrist and fingers straight, don't let me bend them.'
- *Hand grip: C8, T1.* 'Squeeze my fingers hard and stop me pulling them out'. Only allow the patient two of your fingers because he may crush more.

Ulnar nerve tests (fingers)

Abduction of fingers ('spread your fingers apart'). Try to squash them together and note how much effort this requires. Note also the bulk of the first dorsal interosseous muscle.

Adduction of fingers. Hold a piece of paper between straight fingers ('don't let me pull it out').

Median nerve tests (thumb)

Abduction of thumb. The patient places his hand down flat with the palm upwards and the thumb overlying the forefinger. Ask the patient to lift the thumb vertically against resistance.

Opposition of thumb. 'Put your thumb and little finger together and stop me pulling them apart' with your forefinger.

NB   Thenar adduction is ulnar.

Reflexes

Examination
See table 2, page 17

Sensory system

Screening
For light touch (cotton wool) and pain (disposable pin) (figure 4, page 23). As a minimum, you should test once each on the front and back of the upper and lower arms and on each digit. Check vibration and position senses on a finger.

Coordination (page 27)

Finger–nose test with eyes open and eyes closed. You are looking for:
- intention tremor (cerebellar) with the eyes open. Past-pointing may be present
- loss of position sense. These patients need vision to know accurately where their hands are and consequently cannot point back to your finger with their eyes closed whilst they can with their eyes open

Dysdiadochokinesia ('tap rapidly on the back of your hand like this ... and now the other side'). The test is more sensitive if the patient taps alternately with the front and backs of his fingers, i.e. pronates and supinates.

LEGS

'Examine this patient's legs (neurologically)'
The commonest neurological lesions affecting chiefly the legs are:
Peripheral neuropathy (particularly diabetes mellitus).
Lumbar root lesions (prolapsed intervertebral disc).
Lateral popliteal (common peroneal) nerve palsy. Local pressure at the head of the fibula causes paralysis of the peroneal muscles and foot-drop. There may be sensory loss.
Spastic paraparesis.
   Try to identify the problem more precisely by asking the patient about any motor or sensory deficit which he has noticed. If no obvious lesion or syndrome is noted, perform systematic examination. The following scheme is recommended.

Motor system

Examination (page 24)

Look for obvious muscle wasting and test the strength of the appropriate muscles if it is present. Note any fasciculation or tremor.

Test muscle tone. Lift the knee off the bed briskly while the patient is relaxed and see if the heel is lifted. Let it drop: observe how stiffly it falls. Then roll the leg to and fro, and see if the foot is rigid at the ankle or normally loose. Alternatively, bend the knee to and fro with an irregular rhythm (so that he cannot consistently resist the movement) or briskly abduct one leg to observe whether bilateral adductor spasm makes the other leg follow.

Test muscle power in groups. 'I am going to test the strength of some of your muscles.'
- *Hip flexion: L1,2: iliopsoas.* 'Lift your leg up straight.' Push down on his knee

- *Hip extension: L5, S1: glutei.* 'Lift your leg up straight: push my hand down to the bed.' Push up to resist this
- *Knee flexion: L5, S1,2: hamstrings.* 'Bend your knee: don't let me straighten it.' Keep one hand above his patella and pull up on the ankle
- *Knee extension: L3,4: quadriceps* (femoral nerve). 'Keep your knee straight: don't let me bend it.' Put your forearm behind his knee and push down on the ankle
- *Ankle plantar flexion: S1.* 'Push your foot down: don't let me push it up'
- *Ankle dorsiflexion: L4,5* (common peroneal nerve). 'Pull your foot up towards you and don't let me pull it down'

Knee and ankle reflexes
Also examine ankle and patella clonus if these are brisk. Practise the technique.

Plantar response
Gently but firmly draw a key or orange stick up the outer border of the sole and across the heads of the metatarsals.

Sensory system (page 22)
Light touch and pinprick
- once each on the medial and lateral sides of thigh and calf
- on the dorsum of the foot, tip of the big toe and lateral border of the foot

Vibration sense at the medial malleolus and if it is absent there, progress to the knee and hip.

Position sense. Test position sense at the big toes. If absent check it at progressively more proximal joints.

Reduction or absence of vibration and position senses suggests not only dorsal column loss (now usually due to B_{12} deficiency) but also may be part of a peripheral neuropathy (now usually diabetic). However, in peripheral neuropathy you expect the other modalities to be reduced (pin and touch).

Coordination (page 27)
Heel–shin test. 'Put your heel (touching his heel) on your knee (touching his knee) and slide it down your leg (sliding your finger down his shin).' This is primarily a test for intention tremor. If present you should look for other signs of cerebellar disorders (arms, eyes, speech). Then ask the patient to stand and stand near to him (to assist him if he stumbles). Look for:
Rombergism (more unsteady with the eyes closed than with them open) which indicates loss of position sense (posterior column lesion).
Truncal ataxia while standing with his feet together (cerebellar lesion).
Ataxic gait on walking heel to toe—note direction of fall (ipsilateral cerebellar lesion).
Abnormalities of gait on 'normal' walking (including turning).

ABNORMALITY OF GAIT (excluding orthopaedic disorders)

'Watch this patient walk.'

Hemiplegia

The leg is rigid and describes a semicircle with the toe scraping the floor (circumduction).

Aetiology: almost invariably a stroke.

Paraplegia

Scissors or 'wading through mud' gait.

Aetiology: multiple sclerosis, cord compression; rarely congenital spastic diplegia.

Festinant gait of parkinsonism

The patient is rigid, stooped and the gait shuffling. The arms tend to be held flexed and characteristically do not swing. He appears to be continually about to fall forwards and may show propulsion or retropulsion. Turning is poor. There may be 'freezing' in doorways.

Cerebellar gait

The patient walks on a wide base with the arms held wide. He is ataxic, veering and staggering towards the side of the disease.

Aetiology: usually multiple sclerosis. Cerebellar tumour (primary or secondary), the cerebellar syndrome of carcinoma (non-metastatic) and familial degenerations should be remembered.

Sensory (dorsal column) ataxia

A stepping and stamping gait. The patient walks on a wide base and looks at the ground. He tends to fall if he closes his eyes (rombergism).

Aetiology: tabes dorsalis, diabetic pseudotabes, subacute combined degeneration of the cord, Friedreich's ataxia. Ataxia in multiple sclerosis may very rarely be of this kind (it is usually cerebellar).

Steppage (drop-foot) gait

There is no dorsiflexion of the foot as it leaves the ground and the affected legs (or leg) are lifted high to avoid scraping the toe.

Aetiology: usually lateral popliteal nerve palsy (mechanical or diabetic). Less commonly poliomyelitis or peroneal muscular atrophy. Very rarely heavy metal (lead, arsenic) poisoning.

Waddling gait

The pelvis drops on each side as the leg leaves the ground.

Aetiology: wasting disorders of the muscles of the pelvic girdle and proximal lower limb muscles (page 24), and osteomalacia.

NOTES

Sensory testing (vibration and position, touch, pain, temperature)

It is important that the patient understands what sensations you are testing and what is an appropriate response on his part. Two of the stimuli conventionally used (vibration and position senses) are strange ones and the patient needs quickly to be taught about them. If you already have a good and professional system the following suggested scheme will be unnecessary.

Vibration sense

Ensure that the patient can recognise vibration by placing the vibrating tuning fork on to his sternum. 'Now with your eyes closed tell me if you can feel the vibration.' Start at the big toes and work proximally to the medial malleoli, patellae and anterior superior iliac spines comparing right with left (and with yourself if necessary).

Position sense

With the patient looking, hold a big toe or a finger by its sides (holding the top and bottom introduces light touch sensation). Move the toe away from the patient—'this is down'—and then towards the patient—'this is up. Now with your eyes closed tell me whether I move the toe (finger) up or down.'

Light touch (cotton wool) and pinprick

These stimuli should be familiar to the patient. Appropriate instructions might be: 'Say now every time I touch you', and/or 'Say pin when you feel a pinprick'. No person is entirely consistent in sensory testing and a few discrepant responses are to be expected and ignored. Increasingly inconsistent responses are often due to wandering attention. Areas of anaesthesia are easily produced by suggestion. The pin should be safely discarded after use on one patient because of the risks of transmission of infection, especially HIV and hepatitis B.

Ask the patient to outline for you the extent of any numbness or tingling that he feels: you may then confirm and define the extent of sensory loss with the cotton wool or a pin.

You must have an approximate idea of the dermatomes (figure 4). The following points may be found useful:

C4 and T2 are the neighbouring dermatomes over the front of the chest at the level of the first and second ribs.
C5–T1 supply the upper limb.
C7 supplies the middle finger front and back.
T7 supplies the 'lower ribs'.
T10 supplies the umbilical region.
T12 is the 'lowest' nerve of the anterior abdominal wall.
L1 supplies the inguinal region.
L2–3 supply the anterior thigh (lateral and medial).

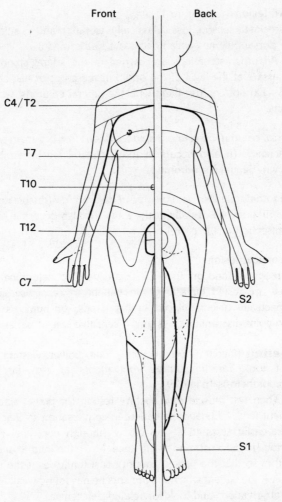

Figure 4. Sensory dermatomes with key points to remember.

L4–5 supply the anterior shin (medial and lateral).
S1 supplies the lateral border of the foot and sole, and the back of the calf up to the knee.

Patterns of sensory loss in limbs

Peripheral sensory neuropathy (page 136)

All modalities tend to be lost symmetrically and initially distally. The loss is more marked in the lower limbs than in the upper. This pattern is seen in diabetes mellitus, carcinomatous neuropathy, vitamin B_{12} deficiency, and drugs or chemicals.

NB 'Glove and stocking' anaesthesia, with a very well demarcated upper border, may occur in hysteria and in malingerers.

Spinal cord lesions (see figure 1)

Dissociated sensory loss. Classically, vibration and position sense are carried in the dorsal columns which decussate in the medulla.

All other sensations are carried in the lateral spinothalamic tracts which decussate at the level of the origin in the cord, or just above it.

NB   Do not confuse them with the 'lateral columns' which are the pyramidal tracts.

Dorsal column loss without spinothalamic loss occurs in both legs in vitamin B_{12} deficiency. (It also occurs in the ipsilateral leg in hemisection of the cord—Brown–Séquard syndrome.)

Spinothalamic loss without dorsal column loss(dissociated anaesthesia) occurs in syringomyelia, usually in the arms. (It also occurs in the contralateral leg in hemisection of the cord.)

Cerebral cortical lesions

Stereognosis and graphaesthesia are used to determine parietal sensory loss. They are tested by asking the patient to recognise, with the eyes closed, respectively objects placed in his hands, or numbers drawn on his palm. Two-point discrimination is also a sensitive test of parietal cortical function.

Motor testing (involuntary movement, tone, power, wasting, coordination)

First look for *involuntary movements* at rest—fasciculation, tremor or choreoathetosis (page 29).

Then test *muscle tone* (before testing for power since this may leave the patient tense). Engage the patient in conversation so that he is relaxed. Tone is most easily assessed at the elbow (though cogwheel rigidity may be more obvious at the wrist) and at the knee. Move the joint to and fro with an irregular rhythm so that the patient cannot consistently resist the movement.

Ask the patient which movements he has found weak and then try to confirm his observations and look for related deficiencies.

Test *muscle power* in groups. Make your instructions slow and precise. Look and feel the bulk of the muscles as you test their strength. You must have an approximate idea of the root values of at least certain movements so that you can perform a rapid 'motor root' screen (upper limb page 17, lower limb page 20).

You must know the root values of the common reflexes (see table 2, page 17).

Patterns of motor loss in limbs

Lower motor neurone lesion

There is reduced or absent power with marked muscle wasting in the established lesion. The muscles are flaccid and the reflexes absent. In the foot there is no plantar response. The lesion affects the motor distribution of the spinal root or peripheral nerve.

Upper motor neurone lesion

There is reduced or absent power with relatively little wasting. The muscle tone and reflexes are increased and clonus often present. In the foot the plantar response is upgoing. There tends to be a characteristic distribution of weakness. Thus in the arms weakness is more marked in elbow extension than flexion and wrist dorsiflexion than palmar flexion. In the legs it is more marked in hip flexion, knee flexion and ankle dorsiflexion than in their antagonist movements. This is most easily remembered by recalling the posture of the limbs in the hemiplegic patient when he is walking.

Proximal myopathy

Proximal muscle wasting and weakness also occur in polymyositis, carcinomatous neuromyopathy, hereditary muscular dystrophies, Cushing's syndrome usually from steroid therapy, thyrotoxicosis, osteomalacia and diabetes (amyotrophy, see page 201). *Trichinella spiralis* infection of muscles may produce acute myositis.

Isolated peripheral nerve lesions

Median nerve lesion (carpal tunnel syndrome)

These patients, often middle-aged and female, may complain of tingling and numbness of the fingers and/or weakness of the thumb, which is at its worst on waking. It is often unilateral at the time of presentation and remains so if idiopathic. Pain at the flexor aspect of the wrist may occasionally radiate up to the elbow and exceptionally as far as the shoulder. You should examine for:
* thenar wasting and weakness of thumb abduction and opposition
* sensory loss, palmar surface only, of the thumb and two and a half fingers (i.e. to the middle of the ring finger)
* Tinel's sign. Percuss over the flexor retinaculum to elicit tingling in the same area
* evidence of pregnancy (or ask if she is on 'the pill'), myxoedema, rheumatoid arthritis and acromegaly. It is commonest in over-weight middle-aged women with none of these

NB Bilateral carpal tunnel syndrome is commonly due to rheumatoid arthritis and also occurs in chronic renal dialysis patients (amyloid deposits). In the examination also consider cervical spondylosis (T1 lesion), motor neurone disease and syringomyelia if you are in doubt about the diagnosis.

Ulnar nerve lesion

The ulnar nerve supplies all the small muscles of the hand except the thenar eminence (but including adductor pollicis). It may be compressed in the ulnar tunnel at the wrist or in the ulnar groove at the elbow (e.g. if the arm has been incorrectly positioned in general anaesthesia). These patients may complain of tingling or 'deadness' and/or weakness of the ring and little fingers. You should examine for:
* flattening of the contours of the hand due to muscle wasting. The ring and

little fingers are held slightly flexed, and there is loss of power in abduction and adduction of the fingers (claw hand)
- sensory loss, back and front, over the one and a half ulnar fingers (i.e. little finger and half the ring finger)
- 'filling in' of the ulnar groove at the elbow and limitation of movement at the elbow. X-rays of the elbow may show osteoarthritis or local fracture

NB   If you are in doubt about the diagnosis consider a lesion in the neck and look for restricted movements of the cervical spine (T1 lesion).

Radial nerve lesion

These are rare and result from local pressure (e.g. an arm over the back of the chair) which causes wristdrop. Sensory loss may be very limited because the median and ulnar nerve territories overlie the radial territory.

Lateral cutaneous nerve of the thigh

Compression causes meralgia paraesthetica, a syndrome characterised by hyperalgesia, burning pain, and numbness in the lateral aspect of the thigh and is associated with tight jeans or obesity.

Lateral popliteal palsy

The lateral popliteal (common peroneal) nerve supplies the peroneal muscles which dorsiflex and evert the foot. The nerve may be damaged as it passes over the head of the fibula resulting in foot-drop. There may be sensory loss over the outer aspect of the leg and foot.

Wasting of the small hand muscles

These are innervated by the T1 root. Wasting of the muscles in both hands occurs with:
- old age and cachexia
- rheumatoid arthritis
- bilateral cervical ribs
- motor neurone disease
- syringomyelia
- bilateral median and ulnar nerve lesions

If present in one hand only, the following should also be considered:
- cervical cord lesions including tumours
- brachial plexus trauma
- a Pancoast tumour

Proximal myopathy

This characteristically produces difficulty in standing from the sitting position and difficulty in raising the arms above the head. It occurs (often slight) in thyrotoxicosis, diabetes mellitus, polymyositis, carcinomatous neuromyopathy, osteomalacia, Cushing's syndrome (usually iatrogenic) and in the hereditary muscular dystrophies.

Mixed motor and sensory neuropathy
   See peripheral neuropathy (page 136) and mononeuritis multiplex (page 137)

Incoordination
   There are two chief patterns of incoordination, one dominated by a failure in controlling accurate limb movements (cerebellar) and the other dominated by an ignorance of limb position without visual or cutaneous clues (proprioceptive).

Cerebellar incoordination

   'Demonstrate some cerebellar signs.' The signs are ipsilateral to a destructive lesion.

   Finger–nose test. The intention tremor is more marked when the patient has to stretch to reach your finger. If you keep your finger still and then ask the patient to repeat the test with the eyes closed, you may bring out 'past-pointing'— deviation of the patient's finger consistently to one side of your own (the same side as the cerebellar lesion). The tremor is not altered by closing the eyes. The heel–shin test has similar significance. Remember that muscular weakness alone may make the patient unsteady in these tests, and that this may resemble an intention tremor.

   Dysdiadochokinesia (page 19). Rapid repetitive alternating movements of the wrists are irregular in both force and rate in cerebellar disease. There also tends to be abnormal movement at elbow and shoulder. Supination/pronation tests are more sensitive than flexion/extension ones.

   Nystagmus (page 11), typically horizontal, is more marked on looking towards the side of the lesion. Do not get the patient to focus on an object too far laterally or too near to the eyes.

   Dysarthria. Slurred and explosive, sometimes as if drunk.

   Truncal ataxia. The gait is reeling and staggering as if drunk with a tendency to fall to the side of the lesion. Heel–toe walking may accentuate the sign. It may be the sole cerebellar sign in midline (vermis) cerebellar lesions.

Causes of cerebellar signs
   Multiple sclerosis.
   Brain-stem vascular disease.
   Anticonvulsant therapy may produce gross nystagmus.
   Rarely brain-stem tumours, posterior fossa tumours (especially acoustic neuroma), degenerative disorders (e.g. alcoholism and hereditary ataxias), the cerebellar syndrome of bronchial carcinoma and (very rarely) hypothyroidism.

Proprioceptive incoordination (dorsal column loss)

The signs are ipsilateral to the lesion. When there is loss of proprioception, the patient can still place the limbs accurately by looking at them. Incoordination is therefore only obviously present when the eyes are closed. Tests are performed with the eyes open and the eyes closed. When the patient's coordination is worse with the eyes closed than with them open, he is said to have loss of position sense (i.e. dorsal column loss or proprioceptive loss). If there is dorsal column loss (vibration and position senses) but no spinothalamic loss (pain and temperature senses), there is said to be a 'dissociated sensory loss'. (This term also describes the rarer reverse situation of spinothalamic loss without dorsal column loss.) Dissociated sensory loss is evidence of spinal cord disease.

Finger–nose test and heel–shin test are normal when the patient can see but incoordinate when he cannot. Rombergism is present when the patient, standing with his feet together, is more unsteady with his eyes closed than when they are open. The gait is ataxic and the patient walks on a wide base with high steps. Muscle tone and the tendon reflexes may be diminished (or increased in B_{12} myelopathy).

Causes of dorsal (posterior) column loss

Subacute combined degeneration of the cord. This may progress sufficiently to give dorsal column loss—peripheral neuropathy is the earliest manifestation. It is very rare in the clinic but patients treated with vitamin B_{12} may be seen in examinations (when the peripheral neuropathy may be considerably recovered though the spinal cord lesions are not).

Tabes dorsalis. This is now very rare though a few cases in older individuals may appear in the examinations.

Hemisection of the cord (see figure 1, page 5).

Tremor

'Look at this patient's tremor.'

There are four common tremors:

- The resting tremor of parkinsonism, maximal at rest and with emotion and inhibited by movement (4–5.5 Hz). It is best demonstrated by passive, slow flexion–extension movements at the wrist. It is mainly distal and asymmetrical
- Essential tremor (5–8 Hz). This is an accentuation of physiological tremor present at rest and brought out by placing a sheet of paper on the outstretched fingers. It increases with age. It is faster (8–12 Hz.) when associated with β2-adrenergic stimulation (bronchodilators), caffeine, anxiety, after exercise and hypoglycaemia. In thyrotoxicosis it is associated with warm moist palms, tachycardia and eye signs of Graves' disease. It is occasionally familial. In alcoholics, the tremor is often reduced by ethanol and exacerbated by its withdrawal. It may improve with β-blockade
- The intention tremor of cerebellar disease (finger–nose test; 3 Hz). It is reduced or absent at rest and associated with past-pointing, nystagmus dysarthria and ataxia, including truncal ataxia. It is rare except in multiple sclerosis

• Flapping tremor occurs in hepatic precoma and in the CO_2 retention of respiratory failure

Athetosis refers to slow sinuous, writhing movements of the face and limbs, especially the distal parts. In torsion spasm (dystonia) the movements are similar but slower and affect the proximal parts of the limbs. The movements are purposeless. Both occur in lesions of the extrapyramidal system. They are rare.

Choreiform movements are non-repetitive, involuntary abrupt jerky movements of face, tongue and limbs. They may be localised or generalised (both are rare). They occur in lesions of the extrapyramidal system and with phenothiazine toxicity. Rheumatic chorea (Sydenham's chorea, page 134) is now very rare. Huntington's chorea is inherited (page 134).

Eyes

'Look at these eyes.'
Unless specifically instructed (i.e. *'Look at the pupils'* or *'Look at the fundi'*) a complete examination is required. There may be obvious exophthalmos (page 182) or squint (page 7) otherwise follow the scheme in table 3.

OPTIC FUNDUS

First check that the ophthalmoscope is adjusted to suit your own eyes (usually no lens) and that the light beam is circular and bright by shining it on your other hand. It is useful to start by observing the patient's eye through the ophthalmoscope from about 2 feet to see if there is any loss of the red light reflex (indicating opacities in the translucent media which may cause difficulty when trying to inspect the retina). You should interpret the fundal findings in the light of the patient's refractive errors (you may discover this from a rapid look at his spectacles) and you should use a similar lens in the ophthalmoscope. Short-sighted (myopic) patients have a negative (concave) lens in their spectacles (objects look smaller through them) and tend to have a deep optic cup and some temporal pallor of the disc. Long-sighted patients (hypermetropic) have a positive lens in their spectacles (convex, magnifying) and their optic disc tends to look small and have ill-defined margins. You should be able to recognise and comment on the following.

Myelinated nerve fibres

A normal variant in which there are bright white streaky irregular patches, usually adjacent to the disc margin.

Diabetic fundus (page 200)

This is characterised by:
- Background retinopathy (capillary leak of proteins, lipids, red cells); micro-aneurysms (dots), most frequent temporal to the macula; retinal haemorrhages (blots); hard exudates
- Maculopathy: oedema and/or background changes at the macula, associated with reduced visual acuity
- Pre-proliferative (secondary to retinal hypoxia): soft exudates (cotton wool spots) of retinal oedema; venous beading and reduplication
- Proliferative (response to retinal hypoxia): new vessel formation; haemorrhage (vitreous, obscuring the retina, and pre-retinal)
- Advanced (secondary to fibrosis): fibrous proliferation; traction retinal detachment
- Results of treatment (photocoagulation): spots of retinal burns

Table 3. Examination of the eyes.

Observe	For	Clinical association
Eyes and eyelids (from in front)	Squint (congenital or acquired) Xanthelasma	Diabetes, atheroma, myxoedema, primary biliary cirrhosis (page 253)
	Ptosis (partial, i.e. third nerve or sympathetic, or complete, i.e. third nerve)	(page 4) If bilateral; myasthenia Dystrophia myotonica
Cornea	Corneal arcus Calcification Kayser–Fleischer rings	Age and hyperlipidaemias Hypercalcaemia (rare) Wilson's disease (very rare)
Visual acuity (Snellen's chart)		May pick up early change in diabetes
Visual fields to confrontation (page 5)		
Eye movements (page 7)	Failure of lateral movements Failure of down and in movement Failure of other movements (with ptosis and fixed dilatation of pupil)	Sixth nerve palsy Fourth nerve palsy Third nerve palsy
	Failure of all movements Nystagmus (page 11)	Usually myasthenia, glass eye Cerebellar, vestibular or brain-stem lesion
Pupils	Dilatation	Homatropine or part of third nerve lesion, Holmes–Adie syndrome
	Constriction	Horner's syndrome, Argyll Robertson pupil Morphine Pilocarpine

NB *Check light and accommodation reflexes* (page 9). *Glass eyes have neither.*

Iris (with ophthalmoscope)	Iritis (page 32)	
Lens	Lens opacities or cataract (shine light obliquely across lens); this is often missed and may make examination of the fundus difficult or impossible	Senility, diabetes, trauma Rare causes include congenital rubella syndrome, hypo-parathyroidism, dystrophia myotonica and drugs (chloroquine amiodarone and steroids)
Fundus (page 30)		

NB   Glaucoma and cataract are commoner in diabetes than in the general population.

Hypertensive fundus

There are usually the changes of arteriosclerosis (grades 1 and 2 including tortuosity, arterial nipping, silver wiring, varying vessel calibre). Hypertension produces haemorrhages and exudates (grade 3) and more severe disease in addition produces papilloedema (grade 4, malignant hypertension). Note that the subhyaloid haemorrhage sometimes seen in subarachnoid haemorrhage may indicate underlying hypertension.

Papilloedema

The earliest findings are redness of the disc and blurring of the nasal margin. Small vessels may appear to dip over the swollen edge, and the optic cup disappears. Later small haemorrhages appear. The blind spot may enlarge.
• raised intracranial pressure (tumour, abscess, meningitis, and the rare benign intracranial hypertension found chiefly in young over-weight women)
• malignant hypertension
• rarely, optic retrobulbar neuritis, venous obstruction, and the hypercapnia of respiratory failure
NB   Papillitis should be distinguished from papilloedema. It is usually due to multiple sclerosis. There may be impaired coloured vision and acuity, a central scotoma, and pain. The disc is red and swollen with a blurred margin, exudates and haemorrhages.

Optic atrophy

• glaucoma
• secondary to papilloedema (disc edge blurred). This is rare
• primary (disc margin sharp with cup and cribriform plate well defined) occurs after papillitis (almost invariably multiple sclerosis), from optic nerve pressure and in retinal artery thrombosis. Rarely methanol abuse, B_{12} deficiency and the hereditary ataxias.

Exudates and haemorrhages

Chiefly in hypertension and diabetes mellitus but also in uraemia, acute leukaemia, raised intracranial pressure, severe anaemia and CO_2 retention.

UVEITIS, IRITIS AND CHOROIDITIS

The uveal tract comprises the choroid (posterior uvea), the ciliary body and the iris (anterior uvea). Uveitis occurs alone or as part of other generalised diseases, some of which tend to involve either the iris (iritis, iridocyclitis or anterior uveitis) or the choroid (choroiditis or posterior uveitis), although virtually all may involve both. Iritis is recognised by ocular pain and blurring of vision with vascularisation around the corneal limbus and a 'muddy' iris. It is usually unilateral. The causes are listed in table 4.

Table 4. Causes of iritis and choroiditis.

Iritis	Choroiditis
Diabetes	Idiopathic (i.e. unexplained), the most frequent in this country
Sarcoid	
Ankylosing spondylitis	Toxoplasmosis (invariably acquired)
Reiter's syndrome	Diabetes
Ulcerative colitis and Crohn's disease	Sarcoid
Still's disease	(Rare causes include toxocara, tuberculosis, syphilis)
(Rare causes include gonorrhoea, toxoplasma, brucella, tuberculosis, syphilis)	

Limbs (joints and peripheral vascular disease)

LEGS

In the legs the usual abnormalities are neurological or vascular. Diabetes mellitis is very common and may cause both, and you may be presented with a 'diabetic foot' (ischaemia, peripheral sensory neuropathy with ulceration and deformity). The skin and joints should also be considered. Many neurological diseases such as multiple sclerosis and strokes are chronic and appear in examinations. Paget's disease commonly shows as an enlarged, hot, bowed tibia. Erythema nodosum occasionally appears in examinations because, although it is short-lived, it is fairly common. Pre-tibial *myxoedema* is occasionally shown. Relatively rare cases include the results of spinal injury or prolapsed intervertebral discs (cervical or lumbar), peripheral nerve damage and subacute combined degeneration. Even patients with motor neurone disease or a carcinomatous neuropathy may be well enough to be included. Syringomyelia and the myopathies are rare but these patients have a better prognosis and are often available for examinations.

'Look at these legs'
Unless attention is directed towards a particular part of the legs such as the feet or knees, the following scheme is recommended:

- Look for obvious *joint deformity*. Also note *bone deformity*, leg shortening and external rotation of fractured neck of femur, Paget's disease, previous rickets (rare except in the elderly), the results of previous poliomyelitis, and Charcot's joints of diabetes and now less commonly, syphilis. Note if *oedema* is present.
- Look at the *skin* (purpura, rash, ulcer) and note cyanosed or necrotic toes.
- Examine abnormal joints.
- *Peripheral vasculature*. Compare and assess the temperature of the dorsa of both feet, noting asymmetry and any interdigital infection and loss of hair. If the feet are cold, feel the dorsalis pedis and posterior tibial pulses, and if these are absent, proceed to feel for the popliteal and femoral pulses, and listen for arterial bruits. Ask the patient about a history of intermittent claudication. If there are ulcers, ask the patient if they are painful. If not, there is a neuropathy, most frequently diabetic.
- Then examine the legs neurologically (page 20).

ARMS

In the arms the usual abnormalities seen are of the joints or the nervous system. The commonest neurological conditions in the upper limbs are the results of multiple sclerosis, stroke or peripheral nerve compression. Rarer conditions which may be seen in examinations are the results of pressure on the cord or brachial plexus (remember cervical spondylosis and cervical rib), motor neurone disease, syringomyelia and dystrophia myotonica.

'Look at the arms' (upper limb, hands)
This may mean primarily the hand which should always be inspected first or the joints (including elbow or wrist). Usually it means a neurological examination (wasting, nerve palsies, root lesions) but:
Observe any tremor at rest (parkinsonism).
Observe the skin for purpura (page 95) and signs of liver disease (liver palms, spider naevi and Dupuytren's contracture).
Look at the fingers and nails for clubbing (page 57) cyanosis, nicotine-staining, anaemia, and the splinter haemorrhages and Osler's nodes of subacute bacterial endocarditis. (Splinter haemorrhages are often occupational and not diagnostic, and Osler's nodes very rare.)
Glance at the patient's face which may provide a further clue, e.g. pallor, exophthalmos, parkinsonian facies, acromegaly, spider naevi, tophi on the ears in gout.
Note any joint swelling (ask if they are painful before touching them) and any associated muscle wasting (often marked in rheumatoid arthritis).

NOTES
If there is evidence of joint disease, look for:

Rheumatoid arthritis (page 168)
This is usually symmetrical, with ulnar deviation at the metacarpophalangeal joints, spindling of the fingers, nail fold infarcts, muscle wasting, and swelling of the joints except the terminal interphalangeal joints. Look for the changes of psoriatic arthritis, including pitting of the nails and onycholysis with involvement of the terminal interphalangeal joints, psoriasis at the elbows and for the skin changes of steriod therapy. Rheumatoid arthritis may produce gross deformity. Nodules (20%) may be present at the elbow and down the radial border of the forearm. Note characteristic proximal inter-phalangeal deformities: boutonnière (flexion and swan-neck (hyper-extension)).

Osteoarthritis (osteoarthrosis) (page 178)
Asymmetrical and most frequently seen in old people as Heberden's nodes—osteophytes around the terminal interphalangeal joints. Any joint of the hand may be involved but it involves especially the terminal interphalangeal and first carpometacarpal joints.

Gout (page 224)
May attack any joint of the body. It may be monoarticular or polyarticular. Usually the metatarsophalangeal joint of the big toe is first involved. It becomes red, hot, shiny and tender. There is often marked soft tissue swelling and there

may be superficial tophi over joints and in the cartilage of the ear. Ask about thiazide diuretics and note any polycythaemia.

NB Osteo-, rheumatoid and gouty arthritis may mimic each other but rheumatoid is usually symmetrical.
Monarticular arthritis may well be purulent: joint aspiration and blood culture are essential.

If a rapid examination as above reveals no abnormality, proceed to examine the upper limbs neurologically (page 16).

Head and neck

HEAD
'Look at this patient's face'

This somewhat unsatisfactory request usually implies either that the patient has an abnormal facies (or neck), or that he has abnormal facial movements, or poverty of movement (parkinsonism and myxoedema). If the abnormality is not immediately obvious, the following check-list of the systems which may be involved might be found useful:

Endocrine and metabolic
Cushing's (iatrogenic)—rare.
Myxoedema; thyrotoxicosis.
Acromegaly.
Pagetic skull.

Neurological
Facial palsy of stroke and Bell's palsy.
Ptosis and ocular palsies (third nerve, sympathetic in Horner's syndrome and myasthenia gravis).
Parkinsonism.
Myopathy (including dystrophia myotonica with cataract and baldness).
Ophthalmic herpes (zoster) includes the conjunctiva.

Cardiorespiratory
Cyanosis of lips (look at the tongue) of chronic obstructive airway (note pursing lips on expiration, and poor expansion), or cardiac failure.
Elevated jugular venous pressure of heart failure (or fluid overload). Kussmaul's sign may be present with cardiac tamponade, and there will be no pulse wave in the extremely elevated pressure due to mediastinal obstruction. Obstructive airways disease gives elevation of the jugular venous pressure during expiration (in proportion to the obstruction).

Gastrointestinal
Jaundice and spider naevi.
Peutz–Jeghers syndrome.
Hereditary haemorrhagic telangiectasia.
Anaemia (white hair, glossitis and lemon yellow skin of pernicious anaemia).
Angular cheilitis is usually caused by over-closure from aged dentures and mandibular resorption rather than anaemia.

Collagen disease
Systemic lupus erythematosus (butterfly rash).
Scleroderma (tight mouth and shiny tight skin of fingers).
Dermatomyositis (periorbital rash).

Skin diseases
Acne vulgaris.
Rosacea.
Psoriasis.
Port wine stain (of Sturge–Weber syndrome).

NECK
'Examine the neck'
This usually means that there is enlargement of the lymph glands, or that a goitre is present, or that the jugular venous pressure is raised (see table 7, page 64).

Cervical lymphadenopathy (page 100)
This is often easier to feel from behind.

Do not forget the occipital group. If lymphadenopathy is present, check for local infection or neoplasm over the whole head and neck . Remember to look into the mouth and pharynx. Check the nose for blood, discharge and patency.

Glands in the root of the neck may be symptomatic of pulmonary, abdominal (including the testes) or breast malignancy.

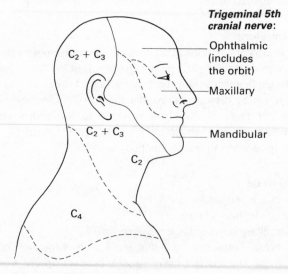

Figure 5.   Head and neck.

Cervical glands may be the presenting symptom of a generalised lymphadeno-pathy. Further examination should include all lymph gland groups and palpation for enlargement of the liver and spleen. Consider secondary carcinoma, the reticuloses, leukaemia, local sepsis, and the granulomatous disorders including tuberculosis, sarcoid, Brucella and infectious mononucleosis. Look for primary ENT carcinoma and do not forget the testes.

NB 'Lump in the neck: look in the mouth.'

Enlarged thyroid

'Look at this patient's thyroid gland'

This means that the patient has a goitre. It is unlikely that the patient is hyperthyroid but this must first be excluded by looking for the evidence such as fine finger tremor, hyperkinesia, eye signs (lid lag, lid retraction, exophthalmos), tachycardia or fast atrial fibrillation and hot, sweaty hands. Similarly check for the characteristic facies, slow movements, dry thick skin, hair changes and croaking voice of hypothyroidism and proceed to test the ankle jerks if indicated.

Look at the patient's neck and ask him to swallow. Palpate the gland first from behind and then from the front. The patient's chin should be flexed to relax the tissues (untrained patients invariably extend the neck). If the patient has to swallow more than two or three times, you should give him a glass of water. Pay special attention to:

• *Character.* Diffuse or multinodular. The gland is diffusely enlarged in Graves' disease, Hashimoto's thyroiditis, iodine deficiency and dyshormonogenesis. Patients with multinodular goitres are usually 'nontoxic' (euthyroid). The usual clinical problem is their bulk, which may produce compression (of trachea, oesophagus or laryngeal nerve) and cause distress from their appearance. Single nodules should be regarded as malignant (though most are not), and removed or biopsied

• *Tenderness.* This is unusual except in viral thyroiditis (very rare) and occasionally in autoimmune thyroiditis and carcinoma

• *Mobility.* Attachment to surrounding tissues suggests carcinoma

• *Retrosternal extension.* Feel in the suprasternal notch and percuss the upper sternum for dullness

• *Lymph glands.* An enlarged chain of lymph glands suggests papillary thyroid carcinoma

• *Trachea.* Central or displaced

• *Thyroidectomy scar.* If present you should suspect hypothyroidism or hypoparathyroidism. Elicit Chvostek's sign (may be present in normal people) and perform Trousseau's test

• Auscultate over the gland for a systolic bruit. Look for vitiligo, acropachy, and pretibial myxoedema if autoimmune thyroid disease is suspected.

You should ask about pressure symptoms of dyspnoea (scabbard trachea), any drugs (especially medicines containing iodine) and take a family history for inborn enzyme deficiency (dyshormonogenesis). If you are asked to suggest investigations you should consider:

Thyroid function tests. These should include as appropriate (and available) serum free T4, T3 and thyroid-stimulating (thyrotrophic) hormone.
Tests for thyroid autoantibodies.
X-rays for tracheal deviation or compression.
Radioiodine tests including a scan for cold nodules.
Ultrasound to distinguish solid from cystic masses.
Laryngoscopy to observe vocal cords if the voice has changed.
Needle biopsy of isolated nodules for cytology; or preferably total removal.

NB The observed incidence of simple goitre, autoimmune thyroiditis and carcinoma in one series was 89%, 10% and 1% respectively. Carcinoma is suggested by a hard fixed gland, lymph gland enlargement, pressure symptoms, vocal cord paralysis, rapid increase in size and evidence of metastasis to bone (page 185).

Abdomen

EXAMINATION

'Examine this patient's abdomen'

The most usual abnormality seen in examinations is a palpable mass or the presence of free fluid, or both. These are relatively rare in the clinic, where the clinician more commonly elicits only areas of maximum tenderness. The commonest conditions suitable for examination purposes are diseases which are chronic and produce enlargement of the spleen or liver such as the chronic leukaemias, myelofibrosis or chronic liver disorders. Other palpable masses include renal swellings, especially polycystic kidneys. Neoplastic or inflammatory swellings may be present and it is usually not possible to distinguish between these on physical examination alone. Patients with acute abdominal disease virtually never appear in clinical examinations. Remember always to look before palpation, to have warm hands and to palpate gently so as to gain the patient's confidence and avoid hurting him. You should ask the patient to let you know if you do hurt him and look at his face periodically during palpation, especially if you elicit guarding or rebound tenderness.

A complete examination of the alimentary system involves inspection of the tongue, mouth, teeth and throat but this is rarely required in examinations. Loss of weight, clubbing, jaundice, anaemia and spider naevi should always be looked for. Hence:

- Look at the hands especially for clubbing, leuconychia, tobacco staining, liver palms, spider naevi and Dupuytren's contracture. Palpate the neck, supraclavicular fossae, axillae and groins for lymph nodes (the testes drain to the para-aortic and cervical glands). Inspect the eyes and conjunctivae for anaemia and jaundice. Lie the patient flat (one pillow) with arms by his sides. Observe the abdomen for:

- General swelling with eversion of the umbilicus in ascites and visible enlargement of internal organs (liver, spleen, kidneys, gall bladder, stomach (in pyloric stenosis), urinary bladder and pelvic organs)

- Abnormal veins or abnormally distended veins usually in cirrhosis with the direction of flow away from the umbilicus (portal hypertension). The flow is upwards from the groin in inferior vena cave obstruction

- Scars of previous operations, striae, skin rashes and purpura

- Pigmentation localised or generalised

- Visible peristalsis suggests obstruction except in very thin patients

- Palpate for internal organs and masses. It is often of value to percuss the liver and spleen areas initially to avoid missing the lower border of a very large liver or spleen. It is essential to start palpation in the right iliac fossa and work upwards towards the hepatic and splenic areas, first superficially and then deeper. Ascites may obscure a liver edge, but firm 'dipping' onto an enlarged liver should always be attempted unless it causes pain.

The 'scratch test' can often help *roughly* to define the extent of hepato-megaly. Place the stethoscope firmly just below the xiphisternal cartilage which is a surface relation of liver in normal people. Sound is conducted through solid objects, so firm stroking of the skin progressing from the right costal margin downwards will be audible until the liver edge is reached.

Liver

Upper border: fourth rib to fifth space on percussion. Moves down on inspiration. If enlarged the edge may be tender, regular or irregular, hard, firm or soft. Note if it is pulsatile (tricuspid incompetence). It may be normal but pushed down by hyperinflated lungs or chronic obstructive airway disease.

Spleen

Smooth rounded swelling in left subcostal region, usually with a distinct lower edge (as compared with the kidney). It enlarges diagonally downward and across the abdomen in line with the ninth rib. The examining hand cannot get above the swelling. Percussion over it is dull. There is a notch on the swelling. It may occasionally be more easily palpated with the patient lying on his right side.

Kidneys

They are palpated in the loin bimanually, i.e. most easily felt by pushing the kidney forwards from behind on to the anterior palpating hand. They move slightly downwards on inspiration. Percussion is resonant over the kidney. The examining hand can easily get between the swelling and the coastal margin. The lower pole of the right kidney can often be felt in thin normal persons.

Abnormal masses

Palpate for abnormal masses particularly in the epigastrium (gastric carcinoma) and suprapubically (an overfilled bladder and ovarian and uterine masses are often missed) and note colonic swellings. The descending colon is commonly palpable in the left iliac fossa (faeces may be indented). The abdominal aorta which is pulsatile and bifurcates at the level of the umbilicus (L4), is easily palpable in thin and lordotic patients. (This is very seldom the only evidence of aortic aneurysm. Abdominal pain and backache are common.)

If general swelling is present, suspect ascites and examine for shifting dullness and ballottement of the liver (dipping). A fluid thrill may be demonstrable in large, tense effusions.

Complete the examination by feeling for inguinal and (if relevant) cervical glands (the drainage from the testes is to the para-aortic and cervical glands), the femoral pulses, checking for leg oedema, and listening for renal bruits and bowel sounds.

External genitalia

It is essential to examine them in practice but rarely required in examinations. Seminoma is a treatable and curable disease of the relatively young and very rarely left-sided varicoele may suggest a left renal carcinoma.

Rectal examination

Essential in practice as rectal carcinoma is common but should not be performed in examinations unless suggested by the examiner. Some examiners will expect the candidates to comment on its desirability particularly in the presence of gastrointestinal disease.

Notes

Splenomegaly

There are two common causes of a very large spleen:
- chronic myeloid leukaemia
- myelofibrosis

NB   Other causes, rare in this country but very common on a world-wide basis, are malaria and kala-azar.

There are two additional causes of a moderately enlarged spleen (4–8 cm):
- reticuloendothelial disease, e.g. Hodgkin's disease and chronic lymphatic leukaemia
- cirrhosis with portal hypertension

But there are many causes of a slightly enlarged spleen:
- any of the above
- glandular fever, brucella and infectious hepatitis (unlikely in the examination)
- subacute septicaemia including subacute bacterial endocarditis and in many infections

Other rare causes include amyloid (rheumatoid arthritis the commonest cause; chronic sepsis is less common), Felty's syndrome, multiple myeloma, sarcoid, collagen disease and storage diseases. Other blood disorders which give splenic enlargement are idiopathic thrombocytopenia, pernicious anaemia, congenital spherocytosis and polycythaemia rubra vera.

Hepatomegaly

There are three common causes:
- congestive cardiac failure
- secondary carcinomatous deposits
- cirrhosis (usually alcoholic)

Other causes include:
- infections—glandular fever, infectious hepatitis
- leukaemia and reticuloendothelial disorders
- tumours (primary hepatoma, amoebic and hydatid cysts)
- amyloid, sarcoid and storage diseases
- primary biliary cirrhosis (large regular liver in women with jaundice and

xanthelasmata)
- haemochromatosis (look for pigmentation)

Hepatosplenomegaly

The list is much the same as for splenomegaly alone since the commonest causes are chronic leukaemia, cirrhosis with portal hypertension, reticuloendothelial disease and myelofibrosis but each of these is usually associated with other clinical signs.

Palpable kidneys

The left kidney is nearly always impalpable but the lower pole of a normal right kidney may be felt in thin people. *Unilateral enlargement* may result from a local lesion, e.g. carcinoma, hydronephrosis, cysts or from hypertrophy of a single functioning kidney. *Bilateral enlargement*, usually gross, occurs in polycystic disease (the liver may also be enlarged) and very rarely in bilateral hydroneph-rosis and amyloidosis. Following *renal transplantation* a kidney may be palpable in the iliac fossa, and the patient may be cushingoid in appearance due to steroid therapy. Look for scars of previous renal surgery and AV shunts.

Mass in right subcostal region

It may be difficult to decide the nature of a mass in this region which may be derived from the liver (including Riedel's lobe), colon, kidney or occasionally gall bladder. If you are uncertain, say so giving the most likely possibilities and the reasons for your conclusions. This will determine the approach to further investigation, which should start with simple studies:

Urine for haematuria and proteinuria.
Stool for occult bleeding.
Ultrasound for solid or cystic masses.

Then proceed as indicated by clinical suspicion and the results of simple studies of one or more of the following:
Liver—liver function tests, isotope scan and biopsy.
Kidney—intravenous urogram.
Colon—sigmoidoscopy, barium enema and colonscopy.
Gall bladder—ultrasound.
CT scan may be helpful for masses which remain obscure and which arise from the pelvis.
Laparotomy

Ascites

The clinical features are abdominal distension, dullness to percussion in the flanks, shifting dullness and a fluid thrill.
The common causes are:
- intra-abdominal neoplasms (remember gynaecological lesions)

- hepatic cirrhosis with portal hypertension (relatively late in the disease (page 256)
- congestive cardiac failure and rarely constrictive pericarditis
- nephrotic syndrome (and other low albumin states)
- tuberculous peritonitis (rare in this country, but should be suspected in Asian and Irish patients)

Paracentesis of a few ml fluid for diagnosis is simple. The specimen should be examined for:

- protein content (> 30 g/litre suggests an exudate; less, a transudate)
- microscopy and bacterial culture (including tuberculosis)
- cytology for malignant cells

Paracentesis may occasionally be required for the relief of severe symptoms but not otherwise because the fluid tends to reaccumulate, and repeated paracentesis leads to excessive protein loss. The suprapubic region is often neglected by physicians examining the abdomen. The commoner causes of a suprapubic mass are the distended bladder (retention from prostatic hypertrophy, tricyclic antidepressants), pregnancy, uterine and ovarian tumours (ovarian fibroids, ovarian cysts, carcinoma)

NB   Management page 257

JAUNDICE

Yellow coloration of the skin and sclerae is usually only apparent when the serum bilirubin is over 35 μmol/litre. Keep in mind the three basic causes of jaundice (haemolytic, hepatocellular, and obstructive) but remember that most cases are due to:

Acute viral hepatitis (page 249): most of these patients are not admitted to hospital unless they are very ill, recovery is unduly prolonged, or intrahepatic cholestasis persists.

Bile duct obstruction from gallstones or carcinoma of the head of the pancreas. Drugs (page 259).

Multiple secondary deposits of carcinoma in the liver (Clinical jaundice is not common when the patient presents but the bilirubin is frequently slightly raised).

Intrahepatic cholestasis (drugs, viral hepatitis, ascending cholangitis and primary biliary cirrhosis).

Infectious mononucleosis.

Gilbert's syndrome (page 49) is intermittent and harmless.

Less common causes include: haemolytic anaemia, congenital hyperbilirubinaemia, stricture or carcinoma of the major bile ducts or ampulla.

'Would you like to ask this (jaundiced) patient some questions?'

Ask about

Age. As a cause of jaundice, carcinoma becomes commoner and hepatitis less common as the patient grows older.

Injections or transfusions in the last 6 months (virus hepatitis) including drug addicts.

Contacts with jaundice and residence abroad.

Occupation. Farm and sewage workers are at risk for leptospirosis.

Presence of dark urine and pale stools of biliary obstruction.

Recent drug therapy especially phenothiazines and 'the pill'.

Period of onset from first symptoms to jaundice. In general hepatitis A is short (1–3 weeks), carcinoma is medium (1–2 months) and cirrhosis is long. Hepatitis B is from 6 weeks to 6 months.

Alcohol consumption.

Recent abdominal pain, surgery anaesthesia (halothane), or a history of chronic dyspepsia may suggest cholecystitis, cholangitis, gallstones or pancreatic carcinoma.

Recent surgery (halothane)

Family history if Gilbert's syndrome is suspected.

'Would you like to examine this (jaundiced) patient?'

Examine

Skin of the face and abdomen and assess the degree of jaundice—deep green suggests long standing obstruction and pale lemon suggests haemolysis. The sclerae often show minor degrees of jaundice not evident elsewhere.

Face, upper chest and hands for spider naevi and the hands for Dupuytren's contracture liver palms and clubbing. Note that xanthelasmata with deep jaundice in a middle-aged woman probably indicates primary biliary cirrhosis.

Neck for lymph node enlargement due to secondary spread of abdominal carcinoma.

Abdomen for:
- recent operation scars which suggest cholecystectomy or surgery for intra-abdominal carcinoma
- hepatomegaly. Irregular when infiltrated with carcinoma, tender in infectious and acute alcoholic hepatitis (and when enlarged in congestive heart failure) and sometimes with carcinoma
- splenomegaly in portal hypertension (and spherocytosis and infectious mononucleosis)
- palpable enlarged gall bladder suggesting bile duct obstruction due to carcinoma of the pancreas (rather than gallstones)
- ascites (which is probably more often due to gynaecological malignancy than to the portal hypertension of cirrhosis, where it occurs late)

Urine if available (see below).

In obstructive jaundice the difficulty is usually to distinguish between benign causes (gallstone obstruction) and malignant causes (carcinoma of the head of the pancreas). Remember that hepatitis A and B, which usually occur in younger patients, and drug jaundice often present with the typical clinical picture of obstructive jaundice from intrahepatic cholestasis and that this may occasionally be persistent.

Drug jaundice should always be reconsidered.

'What investigations would you perform?'
The aims of investigation are:
- to discover the site of any obstruction to the outflow of bile and to determine whether operative interference is necessary
- to determine the degree of impairment of liver cell function and its cause, and to observe its course
- to eliminate rare causes such as haemolysis

Haematology
Including a reticulocyte count and Coombs' test which may give evidence of haemolytic anaemia. A normal reticulocyte count virtually excludes haemolytic jaundice. Leucocytosis may indicate infection (cholangitis) or carcinoma. Abnormal mononuclear cells would suggest infectious mononucleosis (Paul–Bunnell) or, possibly, viral hepatitis.

Urine analysis
Conjugated bilirubin renders the urine yellow.

Urobilinogen is colourless but on standing the urine turns brown as urobilinogen is converted to urobilin by oxidation.

Haemolytic jaundice is acholuric (no bilirubin in the urine) but the urine contains excess urobilinogen because excess bilirubin reaches the intestine and is re-excreted as urobilinogen.

Obstructive jaundice gives urine coloured dark brown with excess bilirubin but a reduction of urinary urobilinogen—because little or no bilirubin reaches the gut due to the obstruction and therefore cannot be reabsorbed and re-excreted. In the early stages of hepatocellular jaundice in acute viral hepatitis, excess urobilinogen may sometimes be present before clinical jaundice becomes apparent. This is due to failure of the liver to take up the excess urobilinogen absorbed from the gut. With increasing severity, biliary obstruction develops and as bilirubin (conjugated) appears in the urine, it disappears from the gut and therefore urobilinogen disappears from the urine. The reciprocal effect also occurs during recovery.

Liver function tests

Protein synthesis
Serum albumin and prothrombin concentrations are reduced in long standing liver disease. The latter is usually partially responsive to vitamin K.

Excretion of alkaline phosphatase

Serum alkaline phosphatase is characteristically greatly elevated in obstructive jaundice and less so in hepatocellular jaundice. A raised level in the absence of other signs of liver disease suggests the presence of malignant secondary deposits in the liver (or bone) or Paget's disease but very seldom in myeloma. The normal range is higher in growing adolescents and in pregnancy.

Bilirubin metabolism

Serum bilirubin is predominantly unconjugated in haemolytic jaundice and the other liver function tests are usually normal. It is mainly conjugated in obstructive jaundice.

Hepatocellular damage

Shown by raised serum level of aminotransferases (transaminases). Very high values suggest viral hepatitis or toxic damage. Slight elevation is consistent with obstructive jaundice. γ-Glutamyl transferase (γ-GT), an inducible microsomal enzyme, is probably the most sensitive index of alcohol ingestion, but it is raised in most forms of liver disease including acute and chronic hepatitis and cirrhosis (or large bile ducts in obstruction) and drugs which induce microsomal enzymes, e.g. phenytoin.

Serology

Always check hepatitis antibodies serology in jaundice cases of unknown cause. Mitochondrial antibodies are detected in 90% of cases of primary biliary cirrhosis. Antinuclear factor and smooth muscle antibodies are detected in over 50% of cases of chronic active hepatitis. Mitochondrial antibodies may also be positive.

X-ray and ultrasound of abdomen

May show gallstones and will put on record the size of the liver and spleen. *Barium swallow* and meal may show oesophageal varices or a distorted duodenal loop from pancreatic carcinoma. *Isotopic liver scans* may demonstrate 'holes' due to carcinomatous secondaries (or large bile ducts in obstruction). *Ultrasound* and *CT scan* may show secondary tumour, stones in the gall bladder and dilated ducts in obstruction (not always shown when the obstruction is due to stones).

Needle liver biopsy

Biliary obstruction is a relative contraindication because of the potential danger of causing biliary peritonitis. Biopsy may provide the histological diagnosis sometimes even in focal lesions. In experienced hands it is a safe procedure provided the prothrombin concentration and platelet counts are normal. Fresh frozen plasma will quickly reverse the prothrombin time for the duration of the procedure.

Other investigation procedures which may be helpful
- for hepatoma: α-fetoprotein and selenomethionine scan

- for carcinoma of the pancreatic head: CT scan
- for obstructive jaundice: endoscopic retrograde cannulation of the pancreatic duct (ERCP) is valuable to define obstruction of the pancreatico-duodenal tree for sphincterotomy to release stones and relieve obstruction by insertion of a stent.

Percutaneous cholangiography. This may be valuable in clinical obstructive jaundice where the cause is in doubt after initial investigations and ultrasound is inconclusive or not available. The needle is inserted up to three times if necessary and contrast medium injected if a dilated bile duct is entered. If not, a liver biopsy is taken.

NB In obstructive jaundice if the cause is not clinically obvious:
- retake the drug history
- perform blood and urine tests as above
- ultrasound, isotope γ scan or abdominal CT scan for large ducts, pancreatic carcinoma, stones, secondary carcinoma
- ERCP if ducts enlarged
- percutaneous cholangiography followed by biopsy if ducts are not entered or, if they are, laparotomy for confirmation and relief of jaundice. If the bile ducts are not enlarged on an ultrasound or CT scan, liver biopsy for histological diagnosis

CONGENITAL NON-HAEMOLYTIC HYPERBILIRUBINAEMIAS

These may explain persistent jaundice in the young after viral hepatitis or slight jaundice in the healthy.

Gilbert's syndrome (autosomal dominant)

This is the only common congenital hyperbilirubinaemia (1–2% of the population). There is impaired glucuronidation of bilirubin (reduced UDPGT—uridine diphosphate glucuronyl transferase) resulting in a raised unconjugated plasma bilirubin and acholuria. About 40% have a reduced red cell survival with a consequent increase in bilirubin production.

The plasma bilirubin is usually <35 µmol/litre.

Diagnosis is by exclusion: there is no haemolysis and the other liver function tests are normal. Fasting, and i.v. nicotinic acid produce a rise in plasma bilirubin.

Liver biopsy is rarely indicated (unless the diagnosis is uncertain) and the liver is histologically normal.

The prognosis is excellent and treatment unnecessary. It is important because it should be not confused with serious liver disease.

Dubin–Johnson (autosomal recessive)

A rare benign disorder usually in adolescents, of failure to excrete conjugated bilirubin. The plasma bilirubin is conjugated. The liver is stained black by centrilobular melanin and there is a late rise in the bromsulphthalein (BSP) elimination curve at 90 min.

Rotor syndrome

A benign disorder with conjugated hyperbilirubinaemia. It is distinguished from the Dubin–Johnson syndrome by a normal liver biopsy.

Crigler–Najjar (autosomal recessive)

It is exceedingly rare and presents in neonates with kernicterus and unconjugated hyperbilirubinaemia (due to absence of uridine diphosphate glucuronyl transferase (UDPGT)). Type I with complete deficiency is fatal in the first year of life, but type II with partial deficiency is not.

URAEMIA (pages 232, 236)

'This patient is uraemic' 'Would you ask him some questions and examine him?'

Ask about

Symptoms of renal failure—thirst, polyuria and nocturia, anorexia, nausea and vomiting, fatigue and itching.
Symptoms of urinary tract infection (dysuria), prostatism (poor stream), renal stone, acute nephritis (haematuria), and nephrotic syndrome (ankle oedema).
Drug therapy, analgesics.

Past history: 'nephritis', diabetes and, in women, pelvic surgery (ureteric obstruction), hypertension and pre-eclamptic toxaemia
Family history: hypertension, polycystic kidneys and gout.

Examine for

Brownish pallor of uraemia and the brown line near the ends of the finger nails.
Bruising.
Hypertension and its consequences, especially cardiac failure.
Hypotension (especially postural) and reduced tissue turgor from dehydration.
Hyperventilation from acidosis (Kussmaul's respiration).
Palpable bladder in outflow obstruction.
Palpable kidneys (polycystic disease and hydronephrosis).
Ankle (or sacral) oedema of nephrotic syndrome or congestive failure.
Signs of dialysis (abdominal scars, vascular shunts).
Peripheral neuropathy.
Pericarditis is usually a late event in uraemia.
Muscular twitching, hiccough, fall in blood pressure and uraemic frost are terminal manifestations.
Rectal examination for prostatic hypertrophy or carcinoma must be performed in practice.

Investigate initially

Urine for microscopy, protein and glucose.
Blood for urea, creatinine, potassium and bicarbonate.
Ultrasound for pelvic dilatation of outflow obstruction and for renal size.

THE RENAL CLINIC

'You are asked to help in a renal transplant or dialysis clinic. What particular features would you check at 3–6 monthly reviews?'

- General wellbeing and weight
- Blood pressure and fundi
- Haemoglobin
- Urea and creatinine, bicarbonate ion and potassium
- Calcium, phosphate, alkaline phosphatase for secondary hyperparathyroidism
- Urine protein output (24 h)
- AV shunts for patency
- Drug dosage (prednisolone, azathioprine, cyclophosphamide, cyclosporin and hypotensive agents) and serum levels as appropriate

DYSPHAGIA

'This patient complains of dysphagia; please question and examine him.'

This term includes both difficulty with swallowing and pain on swallowing. The former symptom is more prominent in obstruction and the latter with inflammatory lesions. The patient can sometimes point to the site of the obstruction.

The history should be taken of the commoner causes remembering that previous reflux oesophagitis suggests peptic stricture and that recurrent chest infections occur with achalasia, bronchial carcinoma or pharyngeal pouches.

Examine the mouth and pharynx (pallor, carcinoma, neurological abnormalities), neck (goitre, and glands from carcinoma) and abdomen (carcinoma) with an initial glance at the hands for koilonychia.

Commonest causes

Carcinoma of the oesophagus and gastric fundus usually give a history of increasing painless difficulty with swallowing foods for the previous 2–3 months. The patient is frequently reduced to taking only soups and drinks by the time of presentation.

Peptic oesophagitis (with pain) proceeds to stricture with difficulty in swallowing.

Rarer causes

- Achalasia of the cardia, mainly in the relatively young. Food 'sticks' and is regurgitated unchanged a short while later (without acid); 25% present with recurrent pulmonary infection
- External pressure. Since the oesophagus is slippery, symptoms of pressure from outside masses (especially carcinoma of the bronchus) are very seldom presenting ones. A retrosternal goitre large enough to produce dysphagia is usually obvious

Very rare causes

Neurological disease: myasthenia gravis (page 153) and bulbar palsies (page 14).

Plummer–Vinson syndrome (Paterson–Kelly–Brown). Sideropenic dysphagia usually occurs in middle-aged women who have iron deficiency anaemia, koilonychia and glossitis. It may be associated with a postcricoid web which is precancerous.

NB Globus hystericus is diagnosed only after full investigation and when positive evidence of psychological stress exists.

Investigation

If you are asked to discuss investigation, suggest:
Hb, serum iron and ferritin.
Endoscopy.
Barium swallow.

NB The postcricoid web occurs in the anterior oesophageal wall and appears on barium swallow as an anterior indentation at the top of the oesophagus at the level of the cricoid cartilage.

Oesophagoscopy and biopsy

May differentiate between benign peptic stricture and carcinoma.

DIARRHOEA

Acute gastroenteritis with diarrhoea and vomiting is the second most common group of disorders affecting the community (second only to acute respiratory infections).

Aetiology

Infectious diarrhoea

Usually *acute,* e.g. winter vomiting disease and travellers' diarrhoea. The aetiology of these syndromes remains unknown with the exception of some outbreaks of diarrhoea due to specific serotypes of E. coli to which the local population may be immune. They may be caused by viruses but none of the common enteroviruses (Coxsackie, polio, echoviruses) can be confidently incriminated. Infant diarrhoea is usually caused by a rotavirus. The vast majority of patients are successfully treated symptomatically.

Food poisoning. Salmonella typhimurium is responsible for 75% of bacterial food poisoning. *S. entertitidis* infection from eggs and poultry is increasing rapidly. Staphylococcal food poisoning results from eating precooked meats and dairy foods, and is produced by the bacterial toxin.

Enteric fevers. Typhoid and paratyphoid must also be considered in patients returning from endemic areas.

Dysentery (see page 377). Results from ingestion of organisms of the genus *Shigella* (bacillary dysentery). Amoebic dysentry and giardiasis should also be considered in patients recently returned from the tropics.

Campylobacter infection may cause bloody diarrhoea.

Clostridium difficile infection (pseudomembranous colitis) usually follows antibiotic therapy.

Cryptosporidium can cause persistent, severe and intractable diarrhoea in AIDS.

Non-infectious diarrhoea

The following conditions must be considered:

Drugs, including purgatives (common), antibiotics, NSAIDs and digoxin (both rare).

Diverticulitis (common).

Colonic carcinoma sometimes with spurious diarrhoea secondary to partial obstruction. Usually alternates with spells of constipation.

Irritable bowel syndrome (page 276) 'nervous diarrhoea' (common).

Ulcerative colitis and Crohn's disease.

Malabsorption syndromes.

Diabetes, thyrotoxicosis (rare).

Post vagotomy.

'This patient has developed diarrhoea. Would you question and examine him?'
In hospital practice, the acute diarrhoeas are seen less frequently than in general practice. It is important to determine whether the recent attack is an isolated one, or part of a chronic or recurrent history. If it is isolated and acute, ask about travel and residence abroad, contact history, previous antibiotic therapy and if food poisoning is suspected, the time relationship to previous food and its effect on other eaters. If the diarrhoea is recurrent or chronic, ask about appetite, weight loss, abdominal pain, blood or mucus in the stools, drug ingestion including purgatives and operations.

Examination

In practice a complete medical examination is required. In examinations, note particularly weight loss, anaemia and clubbing (Crohn's disease). Look for abnormal abdominal masses (usually carcinoma but Crohn's disease should be suspected in young patients). Rectal examination and sigmoidoscopy should invariably be performed in chronic and recurrent diarrhoeas but these should not be attempted in examinations (though the examiner should be told of their necessity).

Investigation

'How would you investigate this patient?'
If it is a single episode of acute diarrhoea and has not settled within 5–7 days or if the patient is ill, perform:

Full blood count for anaemia and blood cultures for *S. typhi*, *S. paratyphi* and *S. enteritidis*, particularly in travellers from abroad.

Stool to laboratory for examination for cysts, ova and parasites *(Amoeba,*

Giardia) and for culture (typhoid and paratyphoid, *Campylobacter*, *Clostridium difficile)*.

Sigmoidoscopy, particularly in suspected ulcerative colitis or carcinoma (or amoebic colitis). Biopsy and history may be diagnostic.

If acute diarrhoea remains undiagnosed or fails to respond to simple symptomatic remedies within 1–2 weeks or in chronic diarrhoea, it is usually necessary (if not previously indicated) to proceed to further investigation, including sigmoidoscopy with biopsy followed after a few days (to allow healing) by barium enema. If the history suggests malabsorption (page 270) perform endoscopic duodenal biopsy and if Crohn's disease is suspected obtain small bowel barium studies.

NB   Dysentery (bacillary and amoebic), typhoid and paratyphoid, and cholera are notifiable to the public health authorities.

Bloody diarrhoea suggests:

- colonic carcinoma
- diverticular disease
- ulcerative colitis
- dysentery
- ischaemic colitis
- *Campylobacter* enteritis

but the most common cause of rectal bleeding is haemorrhoids and fissures. If the cause is not obvious, rectal bleeding needs full investigation with sigmoidoscopy and barium enema, proceeding to colonoscopy if necessary.

Respiratory system

The most usual types of clinical case seen in examinations are those secondary to carcinoma of the bronchus or due to long standing chronic disease. Asthma and chronic bronchitis are very common chronic disabilities. Bronchiectasis is sufficiently common to appear in examinations. Pleural effusions are usually secondary to underlying carcinoma (primary or secondary) or infection. There are still many patients with long standing healed tuberculous fibrosis (mainly of the upper lobes) with mediastinal shift.

EXAMINATION
'Examine the chest' or 'Examine the lungs'.
This means 'Examine the respiratory system' unless otherwise specified.

If allowed to question the patient, enquire about smoking, occupation, dyspnoea, chest pain, cough, sputum, and haemoptysis, allergy, family history of allergy and past history of asbestosis or mining. The diagnosis of chronic bronchitis is made on the history of 3 months' productive cough in 2 consecutive years.

Observation
On approaching the patient note dyspnoea and cyanosis and any evidence of loss of weight.
Examine the hands for clubbing, tobacco-staining and feel for the bounding pulse of carbon dioxide retention if you suspect respiratory failure. Ask the patient his age and occupation (for occupational lung diseases) and assess hoarseness.
Quickly check the height of the jugular venous pressure, and the tongue for cyanosis.
Remove all clothes above the waist and observe the shape of the chest and spine, any scars and the movements for symmetry and expansion (subtle differences are best seen from the end of the bed), and the use of accessory muscles in the neck and shoulders.
Count the respiratory rate.

Palpation
Palpate for chest expansion comparing movements on both sides. *Diminished movement means pathology on that side.*
Palpate the trachea in the suprasternal notch (easier with the head partially extended). Deviation denotes fibrosis or collapse of the upper lobe or whole lung in the direction of deviation, or pneumothorax (or very rarely a large pleural effusion) on the other side.
NB Local causes may produce deviation in the absence of lung disease, e.g.

Table 5. Physical signs in lung disease.

	Movements on side of lesion	Trachea	Percussion	Breath sounds	Tactile frem and vocal resonance
Pleural effusion	Diminished	Usually central May be deviated away from lesion if very large	Dull (stony)	Diminished, often with bronchial breathing at top of effusion	Diminished
Pneumothorax	Diminished	Usually central May be deviated away if very large	Hyperresonant	Diminished	Diminished
Consolidation (pneumonia)	Diminished	Central or deviated towards side of lesion if associated with collapse	Dull	Bronchial (tubular) if airway open Absent if airway obstructed, e.g. carcinoma	Increased if airway open Diminished if airway obstructed
Fibrosis	Diminished	Deviated towards fibrosis if upper lobe affected	Dull	Bronchial	Increased
Chronic obstructive pulmonary disease	Diminshed	Central, possibly with tag	Normal or hyperresonant	Scattered added sounds	Normal

NB All the abnormal signs—bronchial breathing, increased vocal resonance, increased tactile fremitus, whispering pectoriloquoy—occur in consolidation.

goitre and spinal asymmetry. The position of the apex beat is rarely of help in assessing lung disease except if there is marked mediastinal shift.
Palpate for cervical lymphadenopathy.

Percussion

Percuss by moving down the chest comparing both sides. Stony dullness in the axilla usually indicates pleural effusion. Pleural thickening and collapse, consolidation, or fibrosis of the lung also give dullness.
NB Upper lobe fibrosis in an otherwise fit elderly patient is probably due to old tuberculosis.
Diminished movement with resonance on one side usually means pneumothorax (or occasionally a large bulla).

Auscultation

Bronchial breathing occurs in consolidation including that at the top of effusions. Diminished breath sounds occur overlying an effusion, pleural thickening, pneumothorax and, in the obese, due to interposition of abnormal features between the lung surface and the stethoscope. Diminished breath sounds also occur with obstructed airways.

Added sounds are either wheezes (*rhonchi*) or crackles (*crepitations—* sounds like rubbing strands of hair between finger and thumb behind the ear, râles). Wheezing is common in asthma and bronchitis but sometimes occurs in left ventricular failure. Crepitations are fine in pulmonary congestion and fibrosing alveolitis and coarse in the presence of excess bronchial secretions. *Tactile fremitus* and *vocal resonance* are both increased over areas of consolidation. Friction rubs occur with pleurisy.

Whispering pectoriloquy occurs in association with consolidation. The patient is asked to whisper (not phonate) '1–2–3–4' and this is heard by the exploring stethoscope on the chest wall overlying the consolidation. (It can be imitated by whispering with both ears blocked with index fingers.)

NOTES

Clubbing

Associated with diseases in the lungs, heart and abdomen:

Carcinoma of bronchus (the only common cause).
Pus in the pleura (empyema), lung (abscess) or bronchi (bronchiectasis, cystic fibrosis).
Fibrosing alveolitis.
Cyanotic congenital heart disease.
Subacute bacterial endocarditis.
Crohn's disease (less commonly, ulcerative colitis and cirrhosis).

Haemoptysis

Aetiology

Common

Bronchial carcinoma (or rarely other vascular tumours).
Tuberculosis (active or healed). NB Aspergilloma in healed cavity.
Pulmonary embolism with infarction.
Infection (pneumococcal pneumonia, lung abscess and *Klebsiella pneumoniae*).
The presence of chronic bronchitis, a common cause of slight haemoptysis, does not exclude any of the above.

Uncommon

Bronchiectatic cavities or chronic bronchitis.
Mitral stenosis.
Foreign body—history of general anaesthetic, visit to dentist, or inhalation of food.
Coagulation disorders.

Very rare

Wegener's granulomatosis (a generalised vasculitis which may present with rhinitis and round lung shadows with or without ENT masses and/or renal failure).

Goodpasture's syndrome (glomerulonephritis with haemoptysis).

Investigation

The usual clinical problem is to exclude carcinoma and tuberculosis. A full history and clinical examination will usually identify pulmonary infarction, foreign body, bronchiectasis, mitral stenosis and pulmonary oedema.

Chest X-ray

Sputum for culture, including tuberculosis and cytology for malignant cells.

Fibreoptic bronchoscopy with brush biopsy for cytology and culture, and needle biopsy for cytology of peripheral lesions. Visible lesions are biopsied—this is essential in all patients suspected of early bronchial carcinoma, which is amenable to surgery only if diagnosed early.

Isotope lung scan for suspected pulmonary embolism.

Bronchography for suspected bronchiectasis may be diagnostic

CT scanning has largely replaced bronchography.

NB About 40% of patients with haemoptysis have no demonstrable cause. Patients who have had a single small haemoptysis, no other symptoms, and a normal chest X-ray (PA and lateral) probably do not require further investigation, but a follow-up appointment with a chest X-ray is advisable after 1–2 months. Patients who have more than one small haemoptysis should be regarded as having carcinoma or tuberculosis until proved otherwise, and be submitted to fibreoptic bronchoscopy.

Pleural effusion

Aetiology

Carcinoma: primary bronchus (the effusion implies pleural involvement) or secondary (commonly breast).

Cardiac failure.

Pulmonary embolus and infarction.

Tuberculosis.

Other infections (pneumonia).

Rarely, lymphomas, systemic lupus erythematosus, rheumatoid arthritis and transdiaphragmatic spread often including peritoneal dialysis and Meigs' syndrome (usually a right-sided transudate from benign ovarian fibroma).

NB Aspiration of the fluid is usually necessary both for treatment and to assist diagnosis. A pleural biopsy should be performed at the same time. Specimens are sent to the laboratory for:

- microscopy
- bacterial culture including tuberculosis

- histology
- cytology for malignant cells
- protein content. 30 g/litre approximately divides exudates from transudates

Cyanosis

'Cyanosis' is a clinical description and refers to the blue colour of a patient's lips, tongue (central) or fingers (peripheral). Central cyanosis is almost always due to the presence of an excess of reduced haemoglobin in the capillaries. Over 3 g/100 ml is usually present before cyanosis is apparent. Thus, in anaemia severe hypoxaemia may be present without cyanosis. Cyanosis may be central or peripheral.

'Look at this (cyanosed) patient'

It is often difficult to tell whether cyanosis is present or not. Comparison of the colour of the patient's tongue or nail beds with your own nail beds (presumed to be normal) may help if both hands are warm.

Look at the patient's tongue. If it is cyanosed, the cyanosis is central in origin and secondary to:

- chronic bronchitis and emphysema often with cor pulmonale
- congenital heart disease (cyanosis may be present only after exercise)
- polycythaemia
- massive pulmonary embolism

In central cyanosis there is always cyanosis at the periphery.

If the tongue is not cyanosed but the fingers, toes or ear lobes are, the cyanosis is peripheral and:

- physiological due to cold
- pathological in peripheral vascular disease (the cyanosed parts feel cold)

NB Left ventricular failure may produce cyanosis which is partly central (pulmonary) and partly peripheral (poor peripheral circulation).

A rare cause of cyanosis, which is not due to increased circulating reduced haemoglobin, is the presence of methaemoglobin (and/or sulphaemoglobin). The patients are relatively well and not necessarily dyspnoeic. *Methaemoglobin-aemia* and *sulphaemoglobinaemia* are usually the result of taking certain drugs, e.g. phenacetin and sulphonamides. Primaquine (an 8-amino quinoline) and nitrites may cause methaemoglobinaemia.

Cyanosis is an unreliable guide to the degree of hypoxaemia.

BLOOD GASES

'Comment on these blood gases'

The normal arterial values are:

Po_2	12–14 kPa (90–105 mmHg)
Pco_2	4.7–6.0 kPa (35–45 mmHg)
pH	7.37–7.42
Standard HCO_3^-	23–27 mmol/litre

Look at the pH for acidosis or alkalosis.

Look at the $P\text{CO}_2$. If it is raised this may account for an acidosis of respiratory origin (respiratory failure). If it is reduced this may account for an alkalosis due to hyperventilation (pain, stiff lungs, anxiety and hysterical hyperventilation or artificial ventilation).

Look at 'standard HCO_3' (measured at $P\text{CO}_2$ of 40 mmHg, i.e. with simulated normal ventilation). If it is raised this accounts for a metabolic alkalosis. If it is reduced it accounts for a metabolic acidosis (usually renal or ketotic).

Look at $P\text{O}_2$. If it is high, the patient is on added O_2. If low, the patient has lung disease (the $P\text{CO}_2$ is usually high) or a right to left shunt.

Interpretation

$P\text{CO}_2$ reflects alveolar ventilation.
$P\text{O}_2$ reflects ventilation/perfusion imbalance, gas transfer or venous to arterial shunts.

Gas patterns

High $P\text{CO}_2$, low $P\text{O}_2$. Respiratory failure due to chronic bronchitis asthma or chest wall disease (e.g. ankylosing spondylitis and neuromuscular disorders).

Normal or low $P\text{CO}_2$, low $P\text{O}_2$. Hypoxia due to parenchymal lung disease with normal airways. These patients hyperventilate and hence lower the $P\text{CO}_2$ because of hypoxia (and 'stiff lungs'), e.g. pulmonary embolism, fibrosing alveolitis. Another cause is 'venous admixture' from right to left shunts (e.g. Fallot).

Low $P\text{CO}_2$, normal $P\text{O}_2$. A common pattern seen usually after painful arterial puncture (causing hyperventilation), and in hysterical hyperventilation.

Causes of hypoxaemia

- Low inspired oxygen concentration due to altitude or faulty apparatus
- Hypoventilation due to sedative drugs, CNS disease, neuromuscular disease, crushed chest, or obstructive sleep apnoea. The arterial $P\text{CO}_2$ is characteristically high
- Ventilation–perfusion imbalance (V/Q). Hyperventilation of some alveoli cannot compensate for the hypoxaemia which results from the hypoventilation of other alveoli. This is the usual cause of a reduced $T\text{LCO}$
- Physiological shunt (venous admixture) when deoxygenated blood passes straight to left heart without perfusing ventilated alveoli. This occurs in cyanotic congenital heart disease. The arterial $P\text{O}_2$ is not significantly improved by the administration of 2 litres oxygen/min

Type 1 respiratory failure refers to patients with lung disease which produces hyperventilation as well as hypoxaemia such as pulmonary oedema, pneumonia, asthma, pulmonary fibrosis and pulmonary thromboembolism.

Type 2 respiratory failure with a high $P\text{CO}_2$ (and hypoxaemia) implies a defect in ventilation with obstructed airways, reduced chest wall compliance, or CNS disease because normally the excess CO_2 would be blown off.

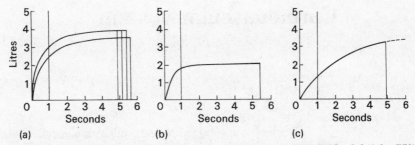

Figure 6. Spirometric patterns. (a) Normal (elderly man) FEV/FVC = 3.0/4.0 = 75%; (b) restrictive, FEV/FVC = 1.8/2.0 = 90%; and (c) obstructive, FEV/FVC = 1.4/3.5 = 40%.

VENTILATORY FUNCTION TESTS (FEV$_1$, FVC, PEFR)

The simplest tests of lung function are spirometric. If a patient exhales as fast and as long as possible from a full inspiration into a spirometer, the volume expired in the first second is the FEV$_1$ (forced expiratory volume in 1 s) and the total expired is the FVC (forced vital capacity). Relaxed (slow) vital capacity may provide a better measure of trapped gas volume in chronic airways obstruction and is as easy to measure as these other values. Constriction of the major airways (e.g. asthma) reduces the FEV$_1$ more than the FVC. Restriction of the lungs (e.g. by fibrosis) reduces the FVC and, to a lesser degree, the FEV$_1$. The ratio of FEV$_1$ to FVC (FEV%) thus tends to be low in obstructive airways disease (e.g. chronic bronchitis and asthma) and normal or high in fibrosing alveolitis (page 306). It is best to see the shape of the actual curve as well as the figures derived from it (figure 6). Spirometry is often performed before and after bronchodilation.

The PEFR (peak expiratory flow rate) measures the rate of flow of exhaled air at the start of a forced expiration. It gives similar information to the FEV$_1$.

Normal values for all these tests vary with age, sex, size and race, and suitable nomograms should be consulted unless the changes observed are gross.

Transfer factor (*T*LCO)

The patient must have a vital capacity of over 1 litre and be able to hold his breath for 15 s. This test measures the transfer of a small concentration of CO in the inspired air on to haemoglobin. It is reduced in diseases which reduce ventilation (V) or perfusion (Q) or alters the balance between them (V/Q). Correction must be made for haemoglobin (Hb) concentration as transfer factor varies directly with Hb. Its chief value is for monitoring progression in interstitial disease including fibrosing alveolitis.

Cardiovascular system

There is no shortage of patients with cardiovascular disease who are suitable for inclusion in examinations. Patients with ischaemic heart disease have few physical signs and the diagnosis of angina of effort will be made on symptoms alone. Valvular disease, whether acquired or congenital, and septal defects often give rise to murmurs which may be diagnostic. The penalties for failing to elicit and describe and interpret these correctly are often disproportionate to their real importance in diagnosis and treatment. A cardiologist rarely reaches a final decision on physical signs alone unsupported by an electrocardiogram, chest X-ray and echocardiogram. Patients with congestive heart failure and cases of myocardial infarction are very common in hospital and during the recovery phase may be suffiently well to be included in an examination list.

ARTERIAL PULSE
'Examine the (arterial) pulse'
If you are asked this, there is frequently an arrhythmia (often atrial fibrillation or multiple ectopic beats). Less commonly you may feel the very slow pulse of complete heart block or there may be a tachycardia such as that associated with thyrotoxicosis, the clinical features of which you may notice on approaching the patient (though not so obvious in the elderly).
Do not attempt to estimate the blood pressure from the pulse.
Examine a carotid, brachial or radial pulse—whichever you are familiar with assessing. Describe as follows:

Approximate rate
Glance at the jugular venous pressure whilst counting, since this may give valuable additional information about cardiac rhythm and failure (see below).

Rhythm
Regular, basically regular with extra or dropped beats, or completely irregular. If it is clinically atrial fibrillation, remember that the pulse rate is different from the heart rate; also listen at the apex.

Volume and character (table 6)
These abnormalities fall into three categories:
- Useful to confirm or assess other findings in the cardiovascular system (plateau, collapsing, small volume)
- Rare and/or difficult (alternans, bisferiens and paradoxus)
- Examination 'catch' (absent radial)

62

Table 6.   Special pulses.

Type	Character	Seen in
Plateau	Low amplitude, slow rise slow fall	Aortic valve stenosis
Collapsing (waterhammer)	Large amplitude, rapid rise and rapid fall	Aortic regurgitation. Also severe anaemia hyperthyroidism AV shunt, heart block, PDA
Small volume	Thready	Low cardiac output due to obstruction: valve stenosis (tricuspid, pulmonary, mitral, aortic) or pulmonary hypertension Shock
Alternans	Alternate large and small amplitude beats rarely noted in pulse; usually on taking blood pressure (note doubling in rate as mercury falls)	Left ventricular failure
Bisferiens	Double-topped	Aortic stenosis with aortic regurgitation
Paradoxus	Pulse volume decreases excessively with inspiration (of little diagnostic value)	Cardiac tamponade, constrictive pericarditis, severe inspiratory airways obstruction (chronic bronchitis and asthma)
Absent radial		Congenital anomaly (check brachials and blood pressure Tied off at surgery or catheterisation Arterial embolism (usually atrial fibrillation)

Notes
1   The state of one vessel wall does not necessarily correlate with the state of the arteries elsewhere.
2   It takes little time to check if the left radial (or brachial) pulse is present.
3   If you think the patient may have hypertension, you should look for radial femoral delay (aortic coarctation).
4   If the character of the pulse is abnormal you should ask whether you may take the blood pressure, to estimate the pulse pressure (and to check alternans).

NB   The rate and rhythm are relatively easy to assess but the character of the pulse extremely difficult.

NECK VEINS

'Look at the veins of the neck' (*'Examine the jugular venous pressure'*).

Raised jugular venous pressure (table 7)

You should comment on the *vertical* height of the top of the column of blood above the sternal angle. The patient will usually be lying at 45° and the neck should be relaxed. The angle of Louis is about 5 cm above the left atrium when the patient is lying at 45°. The normal central venous pressure (CVP) is <7 cm

Table 7. Raised jugular venous pressure.

Character	Compression of neck and abdomen	Conclusion
Non-pulsatile	No change in jugular venous pressure	Superior mediastinal obstruction (usually carcinoma of bronchus), platysmal compression or large goitre
Pulsatile	Jugular vein fills and empties	Right heart failure (page 315) Expiratory airways obstruction (asthma and bronchitis) Fluid overload Cardiac tamponade (very rare)

Notes
1 Large 'a' wave (corresponds with atrial systole) occurs in tricuspid stenosis, pulmonary stenosis, in complete heart block (cannon wave) and rarely in pulmonary hypertension.
2 Large 'v' wave (corresponds with ventricular systole) occurs in tricuspid regurgitation, usually secondary to cardiac failure.
3 There is no 'a' wave atrial fibrillation.

and therefore the jugular vein is normally just visible. The deep venous pulse is seen welling up between the heads of sternomastoid in the front of the neck on expiration, and is a better guide to right atrial pressure than the superficial venous pulse which may rarely be obstructed by the soft tissues of the neck. If you can find neither:

Look at the other side of the neck.
Suspect a low level and press on the abdomen firmly (unless the liver is tender) in order to raise the column. A positive reflux may have no pathophysiological significance and the sole purpose of this manoeuvre is to demonstrate the vein and to show that it can be filled (i.e. the pressure is not high).
Suspect a high level with distension of the veins (not easily seen) with the top of the column above the neck. Check if the ear lobes move with the cardiac cycle and sit the patient vertical to get a greater length of visible jugular vein above the right atrium. The venous pressure can sometimes be demonstrated in dilated veins of an arm or hand held at a suitable height above the right atrium. The level at which pulsation occurs should be determined.

If the jugular venous pressure is raised (especially if >10 cm):
A large 'a' wave occurs in tricuspid stenosis, pulmonary hypertension, pulmonary stenosis, and mitral stenosis. A cannon wave is a massive 'a' wave occurring in complete heart block when the right atrium contracts against a closed tricuspid valve.
Look for a large 'v' wave indicating tricuspid regurgitation: a murmur may be audible on auscultation of the heart.
Examine the abdomen for an enlarged tender pulsatile liver.
Check the ankles for oedema and then sit the patient up and examine the back of the chest for crepitations and for pleural effusions (unilateral or bilateral) and

for sacral oedema. These should be done even if the jugular venous pressure is not raised since oedema of cardiac failure may persist after jugular venous pressure has been reduced by treatment.

Examine for the underlying cause, e.g. heart valve lesion or fluid overload.

HEART
'Examine the heart.'

Most 'heart cases' in an examination have a murmur. Such patients make it easy for an examiner to assess the candidate's ability to elicit and describe accurately the physical signs which are present. You may be watched throughout your examination and you must therefore have devised a system of examination which is second nature to you even in this stressful situation.

A full examination of the heart is not advisable without examining the arterial and venous pulses and this is usually done first. It is important to know not only the auscultatory features of the various heart abnormalities but also to know which of them are found in association with each other and to examine for these with particular care. Thus every patient in whom you have diagnosed mitral stenosis should be examined with special attention to the aortic valve.

Chronic rheumatic heart disease is still the commonest type of 'heart' case in examinations, though many of them have had cardiac surgery. It is becoming progressively less common in clinical practice because rheumatic fever is now a rare disorder. You may see patients with ventricular septal defects; the smaller lesions may not require surgery and often produce loud murmurs (maladie de Roger). For similar reasons you may be shown a patient with an atrial septal defect (ASD)—often not diagnosed until middle age—but the auscultatory findings may be difficult to elicit. Beware of coarctation of the aorta where loud murmurs may originate in collateral vessels over the chest wall.

On approaching the patient note any cyanosis, dyspnoea or malar flush.

Examine the arterial pulses and look for clubbing (page 57)

Examine the jugular venous pulse.

Examine the front of the chest. First look for the scars of previous surgery and then for the localised thrusting apex beat of left ventricular hypertrophy and the parasternal lift of right ventricular hypertrophy. Then palpate for these phenomena and for thrills (palpable murmurs). Note that a tapping apex is thought to be an accentuated mitral first sound and in subsequent examination you will be trying to substantiate a diagnosis of mitral stenosis. Finally listen to the heart, starting at the apex. It may be difficult to establish which are the first and second sounds, but an experienced clinician recognises them by their quality. A thumb on the right carotid artery can help to time the first sound.

Examine each part of the cardiac cycle for murmurs. (Remember to listen for a friction rub of pericarditis and a triple rhythm of cardiac failure. These are easily missed). There is no alternative to experience for this and it is essential to know the character of the murmurs of the commoner cardiac lesions. Their description is formalised and stereotyped so that if you say there is a rumbling

Table 8. Characteristics of murmurs.

Lesion	Murmur and position	Radiation and notes
Aortic stenosis (often with aortic incompetence)	Basal mid-systolic, often loud and with a thrill Possible ejection click	Maximal in 2nd RICS and radiating into neck. Also at apex
Pulmonary stenosis (may be part of Fallot's tetralogy)	Basal mid-systolic with click if stenosis is valvar	Maximal in 2nd LICS. Increase on inspiration (with increased blood flow) Pulmonary component of 2nd sound is quiet and delayed
Aortic regurgitation (often accompanying mitral stenosis in this country because syphilis is now rare)	Early immediate blowing diastolic murmur	Usually maximal in 3rd LICS or less often in 2nd RICS. Radiation between right carotid and cardiac apex Look for Argyll Robertson pupils, etc.
Pulmonary regurgitation very rare	Early immediate blowing diastolic murmur	Maximal in 2nd and 3rd LICS
Mitral stenosis	Mid or late rumbling diastolic murmur at apex	Loud mitral 1st sound. Opening snap. Turn patient on left side (and exercise) to accentuate murmur. Presystolic accentuation if in sinus rhythm
Mitral regurgitation (often mitral stenosis is present as well)	Pan-systolic at apex	Radiation to axilla (but often heard parasternally)
Tricuspid regurgitation	Pan-systolic and lower sternum	'v' wave in neck and pulsatile liver
Ventricular septal defect (small ones are common, severe are rare)	Rough, loud and pan-systolic. Maximal at 3rd–4th LICS parasternally	
Atrial septal defect	Pulmonary systolic murmur with fixed split 2nd sound. (There is no murmur due to blood flow through the defect)	Possible diastolic murmur from tricuspid valve if ASD flow is large
Patent ductus arteriosus	Machinery murmur, maximal in late systole and extending into diastole. Maximal in 2nd–3rd LICS in mid-clavicular line	Audible also posteriorly
Coarctation	Loud rough murmur in systole, maximum over apex of left lung both posteriorly and anteriorly	Murmurs of scapular and internal mammary shunt collaterals Radial femoral delay. Hypertension in arms
Friction rub	Scratchy noise usually systole and diastole	Varies with posture and breathing

Notes: 1 'Base' denotes the 1st and 2nd intercostal spaces. **2** 'RICS' and 'LICS' refer to right and left intercostal spaces.

diastolic murmur at the apex, you have diagnosed mitral stenosis. You should attempt to make whatever you hear fit one of the known patterns (table 8).

Listen to the lungs especially at the bases posteriorly for fine crepitations. Look for sacral and ankle oedema. Establish the blood pressure.

Difficult systolic murmurs

It may be impossible to define the valve lesion causing an apical systolic murmur on auscultation without echocardiography. The possibilities include:
- mitral regurgitation (papillary muscle dysfunction, floppy valve, ruptured chordae tendineae)
- aortic ejection murmur
- ventricular septal defect (VSD) very occasionally

Continuous murmurs

These are murmurs maximal in systole and passing through the second sound into diastole.

They are caused by:
- patent ductus arteriosus (best heard in second left intercostal space).
- aortic stenosis and regurgitation
- arteriovenous malformation in the lung
- coronary arteriovenous fistula
- ruptured sinus of Valsalva (the pockets behind each leaflet of the aortic valve)—a high-pitched murmur because of high pressure

NB The unsatisfactory question, *'listen here or listen at this point'*: usually the apex or aortic area, is used to ensure that the candidate rolls the patient onto the left side for mitral stenotic mumurs, or sits them forward and asks them to exhale fully for aortic regurgitation.

Heart failure (page 315)

The signs of left ventricular failure are tachycardia, triple rhythm, fine basal crepitations of pulmonary oedema and pleural effusion usually associated with signs of right ventricular failure, i.e. raised jugular venous pressure, hepatomegaly, ankle and sacral oedema.

If right ventricular failure is secondary to lung disease (cor pulmonale), there is usually clinical evidence to suggest chronic obstructive pulmonary disease (page 282) or less commonly pulmonary embolism (page 303). Other rare causes include bronchiectasis, fibrosing alveolitis, cystic fibrosis and primary pulmonary hypertension. Treatment is discussed on page 317.

In heart failure resistant to these measures, therapy with diamorphine captopril or isosorbide may be used for improvement in left ventricular function.

HYPERTENSION

'This person has hypertension—please examine him to demonstrate the key signs.'

If you are allowed to question the patient, ask about anginal chest pain, intermittent claudication, headaches, visual changes, family history, salt intake, breathlessness and drugs taken (especially the contraceptive pill, cold cures containing sympathomimetic drugs, and monoamine oxidase inhibitors).

Slight or moderate hypertension usually gives no abnormalities detectable on physical examination. In long standing or severe hypertension there will usually be left ventricular hypertrophy and a loud aortic second sound. The other consequences of sustained hypertension should be looked for, i.e. hypertensive retinopathy, heart failure, renal failure, cerebrovascular disease. It is essential to think of the less common causes of hypertension and therefore to consider the following:
- observe the face for evidence of Cushing's syndrome—usually due to steroid or adrenocorticotrophic hormone (ACTH) administration
- feel both radials and take the blood pressure in both arms for coarctation
- examine for aortic coarctation (radial-femoral delay, weak femoral pulses and the bruits of the coarctation and of the scapular anastomoses and visible pulsation of the anastomoses)
- a renal artery bruit may be present in the epigastrium in renal artery stenosis
- the kidneys are palpable in polycystic disease
- think also of the chronic renal diseases (test the urine), of phaeochromocytoma (rare), and of primary hyperaldosteronism (very rare)

MYOCARDIAL INFARCTION

'This patient has had a myocardial infarction, would you ask him some questions?'

The patient will be in the recovery stage. The history is more important than the physical signs. Symptoms (pain or fatigue) are often present in the preceding weeks.

Ask about

Pain. Onset (rest or exercise), quality (compressing), distribution (including radiation), duration (usually over half an hour). Tearing interscapular pain suggests dissecting aneurysm.

NB Intensity is no guide to the extent of the infarct, especially in the elderly where pain may often be absent.

Breathlessness. About a quarter of all cases describe an acute attack of dyspnoea as a feature of the attack and in the elderly it may be the only feature.

Cold sweat. Also common, and often associated with nausea and vomiting.

Pallor. Normally reported by witnesses.

Previous attacks of angina. If they have had a previous infarct or angina their new pain will usually resemble that which they have had previously.

Past history of hypertension, strokes, symptoms of peripheral vascular disease and, in young women, whether they have diabetes mellitus or are on the contraceptive pill.

Family history of heart attacks, especially if young; diabetes; hypertension; gout.

Other risk factors, e.g. smoking, occupation.

Examination

'Would you like to examine him?'

Evidence of a low cardiac output (hypotension and small volume rapid pulse).

Signs of cardiac failure including crepitations at the lung bases.

Arrhythmias, tachycardia, bradycardia.

Pericardial friction (immediate and post-infarction syndrome).

Evidence of mitral regurgitation (papillary muscle dysfunction).

Evidence of a cardiac aneurysm (double impulse). Rare.

Evidence of septal perforation (acquired VSD). Rare and acute.

Deep venous thrombosis—a complication of immobilisation.

Evidence of hyperlipidaemia, especially xanthelasmata and tendon xanthomata.

Evidence of associated diseases: hypothyroidism, diabetes mellitus, gout, cigarette smoking (smell and finger-staining).

Evidence of the relevant alternatives in the differential diagnosis, especially pulmonary embolism, pericarditis, dissecting aneurysm, pleurisy, cholecystitis, reflux oesophagitis, radicular pain.

Investigation

'What investigations would you perform?'

Ask for an ECG series and a cardiac enzyme series, e.g. hydroxybutyrate dehydrogenase, aspartate transferase or MB isoenzyme of creatine phosphokinase. You may note rises in the white cell count, ESR and temperature. A chest X-ray is necessary in all cardiac investigations.

Management

'Discuss the management'

The following aspects should be considered (see page 311):

Bed rest.

Analgesia and sedation.

Oxygen therapy.

Anticoagulants:

Complications (cardiac failure and shock, arrhythmias, rupture of septum, papillary muscle dysfunction and cardiac aneurysm).

Thrombolytic therapy (aspirin, streptokinase) rt-PA (alteplase), APSAC (onistreplase).

Smoking.

Obesity.

Hyperlipidaemia (page 209).

Advice on discharge from hospital, i.e. work, driving, sexual activities (page 315).

CARDIAC ARREST

Cardiac rescusitation. You may be taken to a dummy (resusci-Annie) and told *'You are the first to arrive, having been called by another patient. Carry on'*

• feel for a major pulse (femoral or carotid) while checking that the patient has lost consciousness. Continued quiet respiration and eyelid flickering suggest a faint, but spasmodic respiration and/or fits may occur immediately after arrest

Table 9. Cardiac arrhythmias.

Rhythm	Rate		Diagnosis
	Atrial	Ventricular	
Regular	90 +	90 +	Sinus tachycardia
	120–200	120–200	Paroxysmal atrial tachycardia
	200–400	100–200	Atrial flutter with block
	80 +	30–45	Complete heart block with cannon 'a' waves in jugular vein pulse, variable intensity 1st sound, wide pulse pressure
	40–50	40–50	Sinus bradycardia
Irregular			Multiple ectopics (including coupled beats) ECG basically regular
		60–100 treated 100 + untreated }	Atrial flutter with varying block Atrial fibrillation (apex rate is only guide to true heart rate. ECG essential)
Cardiac arrest		120–200	Ventricular tachycardia
		No peripheral pulse {	Ventricular fibrillation and sometimes ventricular tachycardia Ventricular asystole

- call for help and resuscitation box
- establish the *Airway* by removing the pillow and extending the neck to the anaesthetic position
- *Breathe* using mouth-to-mask ventilation and an airway
- consider a precordial thump, and establish *Circulation* with external cardiac massage at a rate about 80/min and a ratio to breathing of about 1 : 5 (or 2 : 15 if alone)

NB Advanced life support ideally needs a team of nurses and doctors (including an anaesthetist). If the ECG indicates ventricular fibrillation or ventricular asystole, attempt defibrillation three times (200, 200, 360 joules), then give adrenaline 1 mg by central intravenous line (or 2 mg into the endotracheal tube) if still unsucessful. In ventricular fibrillation, continue 360 joules shocks before and after lignocaine 100 mg i.v. (or 200 mg endotracheal) and later, bretylium. In asystole, give atropine 2 mg i.v. and consider external

Underlying diseases	Therapy (treat underlying disease) (see pages 312–314)
Anxiety, cardiac failure, thyrotoxicosis, fever, anaemia	Treat underlying disease
None (60%), thyrotoxicosis, digitalis, tobacco, caffeine, Wolff–Parkinson–White syndrome	Vagal stimulation (pressure on the carotid sinus), β-blocker or verapamil or digoxin
Ischaemic heart disease, thyrotoxicosis, (digitalis)	Digoxin, DC cardioversion, verapamil
Post-infarction, idiopathic, digitalis, cardiomyopathy	Nil if asymptomatic Atropine, isoprenaline or cardiac pacemaker after myocardial infarction
Athletes, myocardial infarction, myxoedema, hypothermia, sino-atrial disease	As heart block if following infarction
Ischaemia, digitalis, thyrotoxicosis, cardiomyopathy	Stop digitalis and give potassium if necessary. Lignocaine, disopyramide or mexiletine, β-blocker if due to digitalis
Ischaemia, rheumatic heart disease (MS), thyrotoxicosis. Rarely pulmonary embolism, constructive pericarditis, cardiomyopathy or bronchial carcinoma	Digoxin, or DC cardioversion following myocardial infarction and following treated mitral stenosis and thyrotoxicosis
Myocardial infarction and ischaemia (see page 310)	

pacing. Allow 2 min for each drug to act. In prolonged resuscitation, transfer to intensive care and give adrenaline 1 mg i.v. every 5 min, and consider sodium bicarbonate, 50 mmol, according to the blood gases. Also check electrolytes and chest X-ray.

CARDIAC ARRHYTHMIAS (table 9, pages 70–1)
Digitalis may cause almost any arrhythmia especially if the serum potassium is low, e.g. patients in cardiac failure on diuretics.
Consider thyrotoxicosis in any tachyarrhythmia, especially atrial fibrillation.
Confirm the rhythm with an ECG.

ELECTROCARDIOGRAMS
Many physicians approach the interpretation of ECGs with a feeling of insecurity. If you have a system which is quick and which works, you need not

read any further. There are a relatively small number of common patterns (page 76) and these become easily recognisable with experience. Complex dysrhythmias are virtually never shown to examination candidates. You should be able quickly to determine the mean frontal QRS axis (page 85).

Interpretation

'Look at this ECG'
Make sure that you understand the layout of the leads.
Little is lost by ignoring AVr and AVl.
AVf is useful in inferior myocardial infarction.
Whatever your final diagnosis, you should initially comment on the rate and rhythm.

Rate

Assess the rate by counting the large squares between two QRS complexes (and dividing into 300).

RR interval   Rate
2 squares = 150/min
3 squares = 100/mm
4 squares = 75/mm
5 squares = 60/min

Rhythm

Quickly scan *all* the QRS complexes. Check if there is a P wave before *every* QRS complex.

1 *If the rate is fast and rhythm regular*, consider:
• paroxysmal atrial tachycardia (a rate of 150—two big squares—should make you suspect this)
• atrial flutter ('sawtooth baseline'). F(flutter) waves in leads II and V_1
• ventricular tachycardia (page 81)

2 *If the rate is fast and rhythm irregular*, consider:
• atrial fibrillation (total irregularity) with a ragged baseline and absent P waves
• atrial flutter with varying block
• multiple ectopic beats

3 *If the rate is slow and rhythm regular*, consider:
• complete heart block
• sinus bradycardia (β-blockade, myxoedema, hypothermia, sino-atrial disease)

NB It is sometimes difficult to determine whether the complexes are completely regular or not, especially with an unusually regular atrial fibrillation. The easiest and most accurate way to determine this is to put a piece of paper with its edge along the trace and to mark every QRS complex for about five beats. If you then move the paper up by one or two beats, the marks on the paper will still coincide accurately with QRS complexes only if the rhythm is regular. Total irregularity is almost always diagnostic of atrial fibrillation. The same procedure is useful for checking on P waves in suspected supraventricular extra beats; it demonstrates the compensatory pause well.

4   *Extra beats* with:
• normal QRS complexes (supraventricular or 'atrial')
• wide QRS complexes (ventricular or supraventricular with aberration)

5   *Prolonged PR interval*
• partial heart block (look for Wenckebach)

6   *Fast and slow rates and dysrhythmias* in one trace:
• sino-atrial disease (page 84)
Now that you have scanned the total ECG trace you may have found an obvious abnormality such as the changes of an extensive acute anteroseptal myocardial infarction or one of the special patterns (page 76). If not, check the trace for abnormal QRS complexes.

Electrocardiographic deflections
If you have not yet made a diagnosis, methodically work through the cardiac cycle using as many leads as you need for each component.

P wave
Usually most easily seen in leads V_1 and V_2 though the significant shape of it may be best seen in II and the lateral chest leads (V_{4-6}).
The P wave is bifid in left atrial hypertrophy (P mitrale) in leads II and V_{4-6} and biphasic, predominantly negative, in leads V_{1-2}.
The P wave is peaked in right atrial hypertrophy including 'cor pulmonale' (P pulmonale).
The P wave may be 'lost' in nodal rhythm, i.e. when it coincides with the QRS complex.
The P wave may be inverted in nodal rhythm and precede or follow the QRS complex.

PR interval
For first, second or third degree heart block (usually due to ischaemic heart disease) (page 308).
Second degree heart block may be of two kinds:
1   *Möbitz Type 1*. Wenckebach with progressive lengthening of PR interval until one QRS is dropped.
2   *Möbitz Type 2*. A simple pattern of dropped beats but without change of PR

interval in successive cardiac cycles. It is less common and has a worse prognosis.

NB   A short PR interval occurs in nodal rhythm, and in the Wolff–Parkinson–White syndrome (note the Δ wave).

QRS complex

It may now be worth making a rough estimate of the mean frontal QRS axis (page 85).

ST segment

It is raised convexly (domed) in myocardial infarction and raised concavely in pericarditis.

It is depressed, especially leads V_{5-6} in digitalis administration, left ventricular hypertrophy and in ischaemic heart disease (plane depression), particularly on effort.

T wave

It is 'peaked' in hyperkalaemia and sometimes acutely after myocardial infarction.

It is inverted in:

- bundle branch block (T always in the reverse direction to the main QRS complex)
- digitalis effect ('reversed tick' $\vee$)
- ventricular hypertrophy
- ischaemia
- cardiomyopathy

Roughly check the QT interval (from the beginning of the QRS complex to the end of the T wave). It varies as a function of the square root of the RR interval (rate). The upper limit of normal is approximately:

Rate	QT
60	0.43
75	0.39
100	0.34

This may be exceeded in hypocalcaemia, myocardial disease (ischaemic and rheumatic) and with anti-arrhythmic drugs (e.g. procainamide, amiodarone, β-blockade and quinidine). It occurs idiopathically (the long QT syndrome) as an indicator of abnormal ventricular repolarisation and may be a prelude to ventricular tachycardia and ventricular fibrillation with syncope and sudden death.

U wave

It can be normally present, and is maximal in leads V_{3-4}. It is increased in hypokalaemia and may be inverted in ischaemia.

If you have still failed to find any abnormality recheck quickly for the following special patterns:

ST segments for pericarditis, especially in leads II and V_{2-3}—concave elevation of the ST segment in all leads *QT interval* for hypocalcaemia (long) and hypercalcaemia (short). The QT_C is the QT corrected for rate (to a standard of 60).

$S_1 Q_3 T_3$ pattern of pulmonary embolism (very very rare).

General voltage decrease of myxoedema, hypothermia, pericardial effusion and obesity.

Changes of *hypokalaemia* and *hyperkalaemia*.

Digitalis effect, 'reversed tick' depression of ST segment and depression of T. Digitalis can produce almost any arrhythmia particularly in potassium depletion (thiazide diuretics).

Special patterns

Myocardial infarction

Anterior or inferior, old or new. Look for pathological Q waves, convex ST elevation and T inversion. Remember that Q waves in leads III and AVf should be accompanied by Q in II before making a firm diagnosis of inferior myocardial infarction. They may otherwise reflect a change of axis or represent a pulmonary embolus.

Ventricular hypertrophy (right or left)

Large R waves occur over the appropriate ventricle in the chest leads (right ventricle, R in V_{1-2}; left ventricle, R in V_{5-6}). There tends to be large negative S waves in the reciprocal leads, e.g. S in V_{1-2} in left ventricular hypertrophy. **NB** If SV_1 plus RV_5 is more than 35 mm it suggests left ventricular hypertropy.

Bundle branch block (right or left)

This is present if the QRS is over 0.12 s. The diagnosis is as easy as counting small squares. Characteristic patterns are shown on page 78. Partial block is present with QRS durations of less than 0.12 s. Right bundle branch block may or may not be pathological; left bundle branch block invariably is.

NB Some ECGs 'tell a story', for example:
- ECG changes of hypokalaemia with 'digitalis effect'—pattern of 'digitalis and diuretics without potassium'
- ECG changes with hypokalaemia and LV hypertrophy—usually hypertensive heart disease treated with diuretics without potassium, but remember Conn's syndrome and Cushing's syndrome
- paroxysmal atrial tachycardia with intermittent AV block–digitalis intoxication (especially with hypokalaemia)
- Inferior M1 with heart block

Sample electrocardiograms (Figures 7–32)

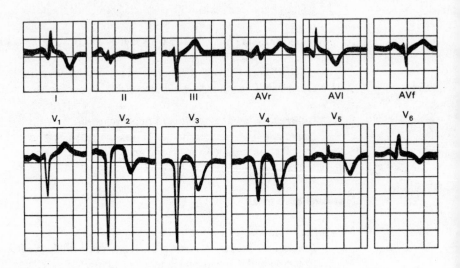

Figure 7. Anterior myocardial infarction. The main Q and STT changes are in the anteroseptal leads V_{2-4}.

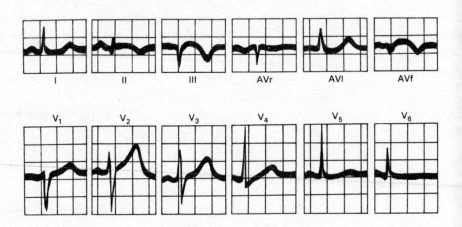

Figure 8. Inferior myocardial infarction. The main changes ar in II, III and AVf. T wave changes in V_{5-6} suggest inferolateral infarction.

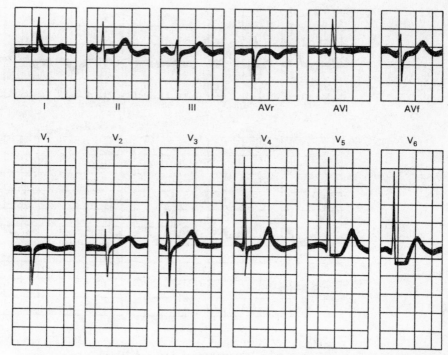

Figure 9. Myocardial ischaemia (clinical history essential). The main characteristic is a depressed ST segment in leads standard II and V_{5-6}. Also not inverted U waves in II, III, AVf and V_{4-6}.

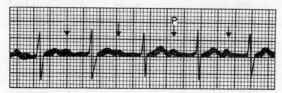

Figure 10. First degree heart block. PR interval 0.30 s.

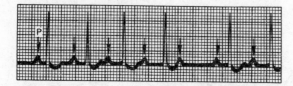

Figure 11. Second degree heart block (Wenckebach or Möbitz Type I).

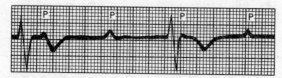

Figure 12. Third degree heart block (complete). A–V dissociation.

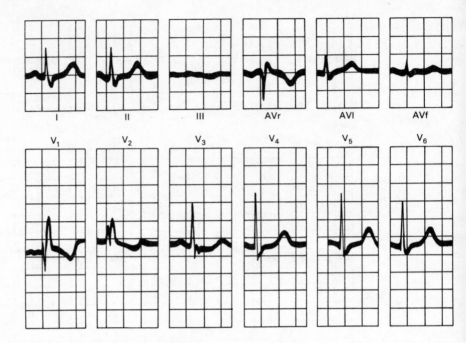

Figure 13. Right bundle branch block. Rsr in the right ventricular leads V_{1-2} and slurred S waves in the left ventricular leads I, AV1 and V_{4-6}.

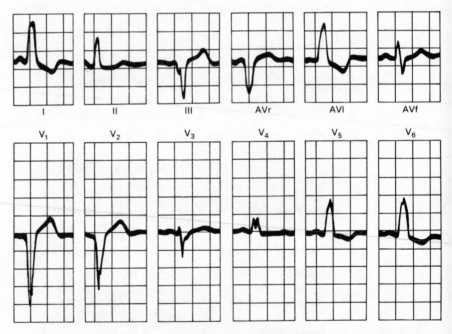

Figure 14. Left bundle branch block. Rsr visible in some of the left ventricular leads, I, AV1 and V_{4-6}; and notched QS complexes in the right ventricular lead, V_{1-2}.

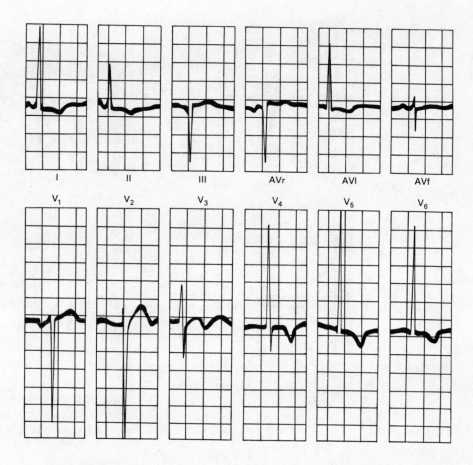

Figure 15.   Left ventricular hypertrophy. Sv_1 and $Rv_{5 \text{ or } 6} > 35$ mm and ST–T 'strain' changes.

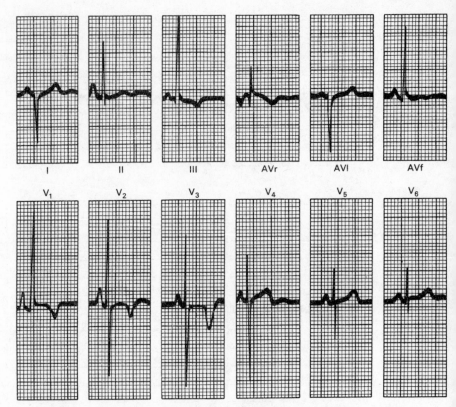

Figure 16.   Right ventricular hypertrophy. Tall R waves and STT 'strain' changes in the right ventricular leads V_{1-3} and a mean frontal QRS axis to the right (+120°).

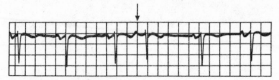

Figure 17.   Atrial extrasystole.

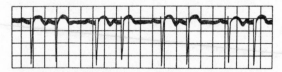

Figure 18.   Atrial coupling or bigeminy: alternate atrial extrasystoles.

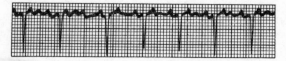

Figure 19.   Supraventricular tachycardia with varying A–V block.

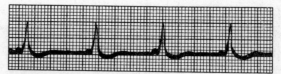

Figure 20. Wolff–Parkinson–White syndrome (WPW). Short PR interval and delta waves. LGL (Lown–Ganong–Levine) has no delta wave but is otherwise identical.

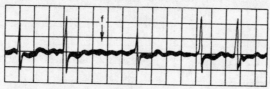

Figure 21. Atrial fibrillation.

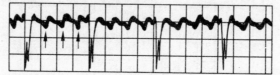

Figure 22. Atrial flutter with 'saw-tooth' atrial waves.

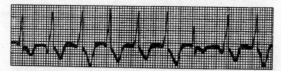

Figure 23. Ventricular tachycardia with slightly irregular 'ventricular' QRS complexes and variable T waves due to dissociated superimposed P waves.

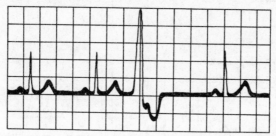

Figure 24. Ventricular ectopic beat. A 'ventricular' bizarre QRS complex. These are more ominous if multifocal, i.e. QRS of varying shape.

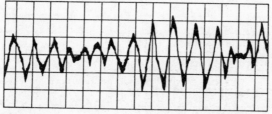

Figure 25. Ventricular fibrillation. This is often seen in 'cardiac arrest' and may be irreversible. It may sometimes alternate with ventricular tachycardia (and sinus rhythm).

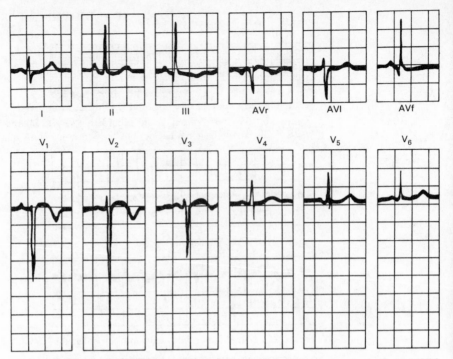

Figure 26. Acute pulmonary embolism with S_1, Q_3, T_3 pattern, a mean frontal QRS axis towards the right ($+90°$) and 'RV strain' pattern in leads V_{1-3}.

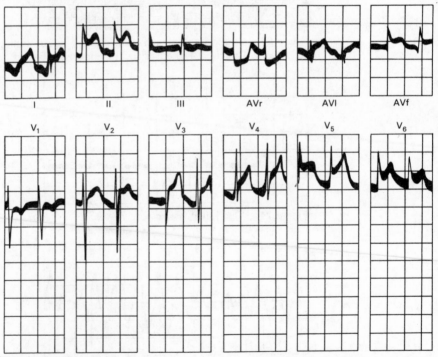

Figure 27. Acute pericarditis. Raised concave-upwards ST segments in most leads, maximal in lead II and V_{5-6}.

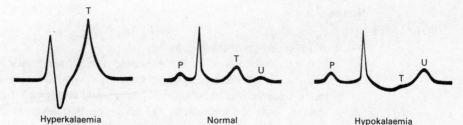

Hyperkalaemia   Normal   Hypokalaemia

Figure 28. Hyperkalaemia and hypokalaemia. The T wave amplitude varies directly with the serum potassium and the U wave inversely (it is often normally present in V_{3-4}). In hyperkalaemia the P waves become smaller and the QRS complex widens into the ST segment. In hypokalaemia the PR interval lengthens and the ST segment becomes depressed.

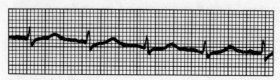

Figure 29. Hypocalcaemia. Normal complexes apart from a prolonged QT_c. (Rate 95/min, QT 0.40, QT_c 0.50.)

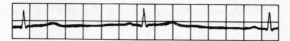

Figure 30. Myxoedema. Sinus bradycardia of 44/min and reduced amplitude of P, QRS and T waves which is present in all leads.

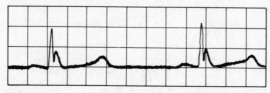

Figure 31. Hypothermia. Sinus bradycardia and J waves (junction of QRS with ST segment).

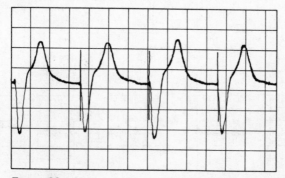

Figure 32. Ventricular pacemaker. Linear pacing artefact immediately preceding the widened 'ventricular' QRS complex.

Notes

Sino-atrial disease (sick sinus syndrome)

This is a chronic disorder often associated with ischaemic heart disease in which sinus bradycardia and/or episodic sinus arrest may alternate with episodes of rapid supraventricular arrhythmia (tachy-brady syndrome). Symptoms include dizziness, syncope, palpitation and dyspnoea. Permanent pacing may become necessary. Diagnosis is often most easily made using 24 h ambulatory monitoring.

Fascicular blocks

There are three fascicles to the bundle of His: right, left anterior, and left posterior. Block of one (unifascicular block) produces the following patterns:

1 Right   RBBsB
2 Left anterior   L anterior hemiblock→ L axis deviation
3 Left posterior   L posterior hemiblock→ R axis deviation

Hemiblock refers to a block in either the anterior or the posterior division of the left bundle. The QRS duration is 'long normal'. Unlike LBBsB, septal depolarisation remains present (q in the anterior leads; and r in the inferior leads—II, III, AVf).

Bifascicular block refers to the combination of two of the unifascicular blocks. The QRS duration is lengthened, but the evidence of septal depolarisation should still be present.
1 + 2 = RBBsB + LAH i.e. RBBsB pattern + L axis deviation (figure 33)

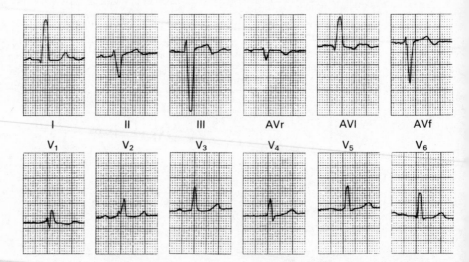

Figure 33. Bifascicular block. Right bundle branch block with left axis deviation.

1 + 3 = RBBsB + RAH i.e. RBBsB pattern + R axis deviation
2 + 3 = LBBsB pattern—more often due to a single proximal lesion

Evidence of first degree heart block—a prolonged PR interval—can be regarded as a separate fascicle for purposes of defining bifascicular blocks. Thus a long PR interval, in combination with a RBBsB or either of the hemiblocks, may be regarded as a bifascicular block when considering the need for pacing.

Broad complex tachycardia

In the differential diagnosis between 'ventricular tachycardia' and 'supraventricular tachycardia with ventricular aberrant conduction', the diagnosis of ventricular tachycardia is favoured by the presence of known myocardial damage e.g. myocardial infarction or a dilated cardiomyopathy. Patients in the ischaemic age group who have a broad complex tachycardia, are very likely (95%) to have ventricular tachycardia. It may produce no clinically detectable haemodynamic signs or symptoms.

Examination in ventricular tachycardia may show signs of atrioventricular dissociation (jugular pulse 'a' waves slower than the apex, jugular cannon waves, variable intensity of the first heart sound, and beat–beat variation in the blood pressure).

The ECG in ventricular tachycardia The ventricular complexes are abnormal in shape and their duration prolonged—usually >120 ms. There is often (50%) AV dissociation (i.e. independent atrial activity) with independent P waves, capture and fusion beats and 2° or intermittent AV conduction block.

Mean frontal QRS axis

If you have a system which is quick and which works, don't read any further. Use leads I, II and III only (i.e. a triaxial reference system) and practise drawing the axes (60° between each). Label them as in figure 34 at the positive ends. The other ends of the axes represent negative QRS deflections.

Look at the three standard leads on your ECG and decide which one has the biggest net deflection (positive or negative). The QRS axis must be lying closer to this lead than any other. If the net deflections in two leads are equally large (e.g. I and II) the QRS axis will be pointing midway between them.

Thus, so far, you should be able to determine the axes shown in figure 35.

You will now have noticed that when a QRS axis is perpendicular to a lead (e.g. a QRS axis of + 90° is perpendicular to lead I), there is no net deflection in that lead. Examples (b), (c) and (d) in figure 35 demonstrate this.

Now draw you own reference system and plot the examples given in figure 35. Check with figure 36.

You can regard the 'biggest deflection' procedure as a rough assessment (to within 60°). The 'smallest deflection' then becomes the 'fine adjustment' (to about 10–15°). Thus if the smallest deflection (in, say, lead I in figure 37) is slightly net positive, the QRS axis must be slightly to the positive side of perpendicular in that lead (say 75° in this example) (compare with (d) in figure 35).

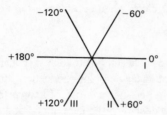

Figure 34.   Main QRS axes for leads I, II and III.

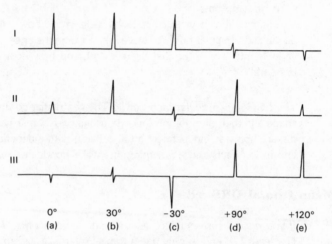

Figure 35.   Determination of main deflection patterns in leads I, II and III.

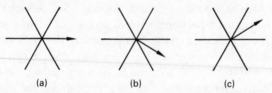

Figure 36.   QRS axes plotted for deflection patterns shown in figure 34 (a), (b) and (c).

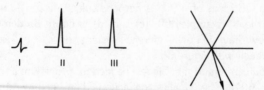

Figure 37.   Fine adjustment of deflection patterns in leads I, II and III.

Now you should be able to determine the axis shown in figure 38.

The normal range is 0° to +90° though significant left axis deviation is usually more negative than −30°. For 'instant' diagnosis you can use the rule:

in significant left axis deviation (LAD) the QRS is negative in II
in significant right axis deviation (RAD) the QRS is negative in I.

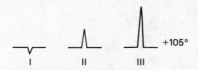

Figure 38. Sample deflection patterns in leads I, II and III.

Right axis deviation occurs in:
• right ventricular hypertrophy or dominance (e.g. cor pulmonale, pulmonary stenosis or hypertension, Fallot's tetralogy and mitral valve disease)
• anterolateral myocardial infarction
• left posterior hemiblock, ostium secumdum ASD and some Wolff–Parkinson–White (WPW) syndrome and (right bundle branch system block (RBBsB)

Left axis deviation occurs in:
• left anterior hemiblock due to ischaemia, infarction, fibrosis or cardiomyopathy
• inferior myocardial infarction
• cardiac pacing, ostium primum, atrial septal defect (ASD) and some WPW and left bundle branch system block (LBBsB)

In atrial septal defect, the ostium primum type tend to have left axis deviation (despite a right bundle branch block) due to involvement of the left branch of the bundle in the lesion. Ostium secundum defects have right axis deviation (with a right bundle branch block).

ECHOCARDIOGRAPHY

Figure 39 is a normal M-mode sweep vertically down the body parasternally from base to apex of the heart, right to left in the figure. Follow the course of blood on the echo through the left heart, starting at left atrium (LA) on the right (a) and pass through the mitral valve (MV) noting the splayed M shape of the movement of the anterior mitral valve leaflet (AMVL) (b). Enter the left ventricle (LV)(c), then reverse direction and go anterior to the anterior MV leaflet (b) and pass through the box shaped echoes from the cusps of the aortic valve (AoV) (a) as they abruptly part and close. Note now the movements of the interventricular septum (IVS) and posterior left ventricular wall (PLVW) towards each other in systole—this can help with timing other events.

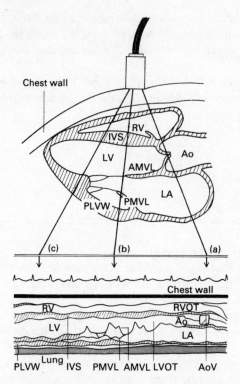

Figure 39. IVS, interventricular septum; RV, right ventricle; LV, left ventricle; AMVL, anterior mitral valve leaflet; Ao, aorta; PLVW, posterior left ventricular wall; PMVL, posterior mitral valve leaflet; LA, left atrium; RVOT, right ventricular outflow tract; LVOT, left ventricular outflow tract; AoV, aortic valve.

Mitral valve disease

Figure 40 shows the normal mitral valve echo. The two points of note are:
1   The diastolic closure rate (EF slope) of the anterior mitral valve leaflet.
2   The mitral valve amplitude (DE).

Rheumatic mitral stenosis. There is early diastolic forward movement of the posterior mitral valve leaflet (PMVL), parallel with the AMVL. The EF slope decreases. The left atrium is large and the valve leaflets are thickened, sometimes with strong echoes from calcification.

Mitral regurgitation (MR). There is increased LV wall movement. The leaflets of a 'floppy valve' (common) are thickened and may prolapse. Weakness or rupture of the chordae may cause prolapse, and ruptured papillary muscle (rare) a flail cusp. Rheumatic MR usually occurs with some degree of stenosis.

Aortic valve disease

Figure 41 shows the normal aortic valve echo and its characteristic square box appearance when open.

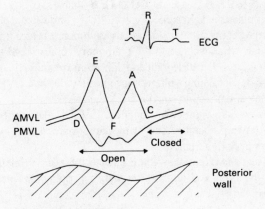

Figure 40. Mitral valve.

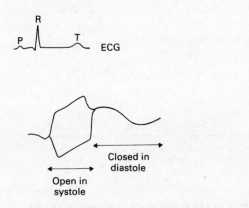

Figure 41. Aortic valve.

The posterior aortic wall echo is continuous with the anterior mitral valve leaflet figure 39.

Aortic stenosis. There may be heavy echoes from calcification and the leaflets may be thickened. The LV wall is thick and the cavity small.

Aortic regurgitation. There is usually fluttering of the anterior mitral valve leaflet in diastole from the regurgitant stream. LV wall movement is increased and the cavity dilated.

Cardiomyopathy

Hypertrophic. There is asymmetrical septal hypertropy (ASH), a small LV cavity and systolic anterior movement (SAM) of the AMVL.

Congestive. The LV is dilated and there is poor movement of the LV wall.

NB Echocardiography is the most sensitive way to detect pericardial effusion, the rare vegetations of endocarditis and left atrial myxomas.

CARDIAC PRESSURE STUDIES (table 10)

CVP lines measure right atrial pressure (RAP) and usually give a good indication of circulating intravascular volume. A pulmonary artery flotation catheter, e.g. Swan–Ganz, when wedged in the pulmonary capillary bed (pulmonary capillary wedge pressure—PCWP), indicates left atrial pressure (LAP). These help:

- To assess circulating volume more accurately than CVP, particularly in low output states, e.g. septic shock
- To assess left ventricular function (LVEDP—left ventricular end diastolic pressure) in cardiogenic shock. It monitors therapy with inotropes and plasma expanders in both situations
- To assess the circulating volume when the normal relationship in pressures between the right and left atria is lost, e.g. pulmonary embolism, myocardial infarction

Table 10.   Normal cardiac pressures (in mmHg).

	SD	Mean
RAP	7/3	<5
RVP	0–25/3–7	—
PAP	25/10	<18
PCWP		
(LAP)	—	<10 or 6–12
(LVEDP)		
LVP	120/7–12	—

RVP = right ventricular pressure
PAP = pulmonary artery pressure
LVP = left ventricular pressure

CARDIAC RADIONUCLEIDE STUDIES

Technetium (^{99m}Tc)-labelled red cells are used to assess left ventricular function by a technique known as gated or equilibrium radionucleide ventriculography (multiple uptake gated acquisition—MUGA). The ejection fraction is derived from stroke volume divided by end-diastolic volume. It remains the same or increases on exercise. Myocardial disease tends to cause dilatation of the heart and the ejection fraction may fall on exercise. This is usually a poor prognostic sign in ischaemic heart disease and in aortic and mitral valve diseases. The isotopic images also record regional abnormalities of the ventricular muscle as areas of akinesia and hypokinesia (broad phase contraction). This is usually evidence of myocardial ischaemia or infarction. Regional paradoxical movement suggests an aneurysm.

Thallium (^{201}Tl) behaves like potassium and is distributed through heart muscle in proportion to coronary artery blood flow. Thus there is a decreased uptake in areas of recent infarction. On exercise there may be areas of decreased perfusion which reverse after rest—this indicates areas of reversible ischaemia.

Haematology

The commoner problems in clinical examinations, as in clinical practice, are to assess the significance of the data provided on a standard blood count (e.g. Coulter count), examine a patient with anaemia, purpura or ecchymosis, or to comment on the coagulation screen of a patient with a bleeding disorder.

ANAEMIA

It is essential to distinguish between pallor and anaemia. Pallor may be due to a deep-lying venous system and opaque skin. In Britain the commonest cause of anaemia is iron deficiency, due to chronic blood loss especially in women during the child-bearing period. The second commonest cause is probably megaloblastic anaemia and most of these are due to intrinsic factor deficiency causing B_{12} deficiency. The malabsorption syndrome, including the postgastrectomy syndrome, can give rise to deficiency in iron, vitamin B_{12} or folic acid. Myxoedema and chronic uraemia may present with a chronic anaemia. Anaemia may be a feature of many chronic conditions in which other clinical features are usually more obvious. These include the leukaemias, reticuloses and rheumatoid arthritis. In tropical countries chronic infections, especially chronic malaria and hookworm infestation, are common and the haemoglobinopathies should be considered.

'This patient is anaemic. What questions would you like to ask and what would you examine for?'

Ask patient

Blood loss: menstrual loss, pregnancy, haemorrhoids, indigestion and melaena, salicylate ingestion.

History of drugs: aplastic anaemia, and megaloblastic anaemia from folate deficiency (anticonvulsants). Non-steroidal drugs and gastric bleeding

H istory of gastric surgery, ulcerative colitis or malabsorption.

Paraesthesiae and sore tongue of pernicious anaemia.

Diet: the elderly pensioner may suffer from iron and/or ascorbic acid deficiency. Vegans may develop B_{12} deficiency and alcoholics folate deficiency.

Observe and assess degree of anaemia

Face and conjunctiva: note the white hair and pale lemon yellow skin of pernicious anaemia.

Tongue: for glossitis of vitamin B_{12} or folate deficiency and angular stomatitis of iron deficiency.

Nails and nail beds: brittle nails and koilonychia of iron deficiency and the

91

splinter haemorrhages (sometimes with clubbing) of infective endocarditis.
Note purpura (aplastic anaemia, leukaemia), mouth ulceration in neutropenia and the leg ulceration of the haemoglobinopathies.
Note rheumatoid arthritis and consider uraemia and myxoedema.
Note racial origin: thalassaemia and sickle-cell anaemia.

Examine also:

Neck for lymph nodes, which may be enlarged in chronic lymphatic leukaemia and reticuloendothelial diseases or be secondaries from carcinoma.
Abdomen for splenomegaly, hepatomegaly and neoplasms (especially of the stomach, colon and uterus).
NB   In the clinic, rectal examination is essential, and sigmoidoscopy should be performed for haemorrhoids, carcinoma and colitis in patients with a history of rectal bleeding.
There may be congestive cardiac failure from severe anaemia.
If you suspect pernicious anaemia, examine for peripheral neuropathy and subacute combined degeneration of the cord.
Retinal haemorrhage may occur in leukaemia and severe B_{12} deficiency.

BLOOD COUNT (table 11)

'Comment on this haemoglobin'
Check the haemoglobin for anaemia or polycythaemia.
NB   A normal white cell and platelet count virtually excludes leukaemia and marrow aplasia.

Hypochromic anaemia

Check the indices for hypochromia (mean corpuscular haemoglobin—MCH and mean corpuscular haemoglobin concentration—MCHC) and microcytosis (mean cell volume—MCV). If present, they suggest iron deficiency.
Perform serum iron, transferrin, ferritin, faecal occult blood and proceed, if indicated, to sigmoidoscopy, barium enema, barium meal and follow-through. A gynaecological examination may be indicated from the clinical history at the outset. Check other possible causes which normally produce normochromic but sometimes hypochromic anaemia (see below).
Exclude thalassaemia and sickle cell anaemia if indicated (haemoglobin electrophoresis and sickling tests).

Macrocytic anaemia

Check the indices for macrocytosis (MCV). In pernicious anaemia there is usually an associated low white blood cell (WBC) and low platelet count.
Perform a serum B_{12} and red cell folate (or serum folate). A bone marrow examination shows megaloblastic change in vitamin B_{12} and folate deficiencies. Parietal cell and intrinsic factor antibodies may be present. An abnormal Schilling test (<6% in 24 h) is corrected by intrinsic factor in pernicious anaemia (page

Table 11. Normal values.

Hb (*men*)	13–17 (g/dl)
Hb (*women*)	11–16 (g/dl)
RBC (*men)*	4.5–6.4 (m/mm^3)
RBC (*women*)	3.9–5.6 (m/mm^3)
Haematocrit (PCV) (*men*)	0.38–0.50
Haematocrit (PCV) (*women*)	0.33–0.45
MCV	80–96 (fl (PCV/RBC))
MCH	27–32 (μg (Hb/RBC))
MCHC	32–36 (% (Hb/PCV))
Reticulocytes	10–100 × 10^9/litre
WBC	4–11 (× 10^9/litre)
Platelets	150–400 × 10^9/litre
Prothrombin time (INR)	Not more than 2 s longer than control
Control time	11–13 s
Partial thromboplastin time	Not more than 7 s longer than control
Control time	30–45 s
Bleeding time	Up to 11 min
Hess (tourniquet) test (80 mmHg for 5 min)	Not more than 5 spots in a square inch
Clotting time	Up to 10 min
Fibrinogen	2–4 g/litre

PCV = packed cell volume

357). Other causes of vitamin B$_{12}$ and folate deficiencies, e.g. alcoholism, malabsorption blind loops and ileal disease (Crohn's); are all rare. In ileal disease, the Schilling test is not corrected by intrinsic factor.

Investigate causes other than vitamin B$_{12}$ and folate deficiencies with liver function tests and γ-glutaryl transferase for alcohol, thyroid function test for hypothyroidism and reticulocyte count (and bilirubin) for haemolysis. Check that the patient is neither pregnant nor using anticonvulsants. Aplastic and haemolytic anaemias are sometimes macrocytic but not megaloblastic.

Normocytic anaemia

If the indices are normal, consider anaemias secondary to other severe disease (such as rheumatoid arthritis, carcinoma, renal failure and chronic infection) and hypothyroidism (which may also give a macrocytic picture).

If the reticulocyte count is raised this denotes marrow hyperactivity and usually (a) haemolytic anaemia, (b) response to vitamin B$_{12}$, folate or occasionally iron therapy, or (c) continued bleeding.

If the WBC and/or platelet counts are low and there is anaemia, this suggests marrow aplasia, usually secondary to drugs (and rarely toxic chemicals) or marrow infiltration (leukaemia, myelofibrosis, multiple myeloma, carcinoma).

Primitive white cells (blast) in the peripheral film indicate an acute leukaemia or occasionally a leukaemoid response to acute infection. The total WBC count is usually raised. The film usually shows whether the leukaemia is myeloid or lymphatic.

Eosinophilia suggests drug sensitivity, intestinal worms, allergy (e.g. asthma), including allergic aspergillosis, and rarely polyarteritis nodosa, pulmonary eosinophilia syndrome and reticulosis such as Hodgkin's disease.

Polycythaemia rubra vera

The red blood cell (RBC), WBC and platelet counts are usually raised. There is an increase in red cell mass and haematocrit. In secondary polycythaemia (secondary to hypoxia) only the RBC count is raised. Polycythaemia is also associated with renal carcinoma and cerebellar haemangioblastoma where there are raised erythropoietin levels.

Notes

Hypochromic anaemia, unresponsive to oral iron therapy, occurs in:
- incorrect diagnosis or mixed deficiency
- patients who do not take their tablets
- continued bleeding (reticulocytosis persists)
- rheumatoid arthritis, SLE, infections (and other chronic illness)
- malabsorption
- thalassaemia
- myelodysplastic syndrome—refractory anaemia (if ringed sideroblasts present = sideroblastic anaemia)

Megaloblasts are found in the marrow and only rarely in the peripheral blood. They are characterised by a large and inactive nucleus (maturation arrest) in a relatively hypermature, and even haemoglobinised, cytoplasm. They are not present in normal marrow and their presence denotes vitamin B_{12} or folate deficiency, which may be secondary to antifolate or phenytoin therapy.

Patients with pernicious anaemia which has been treated with vitamin B_{12} usually have normal peripheral blood, normal marrow (within 24 h) and normal serum folates and B_{12}. They may still be investigated with the Schilling tests and parietal cell and intrinsic factor antibodies are still present.

Vitamin B_{12} and folate deficiencies produce (if sufficiently severe) depression of all the marrow elements including neutrophils and platelets. The polymorph nuclei appear hypersegmented. There is usually some haemolysis with a raised unconjugated serum bilirubin.

In folic acid deficiency consider pregnancy, dietary intake, malabsorption, drugs (phenytoin), alcoholism and haemolytic anaemia.

In haemolytic anaemia (page 358) the serum bilirubin (unconjugated) is raised. There is no bile pigment in the urine (acholuric) but urobilinogen is present in the urine in excess. Reticulocytosis is present and its degree is an indirect measure of the rate of haemolysis. Haptoglobins in the blood are increased. The rate of disappearance of chromium-tagged red cells gives a more accurate measure of the rate of haemolysis. Splenomegaly and pigment stones may occur.

Haemolytic anaemias (page 358) are rare in Britain. They are usually classified as:

1 Intracorpuscular defects (Coombs' negative). (Abnormal RBCs.) Thalassaemia, sickle cell anaemia, hereditary spherocytosis, glucose-6-phosphatase deficiency, haemoglobinopathies.

2 Extracorpuscular defects. (Normal RBCs.)

(*a*) Autoimmune haemolytic anaemias (Coombs' positive) are either primary, or secondary to drugs (methyldopa), leukaemia or reticuloses.

(*b*) Rhesus incompatibility (and mismatched transfusion) is an immune but not autoimmune disorder since the antibody is extrinsic (fetal).

(*c*) Non-immune, e.g. burns, malaria, drugs.

(*d*) Secondary to renal or liver disease.

(*e*) Hypersplenism.

(*f*) Red cell fragmentation.

Primary aplastic anaemia. A pancytopenia with reduction in all the formed elements is rare.

Secondary bone marrow failure. Toxic factors acting on the marrow may affect one or all of the formed elements of the blood, red cells, white cells or platelets. Important recognised causes include drugs (gold, penicillamine, chloramphenicol, carbimazole), radiation and leukaemias.

NB   Very high ESR

(i.e. over 100 mm/h). Suggests (*a*) multiple myeloma, (*b*) systemic lupus erythematosus (SLE), (*c*) temporal arteritis, (*d*) polymyalgia rheumatica, or (*e*) rarely carcinoma or chronic infection including TB.

SKIN HAEMORRHAGE

'Purpura' refers to small (pin head) cutaneous bleeding. 'Ecchymosis' refers to larger lesions (bruises). Bruising is very common, purpura is rare.

A useful working classification of the causes of skin (and other) haemorrhage is shown in table 12. The commonest causes of skin haemorrhage are senile purpura, therapy with steroids or anticoagulants, and less commonly thrombocytopenia due to leukaemia and marrow aplasia.

'Examine this patient's skin' (showing purpura or ecchymosis)

Table 12.   Causes of haemorrhage.

Coagulation defects:
   Haemophilia
   Christmas disease
   Treatment with anticoagulants
   Fibrinogen deficiency (defibrination: disseminated intravascular coagulation—DIC)
Vascular purpuras (increased capillary fragility):
   von Willebrand's disease
   Hereditary haemorrhagic telangiectasia
   Anaphylactic purpura
Thrombocytopenic purpuras:
   Hypersplenism
   Idiopathic thrombocytopenic purpura
   Marrow suppression or replacement
   DIC and microangiopathic haemolytic anaemia

Quickly note

Patient's age (senile purpura).

If he is anaemic (marrow infiltration, aplasia and leukaemia).

If he has rheumatoid arthritis (purpura usually due to drugs, steroids, gold).

Ecchymoses of the lower limbs in the elderly may be due to scurvy. This is seen in persons living alone and on 'ulcer' diet. Potatoes are the usual source of vitamin C in those who cannot afford citrus fruits.

Henoch–Schönlein or anaphylactoid purpura (rare). (This 'purpura' is actually a vasculitis and often most obvious around the buttocks, and upper thighs. It usually follows an upper respiratory tract infection. It is commonest between the ages of 3 and 15 years and is rare in adults (in whom the prognosis is worse). The palpable rash is polymorphic and may be extensive, simulating a skin disease. It is associated with acute nephritic syndrome, arthralgia and abdominal pain.)

If invited to question the patient, ask about drugs (anticoagulant therapy, carbimazole, chloramphenicol, anticoagulants, steroids), about a family history of bleeding (haemophilia and Christmas disease).

Examination

Mouth and pharynx for the ulceration of neutropenia (marrow depression from leukaemia or drugs). For anaemia and lymphadenopathy (marrow aplasia and leukaemia).

For splenomegaly (leukaemia and idiopathic thrombocytopenic purpura).

NB   Platelet deficiency tends to result in multiple small bleeds (purpura, microscopic haematuria) and clotting-factor deficiency in isolated larger bleeds (haemarthrosis, haematemesis, stroke, haematomata in muscles).

COAGULATION DEFECTS

'Comment on this coagulation screen'

If the patient is present, no comment should be made before a good history has been taken and a thorough examination has been performed. You will wish to determine the type (skin, deep tissue, mucosa, joints), degree, precipitation and course of the haemorrhage. Ask about previous dental extractions, surgery, childbirth and trauma. A family and drug history is very important. Physical examination may suggest the underlying cause. Vascular abnormalities and platelet disorders tend to result in minor skin bleeding (purpura and petechia) especially in the lower limbs. Platelet disorders are associated with epistaxis, menorrhagia, and gastrointestinal bleeding. Coagulation defects tend to result in prolonged post-traumatic bleeding (including that due to surgery) and bleeding into joints and muscle. A patient who has a convincing history of considerable haemorrhage and who is at special risk in surgery or biopsy procedures may nevertheless have a normal coagulation screen (table 11). These simple tests cannot always exclude a bleeding abnormality and factors (table 13) may have to be reduced to 10% of their normal level before they can be detected by them. Thus a patient with a bleeding history but a normal coagulation screen will require more detailed investigation including assay of the individual factors.

Apart from those due to anticoagulant administration, 95% of serious coagulation defects are due to von Willebrand's disease and the haemophilias.

Notes

The important factors to remember by number are shown in table 14.

Prothrombin time

Measures the *extrinsic system*. It is the time taken for the patient's citrated plasma to clot when a tissue factor (brain extract) and calcium are added. In a

Table 13. Coagulation mechanism.

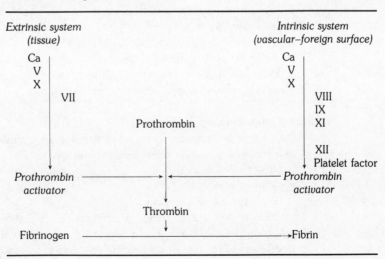

Table 14. Important coagulation factors.

Factor	Defiency states
V	Very rare
VII	Warfarin therapy and liver disease
VIII (= anti-haemophilic globalin)	Haemophilia A and von Willebrand's disease
IX (= Christmas factor)	Haemophilia B, warfarin therapy and liver disease

coagulation screen it is important because it measures deficiencies of V, VII, X, prothrombin and fibrinogen. It is normal in the haemophilias. It is relatively insensitive to reduction in prothrombin.

Partial thromboplastin time

Measures the *intrinsic system*. It is the time taken for the patient's citrated plasma to clot when kaolin (activates XI and XII), platelet substitute and calcium are added. In a coagulation screen it is important because it measures deficiencies of factors V, VIII to XII prothrombin and fibrinogen. It is prolonged in haemophilia.

A normal control is necessary because of the variable potency of the tissue factor.

Thromboplastin generation test

In difficult cases the thromboplastin generation test is used. In this test three components of the clotting mechanism (**1**), (**2**), and (**3**) are mixed together. Of these three, either (**1**) or (**2**) is obtained from the patient. The other two components are either from a normal individual or are laboratory reagents.

1 *Absorbed plasma*: V and VIII are normally present (VII and IX were removed by absorption).

2 *Serum*: VII and IX (and X) are normally present (V and VIII were removed because used up in the clot).

3 *Platelets* (or platelet substitute) and *calcium*.

In classical haemophilia (factor VIII deficiency or haemophilia A) for instance, the mix containing the patient's absorbed plasma (**1**) with normal serum (**2**) would have an abnormal prolonged test.

Vitamin K and anticoagulants

Low levels of vitamin K and administration of coumarins (e.g. warfarin) or indanediones (e.g. phenindione) affect the synthesis of prothrombin and factor X plus:

- VII in the extrinsic system
- IX in the intrinsic system

Similar deficiencies occur in cirrhosis due to hepatocellular failure (often unresponsive to vitamin K). In addition to cirrhosis with portal hypertension, bleeding may be exacerbated by the thrombocytopenia of hypersplenism.

Defibrination syndrome

Synonyms: consumption coagulopathy, disseminated intravascular coagulation (DIC). This occurs in obstetric practice, thoracic surgery and pulmonary embolism, and in shock, especially when associated with infection or bleeding, and following mismatched blood transfusion.

The syndrome may present more chronically as a disorder with intravascular coagulation rather than excessive bleeding. The thrombophlebitis migrans of malignancy may be an example.

Platelets and factor V and VIII are consumed in the pathological coagulation as well as fibrinogen. Fibrinolysis takes place simultaneously with coagulation and produces fibrin degeneration products which can be measured in the serum and urine.

Treatment is primarily that of the underlying disease, usually septicaemia. Replace the platelets and the deficient factors by fresh (12 h) whole blood or fresh frozen plasma and fibrinogen concentrates. Heparin may be given in normal (or lower) doses, progress being monitored by changes in the fibrinogen level.

Haemophilia

Haemophilia A is due to factor VIII deficiency and haemophilia B (Christmas disease) to factor IX deficiency. They are sex-linked recessive disorders of men, carried by women. All carriers who wish to have children should receive genetic counselling. The diseases can be detected *in utero*.

Therapy. As soon as possible after bleeding has started, purified factor VIII or IX is given as required. Cryoprecipitate which contains VIII but not IX is now seldom used. AME concentrate (purified VIII) is also used to raise factor VIII levels in von Willebrand's disease. Fresh frozen plasma contains both factors but is best reserved for when the single factors are not available. Aspirin-containing preparations should be avoided because they impair platelet function and may cause gastric erosion.

von Willebrand's disease

This is an autosomal dominant disease of both sexes with variable clinical severity showing various types of abnormal bleeding, particularly from mucous membranes. There is a prolonged bleeding time, low factor VIII clotting activity and poor platelet adhesion. (von Willebrand factor is a cofactor for this adhesion.)

Thrombocytopenia

May result from decreased production (marrow aplasia, leukaemia or infiltration) or increased destruction (idiopathic thrombocytopenic purpura, hypersplenism and consumption coagulopathy).

Idiopathic thrombocytopenic purpura (ITP) is rare and not to be confused with thrombotic thrombocytopenic purpura (TTP) which is very rare indeed. ITP chiefly occurs in children following a respiratory or gastrointestinal viral infection. Patients present with purpura and a low platelet count. If the platelet count is very low, major bleeding may occur from the nose, gut, or into the brain. The bleeding time is prolonged but coagulation times are normal. Spontaneous recovery is the rule. Platelet counts down to 80 000 mm^3 do not need treatment. Steroids and fresh blood transfusion are required in the more severe cases, occasionally with lasting remission. Danazol, 400–800 mg daily with a maintenance dose of 50 mg daily may be effective. Splenectomy should be avoided if possible especially in children, in view of the risk of pneumococcal septicaemia in asplenic patients, but may be curative when medical management is unsuccessful.

Thrombotic thrombocytopenic purpura is a very rare disease of young adults who present with fever, abdominal pain, purpura and focal neurological signs. Initial haematuria may progress to renal failure. The mechanism is unknown but it may be a disorder of vascular endothelium which is unable to produce a prostacycline platelet inhibitor (hence the widespread intravascular thrombosis). The mortality is high. Treatment consists of plasma exchange and renal dialysis, if indicated, with or without heparin and steroids.

Henoch–Schönlein purpura
See page 96.

Osler's disease (Osler–Weber–Rendu)
Hereditary haemorrhagic telangiectasia: autosomal dominant.
May present as intermittent bleeding, usually gastrointestinal.
There are small capillary angiectases throughout the gastrointestinal tract including the buccal mucosa and tongue.

LYMPHADENOPATHY

Localised
Usually results from:
- local infection (any age)
- carcinoma (usually over 45 years old)
- Hodgkin's disease (usually patients under 35 years) (page 365) and non-Hodgkin's lymphoma

NB Tuberculosis must be considered in all cervical lymphadenopathy. This is also a common site for stage I Hodgkin's disease, and also for neoplastic secondary deposits from the lung, testis, breast and nasopharyngeal carcinomas (ENT examination must be performed before biopsy).

Examine this patient's neck for signs of goitre, and check lymph glands. Consider origin of swelling (including testicles).

Generalised
Usually results from:
- infectious mononucleosis and rubella

- reticuloendothelial disorders
- chronic lymphatic leukaemia
- other less common causes include toxoplasmosis, tuberculosis, sarcoidosis and brucellosis.

NB If glandular enlargement persists blood count is essential particularly to confirm or exclude leukaemia, and a chest X-ray may show hilar lymphadenopathy. A biopsy usually supplies the diagnosis.

Diabetes

'This patient has diabetes mellitus: would you ask him some questions' (also page 198).

A similar approach is advised in the clinic. You should ask his age and occupation and note if he is under- or over-weight. Ask when the diabetes was first diagnosed. Ask about the common presenting symptoms of thirst, polyuria, fatigue and pruritus vulvae. In the young there is often loss of weight even when the appetite is well preserved. This combination also occurs in thyrotoxicosis (common), some malabsorption states, some tumours early in their course (e.g. carcinoma of the bronchus), some hypercatabolic states (e.g. leukaemia), and, to all appearances, in anorexia nervosa.

You should take:
- family history for diabetes
- obstetric history (big babies, stillbirths)
- drug history (corticosteroids and ACTH, thiazide diuretics)

NB Always remember the four endocrine conditions which can present to a diabetic clinic: acromegaly, Cushing's syndrome, haemochromatosis, and phaeochromocytoma.

Go quickly over the systems which can be involved in diabetes, asking questions about relevant symptoms.

Cardiovascular

Angina and myocardial infarct. Intermittent claudication, cold feet, gangrene.

Nervous (page 201)

Legs, feet. Numbness, pain or paraesthesiae, painless ulcers.

Eyes (page 200). Failing vision (transitory with poor control), retinopathy, cataract.

Brain. Ischaemic attacks or strokes. Hypoglycaemia.

Autonomic. Impotence, postural hypotension. Diarrhoea (especially at night) and gastric distension.

Mononeuritis multiplex (pages 137 and 201).

Respiratory

Cough, usually due to chronic bronchitis but tuberculosis is commoner in diabetics than in the general population.

Renal (page 201)

Polyuria (glycosuria, renal failure). Frequency and/or dysuria of infection.

Skin (page 202)

Sepsis, e.g. boils. Xanthelasma (page 210). Necrobiosis lipoidica (rare) (page 202). Vaginitis (usually monilial). Balanitis. Granuloma annulare.

MANAGEMENT

Define the outline of his treatment and assess the adequacy of control (page 202).

Diet

A controlled caloric, low fat, low refined sugar, high fibre diet.

Drugs

Insulin (table 15)

Ask about the type of insulin and the frequency of injection. All insulin-dependent diabetics in the UK use U-100 insulin (100 units/ml), but this may not be so with visitors from other countries.

Human insulin is prepared either by a single amino-acid substitution in a pig insulin molecule (e.m.p.—enzymatic modification of porcine) or by genetic engineering (p.r.b.—pro insulin recombinant bacterial, or p.y.r.—precursor yeast recombinant).

Most patients are best controlled with twice-daily injections of mixed insulins containing short and medium acting preparation, e.g. Actrapid/Monotard, or a premixed preparation, e.g. Mixtard. The basal/bolus technique of tds preprandial Actrapid plus evening Ultratard may be used.

Table 15.   Commonly used insulins.

Name	Onset (h)	Peak (h)	Duration (h)
Neutral soluble	½–1	2–6	6–8
Actrapid			
Velosulin			
Humulin S			
Isophane	2	4–12	12–24
Protaphane			
Insulatard			
Humulin I			
IZS (zinc suspension)	2	2–8	16–24
Monotard			
Humulin Lente			
Ultratard	4–8	12–20	24–28
Biphasic			
Mixtard (30% sol/70% isophane)	½–1	2–8	
Initard (50% sol/50% isophane)	½–1	1–8	12–18
Humulin M1 (10% sol/90% isophane			

Oral therapy

Try to determine the name, tablet size and frequency of administration. You should know whether they are sulphonylureas or the biguanide, metformin.

Assessment of diabetic control

Ask for the patient's routine blood or urine-testing charts. Persistent absence of glucose without hypoglycaemic symptoms suggests a high renal threshold and the charts may be useless for diabetic control. Conversely, persistent glycosuria can mean a low threshold and be similarly unhelpful. It is usually best for the patient to perform his own home blood glucose monitoring accurately and to keep a record. A glucose-oxidase impregnated stick is read on a meter or by eye. Ideally the blood sugar should be normal (4–6 mmol/litre) at all times and the patient symptomless. Realistically aim to keep the blood glucose under 10 mmol/litre at all times whilst avoiding hypoglycaemic symptoms.

Urine glucose measurements are helpful when blood glucose estimations are not available usually because the patient refuses to prick a finger. Since the normal threshold is about 10 mmol/litre, *any* glycosuria suggests poor control.

Glycosylated haemoglobin (HbA$_{1c}$) gives an index of average control over approximately the previous 2–3 months and fructosamine over 2–3 weeks.

Insulin resistance

Hormonal

This is due to an excess level of antagonists such as cortisol (Cushing's syndrome), catecholamines (phaeochromocytoma), growth hormone (acromegaly) thyroxine (hyperthyroidism) or glucagon (glucagonoma).

Non-hormonal

Insulin antibodies (IgG) of about 30% are associated with allergy, usually at the injection site and causing wheals and subcutaneous swelling. Human insulin may prevent these problems.

Symptoms of poor control

Hyperglycaemia

Polyuria (with nocturia) and thirst. Hospital admissions with ketoacidosis. Intermittent blurring of vision. Weight loss.

Hypoglycaemia

'Hypos' or 'reactions'. Determine at what time of day (in relation to food, exercise and insulin) they occur. Early morning headaches may be the only indication of nocturnal hypoglycaemia. Weight gain.

EXAMINATION
'Would you examine him?'
You will probably be directed by the history. Otherwise, examination should include:

Obesity
In the clinic perform routine height and weight measurements.

Injection sites
Thighs, anterior abdominal wall and arms for fat atrophy or hypertrophy.

Eyes (pages 200–201)
Dilate pupil except in patients with lens implants held in place by hooks onto the iris. Cataract and retinopathy (microaneurysms, exudates, retinal vessel proliferation, arteriosclerosis)—page 200.

Legs and feet
Peripheral neuropathy (chiefly sensory). Test the tendon reflexes and for light touch and vibration sense.
Peripheral vascular disease. Check the arterial pulses and temperature of the feet. Even if the pulses are present, the toes may be blue and cold due to 'small vessel disease'.
Remember:
- Necrobiosis (very rare)
- Quadriceps wasting and tenderness (amyotrophy) improved by good control
- Infection

Chest
The history may indicate infection.

Abdomen
Feel for the liver which may often be palpable in the long standing insulin-dependent diabetic due to fatty infiltration.
(**NB**   Haemochromatosis is very rare.)
Test the urine for sugar, protein and ketones.

Autonomic function tests

Parasympathetic
1 Heart rate response to deep breathing.
2 Heart rate response to standing
3 Heart rate response to the Valsalva manoeuvre.

Sympathetic
1 Blood pressure response to standing.
2 Blood pressure response to muscle exercise such as sustained hand grip.

Ask if you may see (a) the result of a recent blood sugar series if control has deteriorated; (b) a recent chest X-ray; (c) the result of a mid-stream urine specimen (MSU) if there is a history of dysuria. The measurement of blood levels of HbA_{1c} (glycosylated Hb) may give a good indication of long-term diabetic control because it reflects the mean blood glucose level over the previous 1–2 months.

Establish the patient on a twice daily mixed insulin or basal/bolus regime using a long-acting formulation such as Ultratard, usually at night, with Actrapid before each of the major meals most conveniently with a cartridge in a pen device. Assess control with home blood glucose monitoring, checking before and after each of the three daily meals plus possibly bedtime and 3 a.m. samples. The patient should be seen regularly.

SCREENING IN DIABETES

'What would you check at annual review?'

- Eyes. Visual acuity (Snellen chart) and examine retinae through dilated pupils (tropicamide and, possibly, pseudephedrine eyedrops)
- Blood pressure
- Feet for sensory neuropathy including ankle jerks, and for arterial disease including the four major arterial foot pulses and evidence of reduced capillary circulation. Note the temperature of the feet and check them for ulcers
- Injection sites for fat atrophy and hypertrophy
- Take blood for creatinine (and/or urea) and glycosylated haemoglobin (HbA_{1c}) or fructosamine. Check the random blood glucose (with the timing of the last meal), and obtain the patient's own estimate of his blood glucose at the same time, using his own technique
- Urine for albumin and microalbumin
- Diet review and patient's understanding of his own diabetes

NB Management of diabetes, see page 202.

Random screening of the whole population is probably not cost-effective, though it does serve to increase its health-conciousness. People particularly at risk include those who have had gestational diabetes (where 60% become diabetic within 16 years), and siblings of Type 2 diabetics particularly after the age of 50.

DIABETES AND PREGNANCY

The risks to the fetus are considerable, with a high perinatal mortality which is related to the degree of diabetic control. If fasting and postprandial blood glucose levels are within normal limits, fetal loss is probably no greater than in the normal population. The more rigid regimes insist on levels below 5.5 mmol/litre for most of the day with a postprandial level below 7–8 mmol/litre. These better levels of control obviate the need for routine Caesarian section. It is usual to monitor maternal plasma or urinary oestrogens and the fetus with ultrasound. In some units amniocentesis at 38 weeks is performed to measure the lecithin/sphingomyelin ratio to assess the risks of the respiratory distress syndrome. Urine testing is not useful because of the fall in renal glucose threshold. Insulin requirements tend to fall in the first trimester, stablise in the second trimester, and rise again in the last trimester only to fall abruptly on delivery. The patient is admitted for accurate diabetic control and delivery at term (see *Diabetes and surgery* below).

DIABETES AND ILLNESS

Even with vomiting, hepatic glycogenolysis can provide enough glucose during most illnesses. Normal doses of insulin are continued and blood glucose estimated 2- to 4-hourly. Soluble insulin is taken 5 units 2-hourly if the blood glucose is in the range 12–20 mmol/litre and not climbing. Ketonuria must be monitored every time urine is passed. Diabetics who have been properly educated in diabetes will know a number of suitable 10 g CHO exchanges, such as a 5 ml spoonful of glucose or sucrose, 50 ml Lucozade or 200 ml whole milk.

DIABETES AND SURGERY

The main danger is that the patient becomes hypoglycaemic whilst anaesthetised. However, with increases in cortisol, glucagon, growth hormone and catecholamines, plus a decrease in insulin, surgery tends to produce hyperglycaemia even in the non-diabetic subject. With elective surgery, the patient should be first on the operating list. No food or insulin is given on the morning of the operation. Bladder catheterisation is not indicated for diabetic control.

Non-insulin dependent diabetes mellitus—NIDDM (Type 2, maturity onset)
- *Before surgery*. Stop drugs 24 h before (48 h for chlorpropamide and glibenclamide).
- *During surgery*. Treat as insulin-dependent if blood glucose >10 mmol/litre, or major surgery. Otherwise, no therapy.
- *After surgery*. Unless now on insulin, or postoperative blood glucose >15 mmol/litre or patient is ill, reinstate oral therapy.

Insulin-dependent diabetes mellitus—IDDM (Type 1)
- *Before surgery*. Continue 'bd mixed' or basal/bolus regimes. Convert others to tds preprandial if well controlled; if not delay surgery and stabilise.
- *During surgery*. Arrange for blood glucose every 2 h. Give 500 ml 4-hourly of 10% glucose with 10 mmol KCl in each. Add as many units soluble insulin to the (500 ml) bag as the patient's current blood glucose (to the nearest 5 units). Adjust KCl dose to suit patient.
- *After surgery*. Slow above regime to 6-hourly and return to normal regime when patient starts eating again.

DIABETES AND DRIVING

The licensing authority and insurance company must be informed when diabetes is diagnosed. Diabetic patients will be given a 'private driver's licence' for up to 3 years depending upon the quality of control, the regularity of medical surveillance and the state of complications. Patients with NIDDM and without complications are given 3-year licences. Patients with IDDM are given a licence when glycaemic control is good, the patient's understanding of the condition is good, and the patient is not subject to frequent or sudden attacks of hypoglycaemia. This implies that the patient must carry glucose tablets (or equivalent) and know and avoid situations in which there is increased risk of hypoglycaemia. The complications of reduction of visual acuity, sensory neuropathy and peripheral vascular disease must be assessed. Patients with IDDM will not normally obtain a 'vocational driving licence' (for HGV and PSV), but NIDDM patients normally will.

Skin

In examinations it is usual to show cases of common disorders such as acne, eczema, athletes foot and drug eruption and those that have complications such as psoriasis and bullous eruptions (page 352). Remember that several skin disorders are manifestations of systemic disease, e.g. purpura and lupus erythematosus.

HISTORY

'What do you think of this rash?'

Diagnosis depends on the history, examination of the skin, examination for underlying systemic disorder with special investigations for this, and special investigations of the skin such as skin biopsy and scrapings for fungi.

If you are allowed to question the patient, pay special attention to:

- When the rash started and whether it has altered in character or progressed
- Where the rash began. This is especially important in contact dermatitis and with pityriasis rosea (herald patch)
- What drugs have been taken especially 'over the counter' drugs. The rash may have been treated topically and as a result may have altered in character and be either better or worse as a result. Discover if possible what drugs, e.g. steroids, antibiotics or antihistamines have been applied to the skin. Some substances in foods can cause urticaria. Many prescription drugs cause rashes
- Does the rash itch? Insect bites and scabies (worse in bed) are relatively common. Dermatitis (page 345) usually gives irritation and itching. Itching is also given by the lesions of urticaria and fibreglass (common) and by lichen planus and flexural psoriasis (rare)
- Enquire about occupation and hobbies particularly with contact dermatitis (page 345) and about changes in life style such as visits abroad or to relatives and friends. Is anyone else in the household affected and what pets does the patient have? Is there a family history, for example, of eczema, psoriasis?
- Ask about the general state of health. Many conditions, some relatively rare, have skin manifestations. Remember the exanthems e.g. rubella, but these are not seen in the clinic or in examination. Ask the patient for his theories about the cause of the rash.

EXAMINATION

You will usually need to look at the entire skin so the patient will have to be completely undressed. Remember the back, buttocks and genitalia (ask the examiner before examining these), and special areas such as scalp, eyes, mouth fingernails and toenails.

- Categorise the type of lesion as macule (flat), papule (slightly raised), nodule, vesicle, bulla, pustule, scaling and crusting, pigmentation, lichenification (thick-ening of the skin with increased skin markings due to continued scratching), purpura

• Determine the distribution of the lesions. Generalised lesions suggest systemic disease or a drug rash. Some diseases, e.g. psoriasis (page 344) acne (page 346) show predilection for certain sites on the body. Localised lesions occur in contact dermatitis and some fungal infections. Fixed drug eruptions recur at the same site every time the drug is taken. The flexures are involved in intertrigo, seborrhoeic dermatitis, psoriasis, and some fungal infections.

• Describe the configuration. Some lesions may be annular, e.g. ringworm, pityriasis rosea. Bullae occur in groups in herpes simplex and dermatitis herpetiformis

• The more common special investigations include:

Inspection under Wood's light which will show green fluorescence in most cases of tinea capitis.

In scabies, extract mite by scraping the burrow and examine with low power microscopy.

Patch testing to chemicals suspected of causing contact dermatitis.

Skin biospy for histology particularly where malignancy is to be excluded, but also for immunofluorescence and electron microscopy.

Part 2
Essential background
information

Neurology

'Headaches' and 'giddiness' constitute the most commonly presenting neurological symptoms. Faints, dizzy turns and blackouts are common and may originate from the cardiovascular system (CVS), e.g. aortic stenosis platelet emboli and dysrhythmias such as complete heart block (CHB) and sick sinus syndrome (page 84). Cerebrovascular accidents are the most common neurological cause for hospital admission. In the Membership examination these are not commonly seen and frequently eliminated on the grounds of being too easy. None the less, it is often difficult to decide when to investigate in depth patients with headache and giddiness, and the management of 'strokes' may not only be difficult but presents a major clinical challenge in terms of numbers of patients alone.

HEADACHE

This is perhaps one of the most common of all presenting symptoms. The aims are to exclude treatable underlying intra- or extracranial disease and to make a definitive diagnosis (e.g. migraine). There are seldom any useful physical signs and the diagnosis is usually made on the history. Commonly the patient's history will correspond with one of the following:

Unilateral facial pain
Including migraine (page 114).

Tension headache
This is characteristically a severe continuous pressure felt bilaterally over the vertex, occiput or eyes. It may be band-like or non-specific in character and of variable intensity. It is commonest in the middle-aged women but may occur at any age in association with stress or depression (ask about family, work, money and for symptoms of depression). The headache may be described with considerable drama and standard analgesics are almost invariably ineffective. Occasionally it may be symptomatic of worry about a brain tumour and relieved by definite reassurance and thorough normal physical examination.

Post-concussion headache
The pain has many features of tension headache but is usually associated with dizziness (not vertigo) and loss of concentration. There is often a history of inadequate recovery following the head injury and of impending litigation.

Raised intracranial pressure
Intracranial tumour, haematoma or abscess. The pain is worst after lying down and is then associated with vomiting. It improves 1–2 h after rising in the

113

morning and is exacerbated by coughing, sneezing or straining. Visual defects may not occur despite severe papilloedema. The patient usually presents within 6 weeks of the onset of symptoms and these usually respond to standard analgesics. Papilloedema is by then usually obvious.

NB   (for teetotallers) Alcoholic hangovers also cause early morning headaches.

Patients whose histories do not fit into one of these categories usually have either an obvious diagnosis (meningitis, subarachnoid haemorrhage, sinusitis, otitis media) or a less obvious local cause (teeth, cervical spine, skull, orbits). Benign hypertension, defects in visual acuity, glaucoma and ocular muscle imbalance seldom present as headache.

Preliminary investigation

Patients with a headache of more than 6 weeks' duration and without abnormal clinical signs probably do not require investigation. Most hospital physicians, when seeing the patient referred from a family practitioner would request:
- full blood count including erythrocyte sedimentation rate (ESR) (to exclude temporal arteritis in the over-fifties)
- chest X-ray for bronchial carcinoma
- skull X-ray may reveal (a) evidence of raised intracranial pressure; (b) shift of midline if the pineal is calcified; and (c) calcification within tumours (meningi-omata and craniopharyngiomata)

In case of doubt it is usually reasonable to see the patient in the clinic at intervals to observe changing symptoms, the development of physical signs or increasing anxiety or depression.

Further investigation

This is rarely necessary but is indicated in the presence of:
- frontal headache on waking with nausea, i.e. symptoms suggestive of raised intracranial pressure
- occipital headache of sudden onset (subarachnoid haemorrhage)
- abnormal, and in particular progressive, neurological signs including confusion and dementia

It should include computerised axial tomography (CT scan) where available and, where not, an isotope brain scan may reveal a space-occupying lesion.

NB   Patients with headache and facial pain may not give histories which fit conveniently into any well-recognised category. They should be seen at intervals to determine:
- symptoms of increasing anxiety or depression
- symptoms of changing pain patterns
- developing abnormal clinical signs

In the absence of these, treatment is with reassurance and simple analgesics.

UNILATERAL FACIAL PAIN

Migraine

Migraine is episodic and affects approximately 10% of population usually mildly. It usually begins around puberty and continues intermittently to middle age. It is commoner in females than males (3 : 1) and there is often a family history. There may have been episodes of unexplained nausea and/or abdominal pain in childhood. It may be associated with periods and 'the pill', with various foods (especially chocolate, cheese and red wine) and emotions (anger, tension, excitement), and with various times of the day or week. A characteristic attack starts with a sense of ill-health and is followed by a visual *aura* (shimmering lights, fortification spectra, scotomas) usually in the field opposite to the side of the succeeding headache. The throbbing *unilateral headache* is associated with anorexia, nausea, vomiting, photophobia and withdrawal. There may be transient hemiparesis or sensory symptoms. It is very rarely associated with organic disease and CT scan with contrast is only indicated if abnormal physical signs persist or progess.

Management

Precipitating causes should be identified and removed—a patient's diary of symptoms and diet may help, and simple analgesics taken early (aspirin, paracetamol). Metoclopramide or domperidone may be given with them to reduce nausea. If attacks are more frequent than, say, two per month or so severe that they interfere with work and social life, treat prophylactically with pizotifen, 1.5 mg nocte, propranolol, 80–160 mg daily, or possibly, methysergide 1–2 mg bd for not more than 3 months. Promethazine and prochlorperazine have also been used.

Cluster headaches (migrainous neuralgia)

These appear to be a form of migraine. Attacks occur in clusters every 12–18 months and consist of very severe pain around an eye occurring often at night for 1–3 weeks. The eye becomes injected and watery and the nostril of the same side blocked up. It often responds to ergotamine.

Neuralgias

Neuralgias are intermittent, brief, severe, lancinating pains occuring along the distribution of a nerve.

Trigeminal neuralgia (tic douloureux)

Occurs almost only in the elderly. (If the syndrome occurs in a patient under 50 years old it may be symptomatic of multiple sclerosis.) The agonising pain is usually triggered from a place on the lips or the side of the nose. Tumour can be a rare cause which can be excluded by CT scan. It tends to get worse with age but may be specifically relieved by carbamazepine (Tegretol). Phenytoin may also be useful. A small aberrant vessel overlying the nerve (or ganglion) can be the cause, and dissection of this completely relieves the symptoms. A patient may need thermocoagulation or section of the sensory root of the fifth nerve. Suicide is a definite risk.

Glossopharyngeal neuralgia

Precipitated by swallowing which produces pain in the pharynx.

Auriculotemporal neuralgia (Costen's syndrome)
Precipitated by swallowing and may be treated by correcting a malocculusion.

Postherpetic neuralgia
Occurs in patients with a history of herpes zoster and the scars of the healed disease are usually obvious. The pain may be almost impossible to relieve.

Temporal arteritis (giant cell arteritis)
Temporal arteritis is a local expression of a connective tissue disease (page 167). The pain is felt in the temples or over the entire scalp and the affected artery is usually dilated and tender. The patient usually feels ill and the ESR is greatly raised. Biopsy is performed if it can be done rapidly and the patient given steroids before sudden blindness supervenes (uncommon).

Atypical facial pain
This refers to a syndrome with episodes of constant ache in the jaw and cheek lasting several hours occurring usually in young to middle-aged women who frequently are depressed. It is often bilateral. Treatment is difficult but patients may respond to antidepressants or antihistamines.

Unilateral pain
Local pathologies involving the eyes, sinuses, teeth or ears may give unilateral pain, as may tumours involving the fifth nerve (cerebellopontine angle tumours). Pain from herpes zoster may occur before the rash appears.

CEREBROVASCULAR DISEASE
Internal capsule (figure 42).
Arterial supply (figure 43).

'Strokes'
Strokes affect about one patient in 500 per year in general practice; 20% are due to intracerebral haemorrhage, and 80% thrombosis or embolism. The mortality from haemorrhage is very high (80% of patients die within 1 month).

Patients particularly at risk include those with hypertension, ischaemic heart disease, cardiomyopathy, diabetes mellitus, peripheral vascular disease and those with polycythaemia or on the contraceptive pill. Other factors include smoking, obesity, hyperlipidaemia, and physical inactivity.

Cerebral haemorrhage usually results from rupture of large intracerebral vessels or of microaneurysms in perforating arteries. Rarely (5%) haemorrhage results from infective endocarditis, tumour, abscess, anticoagulants or blood dyscrasias. Thrombosis *in situ* may follow hypotension which itself may be secondary to myocardial infarction or to cardiac arrhythmias which cause a fall in cardiac output. Rarely, thrombosis follows arteritis, the contraceptive pill, polycythaemia rubra vera or meningovascular syphilis.

Cerebral embolism is caused by emboli arising from the carotid or vertebrobasilar arteries, or from the heart following myocardial infarction, from

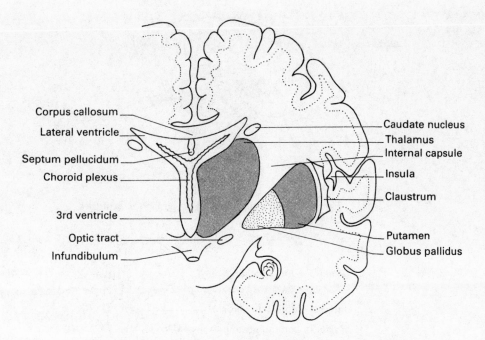

Figure 42.   The internal capsule, thalamus and 3rd ventricle in coronal section.

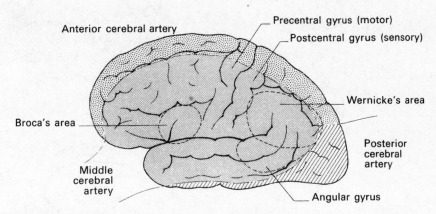

Figure 43.   Lateral surface of the left cerebral hemisphere.

the atrial appendage in atrial fibrillation, and from vegetations in infective endocarditis.

Clinical presentation

It is usually impossible to distinguish between cerebral haemorrhage, thrombosis and embolism except that embolism is more likely if atrial fibrillation is present, after a myocardial infarction, or in infective endocarditis.

The commonest presentation is with hemiplegia but there are many variants and slight weakness of a hand or confusion may be the only evidence of an

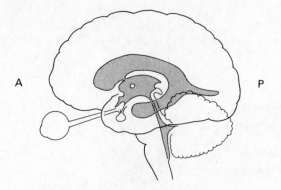

A   P

Figure 44.   Lateral view to show position of ventricles.

(a)

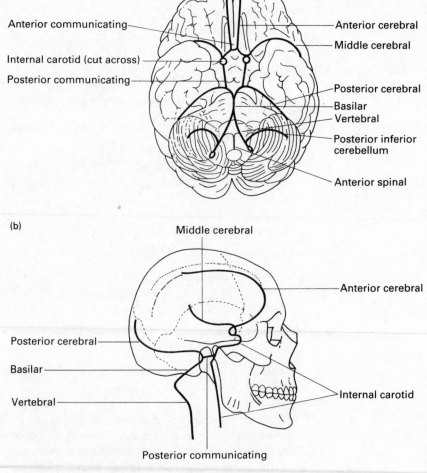

Anterior communicating ——————————————— Anterior cerebral

—————— Middle cerebral

Internal carotid (cut across) ————

Posterior communicating ————

—————— Posterior cerebral

—————— Basilar

—————— Vertebral

—————— Posterior inferior
cerebellum

—————— Anterior spinal

(b)

Middle cerebral

—————— Anterior cerebral

Posterior cerebral ————

Basilar ————

Vertebral ————

—————— Internal carotid

Posterior communicating

Figure 45.   Cerebral arteries (a) basal view (b) Lateral view.

attack. Cerebal oedema with clinical evidence of raised intracranial pressure may be secondary to brain infarction. Expressive dysphasia occurs with lesions affecting Broca's area and there is often an upper motor neurone seventh nerve lesion on the same side as the hemianopia and hemiplegia (left-sided cerebral lesion leads to right-sided homonymous hemianopia, right-sided upper motor neurone seventh nerve lesion and right-sided hemiplegia.)

Investigation

Haemoglobin, haematocrit, ESR, blood glucose, ECG, chest X-ray, and carotid Doppler if indicated. CT scan may help determine antihaemostatic therapy, and guide surgical intervention if the patient shows evidence of raised intracranial pressure.

Management

Act on risk factors such as smoking, blood lipids, diabetes, cardiac dysrrhythmias. Control severe hypertension if present and stop the contraceptive pill.

During the unconscious phase, evidence of continued raised intracranial pressure is shown by a rising blood pressure, falling pulse rate and papilloedema. One enlarging pupil which finally becomes fixed and dilated indicates ipsilateral pressure on the third cranial nerve as it passes over the tentorium cerebelli. Surgical evacuation of a blood clot may prevent pressure damage to the contralateral cortex.

In any one patient it is impossible to assess how much recovery will occur, and attention must be paid to the airway, hydration and nutrition during the unconscious phase. The patient must be turned regularly to prevent sores, and catheterisation is usually necessary. Passive and active physiotherapy are started early, together with speech therapy, and later occupational therapy. Full recovery is often hindered in non-dominant cerebral lesions which control drive and motivation and the ability to perform usual if complex routines, e.g. dressing.

Some features are associated with a poorer prognosis: age, complete paralysis, low level of consciousness, incontinence and combinations of hemiplegia with hemianaesthesia and hemianopia, and higher cerebral dysfunction.

Transient ischaemic attacks (TIAs)

These are sudden focal neurological abnormalities which settle rapidly within 24 h with complete clinical recovery. They are caused by platelet emboli from the carotid or vertebrobasilar arteries. UK incidence is 0.5–1000 per annum.

Carotid TIAs

Internal carotid artery stenosis. Platelets aggregate at a critical stenosis and obstruct blood flow before subsequently breaking up, when blood flow is restored and symptoms remit. This may result in a typical hemiplegic stroke (middle cerebral artery), or a transient episode of: mono- or hemiparesis, dysphasia if the dominant hemisphere is involved, hemianaesthesia, facial palsy, or ipsilateral blindness (amaurosis fugax). Emboli tend to break up where they lodge and symptoms tend to be transient but recurrent. About 40% of patients develop complete strokes or myocardial infarction within 3 years.

Investigation As for stroke.

Management. Stop smoking. Control hypertension and hyperlipidaemia if present. Aspirin (150–300 mg/day) reduces the long term risk of nonfatal stroke and myocardial infarction. Anticoagulants, dipyridamole and surgery to the carotid artery are all of unproven value. There is usually atheroma in all of the cerebral vessels and carotid surgery carries a high operative mortality.

Vertebrobasilar TIAs

This presents as transient episodes of vertigo with ataxia, dysarthria and nystagmus, visual loss and occasionally 'drop attacks'. These may result from emboli to the brain-stem or may follow nipping of the vertebral arteries by osteophytic cervical vertebrae in the presence of an 'incompetent' circle of Willis. It carries a relatively good prognosis compared with disease of the internal carotid arteries.

Thrombosis in the vertebrobasilar distribution is rare. It affects the upper medulla, cerebellum and cranial nerves and gives rise to a variety of syndromes. **NB** Driving is not permitted for 6 months after recurrent TIAs and for 3 months after an isolated TIA or a stroke.

Anticoagulation in cerebrovascular disease

Anticoagulants may be indicated if there is:
- A known cardiac source of embolism
- An evolving stroke due to thrombosis—best assessed by the absence of haemorrhage or tumour on CT scan (or by the absence of red cells in the CSF on lumbar puncture—which usually excludes haemorrhage). Anticoagulants are not indicated in a completed stroke in the absence of an obvious source of embolism
- A history of transient ischaemic attacks otherwise unresponsive to therapy

Arteriography may be indicated in patients with multiple carotid TIAs who are normotensive, unresponsive to aspirin and have a carotid bruit. It is not indicated in hypertensives or in patients with vertebrobasilar disease because surgery is not feasible.

Lateral medullary syndrome (figure 2, page 6)

This is the commonest brain-stem vascular syndrome and presents acutely with vertigo, vomiting, hiccoughs and ipsilateral facial pain. Dysphagia and dysarthria may occur.

The following features may be present:

Ipsilateral:
Palatal paralysis.
Horner's syndrome.
Spinothalamic sensory loss in the face.
Cerebellar signs in the limbs.

Contralateral:
Spinothalamic loss in the body.

Extracerebral haemorrhage

Extradural

This results from traumatic damage to the middle meningeal artery as it passes upward on the inside of the temporal bone. Classically, momenetary loss of consciousness is followed by apparent recovery and death 1–7 days later. Not every fracture of the temporal bone results in middle meningeal haemorrhage but suspicion alone warrants skull X-rays and admission of the patient to observe his conscious level. Should signs of local haemorrhage ensue, burr holes are performed, the clot removed and the vessel tied.

Subdural

This occurs most frequently in the elderly, alcoholics and children. It often follows trauma. A small venous haemorrhage occurs and the clot slowly enlarges in size by absorbing fluid osmotically from the CSF.

Clinical presentation. The symptoms may develop over a period of weeks to months. Headache, confusion and progressive loss of conscious level occur and there may be fluctuation of consciousness. The other signs are of a one-side intracranial mass with contralateral weakness and hemiplegia, possibly with signs of raised intracranial pressure (falling pulse rate, rising blood pressure and papilloedema).

Management. Full recovery may follow removal of the haematoma, irrespective of the patient's age. Subdural haematomata may be bilateral.

Subarachnoid

This usually results from rupture of a berry aneurysm from the vessels of the circle of Willis (figures 45 and 46).
Rupture is more common in the presence of hypertension. Subarachnoid haemorrhage may result from leakage or rupture of an angioma or arteriovenous malformation (AVM) and severe intracerebral haemorrhage may spread into the subarachnoid space.

Clinical presentation. Consciousness may or may not be lost. If not, a history of headache described as 'a severe blow in the back of the neck' may be obtained. There may be associated nausea and vomiting.
On examination, photophobia and neck stiffness are present. The level of consciousness progressively decreases if haemorrhage continues, with signs of

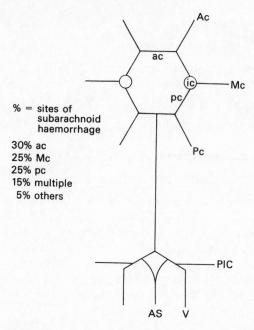

% = sites of
   subarachnoid
   haemorrhage

30% ac
25% Mc
25% pc
15% multiple
 5% others

Figure 46. Cirle of Willis: cerebral arteries and incidence of subarachnoid haemorrhage. ac, anterior communicating; pc, posterior communicating; Ac, anterior cerebral; Mc, middle cerebral; Pc, posterior cerebral; ic, internal carotid; PIC, posterior inferior cerebellar; AS, anterior spinal; V, vertebral.

rising intracranial pressure (rising blood pressure, falling pulse rate, papilloedema). There may be localising signs in the cranial nerves. Remember to listen to the skull for the bruit of a congenital AVM.

Lumbar puncture shows raised pressure and uniform blood staining and later, xanthochromia. Proteinuria and glycosuria may occur. CT scan, where available, should be performed in preference to lumbar puncture and is particularly important where focal neurological signs suggest an intracerebral haematoma or raised intracranial pressure.

Management. Surgery is dangerous in those patients who do not recover fully. Then arteriography and/or CT scan is indicated to determine the site of haemorhage (25% show multiple aneurysm and 10% are negative). The optimum time after haemorrhage to perform arteriography is not agreed though it is usually delayed 7–10 days to ensure that the patient has recovered consciousness. When haemorrhage has stopped spontaneously, some surgeons prefer to delay arteriography to allow arterial spasm to subside but it should be performed before the second week—the time of potential re-bleed. Nimodipine, 60 mg 4-hourly, started within 4 days of onset and continued for 3 weeks appears to reduce the incidence of cerebral infarction and improves outcome. Hypertension immediately after a subarachnoid haemorrhage (SAH) does not usually require therapy. Single aneurysms can be clipped.

Prognosis. This can be considered 'in thirds'. One-third of the patients die in the first attack. Another third have a recurrence (normally between the first and second weeks), and a third of these survive. Of those who survive a year, about a third remain well and symptom-free.

BRAIN DEATH (two independent medical opinions are required)

The three main criteria essential to this medico-legal diagnosis are:

1 A known untreatable cause such as cardiac arrest, intracerebral haemorrhage or severe trauma. Patients with hypothermia or drug overdose are not acceptable.

2 Absent cortical function. Deep coma as shown by absent response to any stimulus (other than spinal reflexes).

3 Absent brain-stem function. This is demonstrated by:
- fixed dilated pupils
- absent corneal, gag and cough reflexes
- absent eye movements and no movement on rolling the head (i.e. the normal 'doll's eye movements' in which the eyes lag behind head movement are absent)
- absent caloric responses. Ice-cold water into an external auditory meatus causes eye movements towards the stimulated ear in normal people
- lack of spontaneous respiration

EPILEPSY

The word describes a wide variety of clinical patterns which have in common a continuing tendency to experience episodes of altered movements, sensory phenomena and odd behaviour, usually with altered consciousness. All are thought to be due to abnormal paroxysmal electrical discharges in the cerebral neurones. Many patients who present following a 'fit' have only had an episode of unconsciousness. It is important to consider and exclude other conditions which are commonly confused with epilepsy. Remember that epilepsy is a clinical diagnosis not an electrical one.

Classification of seizures

Partial (single cortical focus of activity)
- Simple. Symptoms only. No impairment of consciousness. Symptoms may be illusional, olfactory, psychic, cognitive, aphasic, sensory, or motor (Jacksonian)
- Complex. As partial but with impairment of consciousness

NB Partial siezures may proceed to tonic/clonic seizures (grand mal): see below.

Generalised (symmetrical cortical activity)
- Tonic/clonic seizures (grand mal): see below. Also: tonic (spasm), clonic (jerking), or atonic seizures
- Absence attacks (petit mal): see below
- Myoclonic jerks: single or multiple

NB Many seizure patterns remain unclassified.

An account of the fit from a witness is invaluable. In the differential diagnosis from faints, epileptics are stiff and not floppy in the fall, usually have staring open eyes rather than half-closed, have no memory of the fall and take over 30s to recover. Drop attacks occur only past middle age, usually in women in whom there is no loss of consciousness with a sense of surprise about the lack of external cause. A hysterial episode is exacerbated by witnesses, is associated with coarse dramatic movement rather than neat jerking, and clenched flickering eyelids with the eye rolled up (if the lids can be prised apart). Also, recovery is rapid with full mental alertness ('What happened, where am I?') and no neurological signs.

Aetiology

Usually no cause can be demonstrated (idiopathic epilepsy), though the following should be considered:

Syncope

- Vaso-vagal fainting attacks
- Cerebral arterial disease—carotid artery stenosis and vertebro basilar ischaemia. Transient ischaemic attacks (TIAs)
- Low cardiac output—Stokes–Adams attacks in heart block, sino-atrial disease (page 84) and aortic stenosis
- Postmicturition and cough syncope. Syncope of emotional distress and carotid sinus syncope
- Postural hypotension may be due to hypotensive or sedative drugs, particularly in the elderly

Cerebral disorders

- Cerebral tumour (especially in middle or old age), abscess or angioma
- Sequel of severe head injury and birth injury
- Cerebral atherosclerosis
- Other rare causes include toxoplasmosis (the commonest intracranial lesion in AIDS), cysticercosis, syphilis and systemic lupus erythematosus
- Falciparum malaria should be considered in travellers (examine blood film)

Metabolic disorders

- Hypoglycaemia
- Hypocalcaemia
- Renal or hepatic failure
- Drug poisoning
- Alcohol: severe intoxication, rapid withdrawal by habitual heavy drinkers, or following head injury while intoxicated

Apart from simple faints and emotional syncope, each of these syncopal and metabolic situations can be followed by true epilepsy. Even after syncopal attacks, patients may proceed to true epilepsy if propped up.

Individual attacks may be triggered by television, disco strobes, stress, and anxiety of fatigue, the premenstrual syndrome, alcohol (sometimes due to hypoglycaemia especially in diabetics), and water intoxication.

Clinical presentation and management

Grand mal (generalised tonic/clonic seizures)
In over 50% of cases, a fit is preceded by an aura. This is followed by loss of consciousness and the tonic phase. This lasts up to 30 s and cyanosis may occur as the respiratory muscles are also tonically contracted. The clonic phase follows in all limbs and micturition and tongue biting and fingers if unwisely inserted into the mouth to pull the tongue forward occur in this stage, which is followed by sleep lasting for 1–3 h. During sleep the corneal and limb reflexes may be absent and the plantar responses up-going.

Management of acute phase. Protect the patient from injury during convulsion. Intravenous diazepam (5 mg/min for 2–4 min) will control most fits. Status epilepticus may require continued diazepam, or a chlormethiazole or phenytoin infusion with close attention to breathing. General anaesthesia with muscle relaxants and artificial ventilation are sometimes needed to suppress abnormal cerebal electrical activity.

Long-term therapy. The object is to decrease the number and intensity of fits and if possible to abolish them with the least side-effects (chiefly sedation). In patients who are flicker-sensitive, pay attention to the viewing habits when watching television: it is important to keep back from the screen. The standard drugs are carbamazepine 600–1200 mg daily or phenytoin usually taken 100–300 mg daily with the serum level measured 2 weeks after starting and the dose adjusted to maintain therapeutic blood levels. Lower doses, if effective, should be used. Sodium valproate is an alternative first-choice drug. Other drugs include vigabatrin (in refractory grand mal), clobazam, clonazepam and primidone.
NB Sometimes it is not possible to stop all fits without unacceptable sedation. After a single isolated grand mal fit the patient should not drive for 1 year.

Petit mal (absence attacks)
This presents in childhood and is characterised by moments of absence without warning and with immediate recovery. Movements are few and falls rare. The EEG shows typical spike and wave complexes at 3 per second. It virtually never continues beyond adolescence but may be superseded by adult epilepsy.

Management. Normal schooling. Sodium valproate is the drug of first choice though some continue to prefer ethosuximide.

Temporal lobe epilepsy
This is characterised by temporary disturbances of the content of consciousness. Hallucinations may occur (déjà vu phenomenon) as may visual disturbances such as macropsia and micropsia. Unreasoning fear or depersonalisation may be present. Olfactory or gustatory auras may be the only symptom and are related to abnormal foci in the uncinate lobe (uncinate attacks). Automatism may follow the aura. In these, patients perform a complex movement pattern, repeated with

each attack (psychomotor epilepsy). Treatment is similar to that of grand mal. In refractory temporal lobe epilepsy, consider vigabatrin.

In adults intracerebral tumour should be suspected.

Jacksonian (focal) epilepsy

Convulsions originate in one part of the precentral motor cortex. Fits begin in one part of the body (e.g. the thumb) and may proceed to involve that side of the body and then the whole body. Subsequent paresis of the affected limb may last up to 3 days (Todd's paralysis). Sensory epilepsy is a parallel condition originating in the sensory cortex. Treatment is similar to that of grand mal.

Investigation of 'fits'

The object is to detect treatable underlying brain disease and to exclude 'provoked' attacks where the treatment is to avoid the provoking factor, not anticonvulsant therapy, e.g. Stokes–Adams, vaso-vagal syncope.

A full history and clinical examination is taken to exclude other causes of loss of consciousness (see above).

Check blood for evidence of alcohol (mean corpuscular volume, γ-glutamyltransferase and alcohol levels), for hypoglycaemia, and rarely calcium and magnesium.

All patients should have chest X-ray. If a CT scan is available, most doctors would now perform a brain CT scan at this stage. An EEG may be helpful by demonstrating the type of epilepsy, site of an epileptic focus (slow activity may suggest the presence of a tumour) and guide drug therapy. An abnormal EEG does not alone refute or establish a diagnosis of epilepsy.

Epilepsy, if starting in adult life and particularly if Jacksonian, is more likely to be due to a space-occupying lesion.

If CT scanning is not available after a single isolated fit and in the absence of neurological signs with a normal chest X-ray, skull X-ray and EEG, no further investigation is usually necessary and the patient should not normally be diagnosed as 'epileptic'. The patient is seen at regular intervals and if he has a further fit or develops neurological signs (particularly if they are progressive) detailed investigations are indicated. Investigations should include a CT scan and possibly examination of the cerebrospinal fluid. If there is a possibility of a transient cardiac dysrhythmia as a cause of the fits, 24-h ambulatory ECG monitoring should be performed.

Transmission of epileptic tendency

The presence of cortical dysrhythmia on EEG does not mean epileptic attacks will definitely occur. In 35% of cases both parents have EEG dysrhythmias, whereas only in 5% of cases do both parents have normal EEGs.

Prognosis in epilepsy

Six years after diagnosis, 40% of patients will have been fit free for 5 years. Relatively poor prognoses are associated with combinations of grand mal with other seizures, traumatic epilepsy, clustering of episodes, physical signs and mental retardation.

Epilepsy and driving

Epilepsy (a continuing liability to seizures) is an absolute bar to holding a driving licence for not less than 2 years from the last episode, or 3 years of an established pattern of asleep attacks unbroken by any awake attacks. This applies to any epileptic manifestation, e.g. déjà vu phenomenon or absences on or off treatment.

Epilepsy and pregnancy

The risks of fits in pregnancy are greater than complications of anticonvulsants including phenytoin therapy (hare-lip and cleft palate). Patients should be delivered in hospital.

Advice to the patient with epilepsy

There are no rules, but it seems sensible to avoid heights, ladders, unsupervised swimming, and cycling for 2 years from the last episode. Fires should be guarded and children should not be left in the bath unattended.

NARCOLEPSY

This is a rare condition which usually starts in late puberty. There is sudden onset with episodes of irresistible and inappropriate sleep usually without fatigue, though often in sleep-provoking circumstances such as medical lectures. It is associated with cataplexy—attacks of sudden, brief muscle atonia without loss of consciousness often precipitated by laughter (also in medical lectures?) There may be abnormal mental states while passing between awake and asleep: sleep paralysis like cataplexy, and pre-sleep hallucinations like vivid dreams. These are disorders of REM sleep and are strongly associated with HLA DR2. Narcolepsy may respond to amphetamines, and cataplexy to clomipramine.

MULTIPLE SCLEROSIS (MS)

A disease characterised by acute episodes of neurological deficit appearing irregularly throughout the central nervous system both in place and time, with spontaneous but partial remission. Prevalence is 50–80/100 000, with a slight preponderance of females (3 : 2). It is a demyelinating disease with first episodes occurring in young adulthood. The aetiology is unknown; currently 'slow viruses' have been postulated, on the 'kuru', Jakob–Creutzfeld, bovine spongiform encephalopathy (BSE) and scrapie models. The patches of demyelination occur in the white matter of the brain and spinal cord, especially in

- optic nerves—the commonest initial site
- brain-stem
- cerebellar peduncles
- dorsal and pyramidal (lateral) tracts

Clinical presentation

In order of frequency:

Upper motor neurone motor deficit (50%) with weakness, as a paraparesis, hemiparesis, or monoparesis.

Retrobulbar neuritis with ocular pain and dimming of vision.

After recovery 'optic atrophy' or temporal pallor of the disc are characteristic.

Up to 50% of patients with retrobulbar neuritis subsequently develop MS.
Sensory deficit with paraesthesiae and proprioceptive loss in a limb or half of the body.
Cerebellar signs with intention tremor, nystagmus and dysarthria.
Diplopia due to an ocular nerve (third, fourth or sixth) or internuclear paralysis.
After recovery, ataxic nystagmus (i.e. with nystagmus greater in the abducting eye than in the adducting eye) is characteristic.
Acute vertigo and vomiting.
Disturbed micturition (5%). Precipitancy is common.
Eventually there is remaining evidence of optic atrophy, cerebellar lesions, and spastic paraparesis, frequently with posterior column loss. There is some dementia with change of mood, and euphoria is characteristic.

The symptoms are commonly made worse by exertion and heat (patients may be able to get into a hot bath but not out of it).

Cognitive impairment. IQ and language skills often remain normal till late in the disease. However, memory, learning and the ability to deal with abstract concepts often deteriorate particularly in chronic progressive forms.
NB Multiple sclerosis may present differently in middle age as a slowly progressive spastic paraparesis, with or without some posterior column loss, i.e. as spinal cord disease. It must be distinguised from cord compression.

Diagnosis

The clinical diagnosis is made on the basis of a minimum of two characteristic episodes. Other causes of spastic paraparesis may have to be excluded, particularly in patients presenting in middle age.

Lumbar puncture is usually sufficient to establish a diagnosis. The cell count is normal *or* there may be a lymphocytosis. In half of MS patients the protein is increased up to 1 g/litre. The most useful test in CSF is immunoelectrophoresis which shows an increased proportion of IgG in 60% and oligoclonal bands in 90%.

Visually evoked potentials (VEP) test the integrity of the visual pathways: there is a delay and abnormality in occipital EEG tracings in response to a chessboard pattern presented to the eyes. It is positive in 95% of patients with MS but is not specific. Sensory and auditory evoked potentials may also show delay.

Nuclear magnetic resonance (NMR) shows plaques of demyelination as bright lesions especially numerous in the periventricular area (difficult to distinguish from vascular irregularities in the elderly).

Prognosis

The average duration of life from onset is about 20 years. It is an intermittent disease. Overall, 80% experience steadily progressive disability, 15% follow a relatively benign course and 5% die in 5 years. There may be a long latent period (15–30 years) after an episode of retrobulbar neuritis before further neurological symptoms occur and, in most patients (about 80%), further demyelination never occurs. Patients whose disease onset is sensory rather than motor tend to have a better prognosis. A worse prognosis is associated with poor recovery from the first attack, early cerebellar involvement, and loss of mental acuity.

In the middle-aged, multiple sclerosis progresses more slowly and is less intermittent. The patient may never be seriously incapacitated.

Management

Psychological support is essential throughout the illness. Patients often remain surprisingly euphoric but not infrequently there is marked depression.

Physiotherapy and occupational therapy to maintain mobilility of joints and allow mobilisation. This is particularly important in later stages of the disease. Adrenocorticotrophic hormone—ACTH (ACTH gel 80 units daily with gradual dose reduction over 4 weeks) helps to shorten the acute episodes of demyelination, but probably has no effect on the degree of residual disability. Baclofen, a γ amino butyric acid (GABA) agonist acting at spinal cord level, can reduce high tone and improve painful spasms. Dantrolene sodium acts directly on skeletal muscle to reduce spasticity. Terodiline, an antimuscarinic drug, relaxes detrusor and helps with bladder symptoms in upper motor neurone lesions.

MOTOR NEURONE DISEASE

This disease involves progressive degeneration of:
- anterior horn cells in the spinal cord
- cells of the lower cranial motor nuclei
- neurones of the motor cortex with secondary degeneration of the pyramidal tracts

Clinical presentation

Motor neurone disease presents usually in patients between the ages of 50 and 70 years, slightly more frequently in men than women (1.5 : 1), with the clinical features of one of the above groups but usually progresses to produce features of the other two as well. It is rare in all its forms: UK prevalence is 5/100 000 of the population (incidence 1.5/100 000). It is characterised by:
- muscular weakness and fasciculation
- absence of sensory signs

There are three classical forms of clinical presentation:

1   Patients may present with lower motor neurone weakness, wasting and fasciculation of the small muscles of the hand. This is followed by wasting of the upper and the lower limb muscles. This lower motor neurone wasting and fasciculation is termed 'progressive muscular atrophy'.

2   Patients may present with lower motor neurone weakness, fasciculation and wasting of the tongue and pharynx producing dysarthria, dysphagia, choking and nasal regurgitation ('progressive bulbar palsy').

3   Patients may present with upper motor neurone spastic weakness starting in the legs, and later spreading to the arms ('amyotrophic lateral sclerosis').

Any combination of the above three groups can occur. In most cases upper and lower motor neurone lesions are combined at the time of presentation. Fasciculation of some limb musculature is a hallmark of this disease. Lower limb lesions are usually of upper motor neurone type, and the upper limb lesions of lower motor neurone type. The limbs may demonstrate marked muscular wasting but still have exaggerated reflexes. The abdominal reflexes are usually preserved until late in the disease. Pseudobulbar palsy (page 14) may occur but is very uncommon. The bladder is not affected.

Differential diagnosis

The syndrome may be the presenting feature of underlying carcinoma but in these cases sensory changes are usually also present.
Cervical myelopathy may present similarly, but also usually with sensory changes.

Investigations

Creatine phosphokinase (CPK) and/or CSF protein may be raised in some patients. The EMG shows a denervation pattern with normal nerve conduction. Cervical myelography, if necessary, shows no relevant pathology.

Prognosis

Death usually occurs within 2 years of presentation if there are bulbar features and a little later if there are not. Mental alertness is preserved. Death is usually from aspiration pneumonia.

PARKINSON'S DISEASE AND EXTRAPYRAMIDAL DISORDERS

Parkinson's disease

James Parkinson, 1755–1824, London
Prevalence: 1–1.5/1000 in the UK (1/200 in those over 70 years).

Clinical presentation

This is a disturbance of voluntary motor function characterised by the triad of rigidity, tremor and bradykinesia (slow movements) plus postural abnormalities. Vague muscle ache and clumsiness with physical and mental fatigue may be seen, in retrospect, to have been early evidence.

The classical picture of parkinsonism is of immobile flexion at all joints (neck, trunk, shoulders, elbows, wrists and metacarpophalangeal joints) except the interphalangeal. Even in the early case, on walking, the arms do not swing fully and later in the disease the gait is 'stuttering' and shuffling and the patient may show festination. He is slow and unstable on the turn and may 'freeze'. The face is expressionless and unblinking, and speech slurred and monotonous. In the longstanding case, other symptoms are commonly present: difficulty in initiating movement (starting to walk, rising from a chair or turning in bed), poor balance with a tendency to fall because of slow correcting movements, small handwriting, seborrhoea especially of the face, rarely increased salivation (which, with dysphagia, may give rise to drooling), and a soft unintelligible voice (dysarthria). Constipation and urinary frequency occur, sometimes with incontinence.

Oculogyric crises (forced upward deviation of the eyes) occur characteristically in drug-induced and postencephalitic parkinsonism. These patients may also have symptoms of the side-effects of treatment (see below).

The tremor (4–6/s) is usually most obvious in the hands ('pill-rolling'), improved by voluntary movement and made worse by anxiety. Titubation refers to tremor involving the head. Repeated movements, such as tapping with the fingers, though regular in rate and amplitude (unlike those with cerebellar disorders) are reduced in both amplitude and speed. The rigidity may be leadpipe or, with the tremor superimposed, cogwheel. The patient may demonstrate a glabellar tap sign, i.e. the patient continues to blink when the mid-forehead between the eyebrows is repeatedly tapped. False positives are fairly common. Parkinsonism is usually asymmetrical. Patients are frequently, and understandably, depressed. Dementia with confusion and hallucination may supervene later.

Aetiology of Parkinsonism

Idiopathic Parkinson's disease (paralysis agitans). This is of slow onset and inexorably progressive. It presents in the 50–60 year age group and in males more often than females. It results from deficiency of dopamine in the substantia nigra and relative excess of acetylcholine stimulation in the corpus striatum as a consequence. Dopamine granules are reduced in the cells of the substantia nigra. It is asymmetrical, particularly at first, and may be familial.

Atherosclerosis. This is often associated with other manifestations of vascular disease (stroke, dementia, ischaemic heart disease, intermittent claudication and hypertension). There tends to be less tremor and more festination than in idiopathic parkinsonism.

Drugs. Neuroleptics, e.g. chlorpromazine and, less commonly, reserpine, may produce parkinsonism. The high doses used in psychiatry make it relatively common in schizophrenics. Dystonic movements—facial grimacing, involuntary movements of the tongue and oculogyric crises—are more common than in idiopathic parkinsonism, and are usually symmetrical. Tremor is less common. **NB** Acute extrapyramidal syndromes (grinding teeth, masseter spasm) may result from phenothiazines used as sedatives (e.g. perphenazine) and other dopa antagonists such as metoclopramide. They respond rapidly to intravenous procyclidine.

Poisoning. Rarely, Parkinson-like disorders may result from poisoning with heavy metals—manganese and copper (**NB** Wilson's disease, page 133)—after carbon monoxide poisoning, and MPTP injections.

Postencephalitic. Parkinsonism occurred following outbreaks of encephalitis lethargica (between 1917 and 1925, i.e. before even we were born) and still occurs sporadically.

Punch drunk syndrome (from brain damage in boxers).

Management

The object is to reduce each of the symptoms—rigidity, tremor and bradykinesia.

Physiotherapy and occupational therapy

Levodopa is the drug of choice for idiopathic parkinsonism. It is effective in 75% of patients (excellent in 20%), particularly in those with bradykinesia, less so in those with tremor. It is not used in drug-induced parkinsonism. It is now seldom given alone because the side-effects of levodopa (anorexia, nausea and vomiting) are reduced by concomitant administration of a peripheral dopa-decarboxylase inhibitor. It is therefore usually given as Madopar (with benserazide) or Sinemet (with carbidopa). Madopar may be started at '62.5' bd increasing to '250' qds. The monoamine oxidase (B) inhibitor, selegiline, used in conjunction with levodopa may slow the disease process.

Late side-effects of levodopa include the sudden unpredictable swings of the on/off syndrome, peak-dose dyskinesias (often welcomed), early morning akinesia, and end-of-dose failure. This is managed by increasing the dose-frequency (but not the total daily dose) of the levodopa preparation (which will include a dopa-decarboxylase inhibitor) using a slow-release preparation and adding selegiline and/or bromocriptine. Hallucinatory psychosis and dementia may develop. Anticholinergic therapy can be effective in the elderly who are at risk of confusion.

Transplantation of fetal neuronal tissue (high in dopa) into the caudate lobe of patients with Parkinson's disease has produced variable and more recently disappointing results.

Notes

- *Anticholinergic drugs.* Standard atropine-like drugs can be used first in mild disease and patients intolerant of dopa, e.g. benzhexol (Artane 2 mg bd increasing to 5 mg bd), benztropine (Cogentin) and orphenadrine (Disipal). They have more effect on tremor. Side-effects include blurred vision, dry mouth, tachycardia, urinary retention, constipation and glaucoma. There may be confusion and loss of concentration, especially in the elderly
- *Amantadine* may be added to the other two groups of drugs in a dose of 100 mg bd, but helps only a few and tolerance quickly develops
- *Bromocriptine*, a dopamine agonist, can be of value in those patients who cannot tolerate levodopa or those in whom control is unsatisfactory. It tends to be ineffective in those who are not primarily improved by levodopa. Its chief indication therefore is for late failure of levodopa. It is started in small doses (1.25 mg) before bed and the dose is gradually increased. The commonest side-effect is nausea. Domperidone can be added to control the nausea if necessary
- *Stereotactic thalamotomy* is seldom used and only for intractable symptoms of rigidity and tremor in the nondominant limbs on the contralateral side
- *Depression* is easy to overlook in parkinsonism due to reduced emotional expression. It should be treated with a tricyclic antidepressant but not with

monoamine oxidase inhibitors since the combination with levodopa may induce acute hypertension

The remaining extrapyramidal disorders are very uncommon.

Neurodegenerative diseases

A number of these have Parkinsonism as a component.

1   Alzheimer's disease with gross early cognitive impairment.

2   The 'Parkinson-plus' syndromes:

• Steele–Richardson–Olszewski syndrome with failure of voluntary gaze (see below)

• Shy–Drager syndrome with autonomic failure and postural hypotension

• Multi-system atrophy with cerebellar and pyramidal involvement.

Steele–Richardson–Olszewski syndrome

This is a very rare condition which affects males more than females (2 : 1) in late middle age. It is a degenerative condition of the upper brain stem akin to parkinson's disease and often confused with it in the early stages. It may start with no more than an expressionless facies and a rigidly-held spine, though the patients should stand straight rather than stooped. There may be lead-pipe rigidity and cog-wheeling. Characteristically, voluntary vertical eye movements become progressively more fixed, and then laterally and with convergence. Pseudobulbar palsy leads to dysphagia, dysarthria and emotional lability. Falls are common. As with Parkinsonism, there may be some mild dementia.

Hepatolenticular degeneration

(Wilson's disease—page 258).

Aetiology

It is an autosomal recessive disorder where the primary defect is a failure to excrete copper into the bile. Accumulation of hepatic copper inhibits the formation of caeruloplasmin, the copper-binding serum protein. When the storage capacity of the hepatocytes is exceeded, copper is released into the blood and is deposited in:

• liver producing cirrhosis, hepatosplenomegaly and jaundice

• basal ganglia producing choreo-athetosis

• cerebrum producing dementia and emotional lability

• eyes producing Kayser–Fleischer rings (a green–gold 'fuzz') around the cornea, and cataract in the lens and rarely

• renal tubules producing the effects of heavy metal poisoning and renal tubular acidosis (aminoaciduria, phosphaturia, glycosuria and hypercalciuria)

• bones to produce osteoporosis and osteoarthritis

• red cells to produce haemolytic anaemia

The cerebral type is commoner than the hepatic type.

Management

Low dietary copper intake

D-penicillamine (1–2 g daily for 6 months to 2 years followed by maintenance treatment)—a chelating agent to increase 24 hour urinary copper excretion.

The prognosis for improvement is very good. Siblings should be examined and screened for low serum copper and caeruloplasmin plus increased 24 hour urinary copper output.

Chorea

This term describes jerky, explosive involuntary movements, usually of the face and/or arms which appear pseudo-purposive unless very marked. They may interfere with voluntary movements of limbs and with speech, eating and respiration. They cease during sleep.

Chorea may follow a stroke or kernicterus. It may occur in pregnancy (chorea gravidarum) and with the oral contraceptive, and may be congenital.

Huntington's chorea

George Sumner Huntington 1851–1916, American.

This is a Mendelian dominant disorder on the short arm of chromosome 4 and there is usually a family history. GABA (γ-aminobutyric acid) and acetylcholine are reduced in the substantia nigra and globus pallidus. The symptoms usually start between 30 and 45 years of age. The chorea is distal initially and involves the legs (with ataxia), arms (with clumsiness) and face. The movements are rapid and jerky. Epilepsy occurs. Mental changes develop gradually, usually without insight and progress to dementia and death in about 10–15 years. The chorea may respond to tetrabenazine. It is rarely seen outside mental hospitals. Genetic counselling is advised.

Sydenham's chorea

Thomas Sydenham 1624–1689, English.

A child of 5–15 years (female more often than male) is described as restless, clumsy or fidgety. There is proximal chorea of the arms (and less so, the legs) and grimacing. It is associated with rheumatic fever and usually recovers completely in 2–3 months. It must be differentiated from a nervous tic. It is very rare now in the UK.

CEREBRAL TUMOURS

They are rare with a UK incidence of 1/20 000 and may be primary (20%) or secondary (80% from bronchus, breasts, kidney, colon, ovary, prostate or thyroid). Primary tumours originate from:

- supporting tissues such as gliomas (50%) (or astrocytomas), oligodendro-gliomas and ependymomas (both benign)
- meninges producing meningiomas (25%)
- blood vessels—angiomas and angioblastomas
- nervous tissue (very rare)

Symptoms and signs

Caused by raised intracranial pressure

Headache, classically throbbing bilateral frontal and early morning associated with nausea, vomiting and later papilloedema and increased by stooping.
Mental confusion, change in personality, apathy, drowsiness and dementia.
Sixth nerve palsy results from pressure on the nerve as it crosses the petrous temporal bone (a 'false localising sign').

Epilepsy

Occurs in 30% of tumours, particularly of the frontal or temporal lobe.

Progressive focal signs

These depend upon the site of the tumour:
* *Prefrontal.* Progressive dementia with loss of affect and social responsibility. Anosmia may be present and the grasp reflex present in the contralateral hand
* *Precentral.* Contralateral hemiplegia and Jacksonian epilepsy
* *Parietal.* The chief parietal signs are falling away of the contralateral outstretched arm, astereognosis and tactile inattention. Apraxia and spatial disorientation may occur. Low-sited tumours may produce upper quadrantic homonymous hemianopia rather than complete homonymous hemianopia (or visual inattention). Dysphasia occurs with lesions in the dominant temporoparietal region
* *Temporal lobe.* Symptoms of temporal lobe epilepsy with aphasia (if on the dominant side) and an upper quadrantic homonymous hemianopia
* *Occipital lobe.* Lesions produce homonymous hemianopia either complete or quandrantic with macular sparing

Investigation

Screen for primary neoplasms at the sites which most frequently metastasise to the brain (bronchus, breast and kidney). Perform Fluorescent Treponemal, Antibody Absorption (FTAA), and Treponema Pallidum Haemagglutin (TPHA) tests for syphilis and plasma protein electrophoresis for myeloma. Alkaline phosphatase, calcium and ESR on blood can be helpful screening tests. An EEG may show delta waves (4 cps). CT scanning is the investigation of choice where available, and isotope scans may show tumours over 2 cm in diameter. Angiography can show the tumour circulation which may help the surgical approach.

Lumbar puncture is rarely helpful and may be dangerous because of the risk of 'coning'.

Acoustic neuroma

A neurofibroma of the acoustic (eighth) nerve. It is relatively rare and is more common in neurofibromatosis.

Clinical presentation

Typically, symptoms begin at 35–45 years with progressive deafness and diminished reaction on caloric testing, sometimes with tinnitus and mild vertigo. Pressure on other nerves and the brain-stem of the same side at the cerebello-pontine angle produce:

- Seventh nerve: facial palsy
- Fifth nerve: weakness of mastication, loss of corneal reflex and facial sensory loss
- Sixth nerve: lateral rectus palsy
- Cerebellar syndrome (ipsilateral)

Investigation

Skull radiology may reveal erosion of the internal auditory meatus and/or petrous temporal bone. CT scanning will confirm the diagnosis. Cerebospinal fluid (CSF) protein is usually considerably raised to above 1 g/litre. It is a slowly enlarging tumour and by the time it presents may be large (3–6 cm in diameter). Because of this and its vascularity, it is easily seen on an enhanced CT scan.

NB Check for associated neurofibromata especially of adrenal medulla, thyroid, parathyroid, cranial nerves, spinal nerve roots and meninges.

Benign intracranial hypertension

This mimics cerebral tumour with headaches and papilloedema. It may be due to impaired absorption of CSF by the arachinoid villi. It is commoner in obese young women and is associated with the oral contraceptive and pregnancy, and may follow head injury and treatment of infection (e.g. otitis media). The blind spot may enlarge and sight may be threatened. Lumbar puncture shows normal CSF under high pressure. CSF pressure is uniform in the cerebrum, so a CT scan shows normal ventricles and sulci. The absence of pressure gradient reduces the risk of coning on LP. It tends to recover spontaneously in a few months, but carbonic anhydrase inhibitors (e.g. acetazolamide) or peritoneal shunting may be used. Weight should be reduced. Successive removal of CSF may reduce symptom. Steroids are sometimes given.

PERIPHERAL NEUROPATHY

A disorder of peripheral nerves, either sensory, motor or mixed, usually symmetrical and affecting distal more than proximal parts of the limbs. By convention isolated cranial nerve palsies and isolated and multiple peripheral nerve lesions (median, ulnar, lateral popliteal palsies, and mononeuritis multiplex) are excluded.

Aetiology

In general medical practice four disorders must be considered: diabetes mellitus, carcinomatous neuropathy, vitamin B deficiency (including B_{12}) and drugs or chemicals. Only the first is common.

Diabetic neuropathy

Apart from causing isolated cranial and peripheral nerve lesions (including mononeuritis multiplex), diabetes causes a distal, predominantly sensory, neuropathy affecting commonly the distal lower limbs in a 'stocking' distribution. Symptoms of numbness, paraesthesiae and sometimes pain in the feet are associated with loss of vibration and position sense. Characteristically the ankle reflex is also lost (see page 201).

Carcinomatous neuropathy

Carcinoma may be associated with either a sensory neuropathy affecting the 'glove' and 'stocking' regions or motor neuropathy in which there is muscle weakness and wasting usually of the proximal limb muscles. The neuropathy may be mixed. If distal muscles are affected, the neuropathy may be indistinguishable from any motor neurone disease.

Vitamin B deficiency

Sensory neuropathy characterises deficiency of vitamin B_1. Patients, often alcoholics, present with numbness ('walking on cotton wool') and paraesthesiae. Pain and soreness of the feet may be a feature. In vitamin B_{12} deficiency the peripheral neuropathy may be associated with subacute combined degeneration of the cord (page 148) and megaloblastic anaemia (page 357).

Drugs

Peripheral neuropathy may result from treatment for tuberculosis with isonicotinic acid hydrazide (INAH) which is pyridoxine dependent and occurs in 'slow acetylators'. Other drugs include vincristine, vinblastine, phenytoin and nitrofurantoin.

Other rare causes

Uraemia, myxoedema, polyarteritis nodosa, heavy metal and industrial poisoning (e.g. lead, triorthocresyl phosphate), infectious disorders (leprosy, diphtheria, Guillain–Barré syndrome), amyloidosis, sarcoidosis and porphyria.

NB Investigation of patients with peripheral neuropathy is aimed at excluding underlying carinoma and confirming the other common and treatable disorders. In about 50% of cases the aetiology remains unknown.

BRACHIAL NEURALGIA (neuralgic amyotrophy)

This may follow a virus infection and presents with pain in a shoulder (C5 dermatome) and root pain down the arm with rapidly progressive weakness and wasting (usually of C5–6 innervated muscles). Sensory loss is segmental in distribution. Adjacent nerve roots may be involved. The sensory symptoms usually resolve completely but the weakness and wasting may not.

MONONEURITIS MULTIPLEX

A disorder affecting two or more peripheral nerves at one time, producing symptoms of numbness, paraesthesiae and sometimes pain in their sensory distribution with associated muscle weakness and wasting. The lower limbs are more commonly affected and the neuropathy is asymmetrical. This uncommon syndrome occurs in diabetes mellitus, carcinoma, amyloidosis, polyarteritis nodosa and less commonly in other collagen diseases. Leprosy is the commonest cause world-wide but the diagnosis is then usually obvious.

HEREDITARY ATAXIAS

These are familial disorders usually transmitted as Mendelian dominants. Pathological changes of degeneration are present in one or more of the optic nerves, cerebellum, olives and long ascending tracts of the spinal cord. Each family presents its own particular variants. All are rare.

Friedreich's ataxia

Pathology

Degeneration is maximal in the dorsal and lateral (pyramidal) columns of the cord and the spinocerebellar tracts. It is autosomal recessive.

Clinical presentation

Cerebellar ataxia is noted at 5–15 years affecting first the lower and then upper limbs. Pes cavus and spinal scoliosis may be present. Pyramidal tract involvement produces upper motor neurone lesions of the legs, and dorsal column involvement sensory changes and absent ankle jerks. Arrhythmias and heart failure are common due to cardiomyopathy. There may be optic atrophy. Mild dementia occurs late in the disease and patients die from cardiac disease in their forties.

Cerebellar degenerations

This group of hereditary ataxias affect primarily the cerebellum and the cerebellar connections of the brain-stem. All are rare. These disorders may present in late middle age and must be distinguished from:

- tumours of the posterior fossa
- primary degeneration secondary to bronchial carcinomas
- myxoedema

Hereditary spastic paraplegia

The pyramidal tracts are affected and the patients develop progressive spasticity. The onset occurs from childhood to middle age. The disorder, when first seen, must be distinguished from cord compression (which may require emergency decompression) and multiple sclerosis in the elderly. Dantrolene sodium or baclofen reduce spasticity.

MENINGITIS

Aetiology

Besides the bacterial and viral causes listed in table 16 the following points should be considered:

Tuberculosis meningitis is easily missed and should be considered in the differential diagnosis of all cases of viral meningitis.

Cerebral tumours, lymphomatous infiltration abscesses and venous sinus thrombosis may produce a lymphocytosis and raised protein in the CSF.

Neck stiffness and headache without more severe signs may follow a small subarachnoid haemorrhage. Diabetics may be precipitated into coma by meningitis.

The confident diagnosis of 'meningism' may mean failure to diagnose meningitis. If in doubt lumbar puncture should be performed.

Pneumococcal meningitis is often secondary to underlying pneumococcal infection in the lung, sinuses, or ear.

Clinical features

These are:

- of infection
- of meningism (± mild encephalitic features)
- of raised intracranial pressure

Meningococcal meningitis

The meningitis is part of a septicaemia. The meningococcus is carried in the nasopharynx often asymptomatically (carriers) and tends to produce epidemics of infection chiefly in children and young adults. These occur in conditions of overcrowding and in closed communities. After a short incubation period of 1–3 days the disease begins abruptly with fever, headache, nausea, vomiting and neck stiffness. Mental confusion and coma may follow. There may be a characteristic rash with widespread irregular petechiae of variable size. There is risk of cardio-respiratory collapse and consumption coagulopathy (page 99).

Lumbar puncture

The CSF is purulent and shows a raised protein to about 1–3 g/litre (100–300 mg/100 ml), 500–2000 polymorphs/mm^3 and a low or almost absent sugar. Intracellular and extracellular Gram-negative diplococci are present. The organism can also be isolated in blood culture.

Treatment

Drug of choice. Benzylpencillin initially 12–20 megaunits intravenously per day in divided doses.

Secondline treatment (when the patient is allergic to penicillins)
Cefotaxime (1–2 g, 8 hourly) or chloramphenicol (20 mg/kg body weight, 6 hourly)

Supportive therapy with fluids, inotropes and clotting factors may be needed.

In hospital they should be isolated for 24 from the onset of treatment and close family contacts should be given rifampicin.

Table 16. Bacterial and viral causes of meningitis.

Organism	Special clinical features	CSF	Microbiology	Antibiotic of choice
Common causes				
Meningococcus	Purpuric rash Septicaemic shock	Polymorphs: $0.5–2.0 \times 10^9$/litre Protein: 1–3 g/litre Glucose: very low	Gram-negative intra-cellular diplococci Positive blood culture Positive CSF immunoelectrophoresis	Penicillin
Pneumococcus	Cranial nerve damage Otitis media Lobar pneumonia High mortality (10–20%)	Polymorphs: $0.5–2.0 \times 10^9$/litre Protein: 1–3 g/litre Glucose: very low	Gram-positive diplococci Positive blood culture Positive CSF immunoelectrophoresis	Penicillin
Haemophilus influenzae	Commonest in children under 5 years	Polymorphs: $0.5–2.0 \times 10^9$/litre Protein: 1–3 g/litre Glucose: very low	Gram-negative bacilli	Cefotaxime (ampicillin)
Coxsackie virus and echovirus	Paralysis (very rare)	Lymphocytes: $0.05–0.5 \times 10^9$/litre Protein: 0.5–1 g/litre Glucose: normal	Positive throat swab Positive stool culture Serum antibody: rising titre	None
Mumps virus		Lymphocytes: $0.05–0.5 \times 10^9$/litre Protein: 0.5–1 g/litre Glucose: normal	Positive throat swab Positive stool culture Serum antibody: rising titre	None

Rare causes

Organism	Clinical features	CSF	Diagnosis	Treatment
Mycobacterium tuberculosis	Subacute onset / Altered personality / Strokes / Cranial nerve lesions / Fits in children / Pyrexia of unknown origin (PUO)	Lymphocytes $0.1-0.6 \times 10^9$/litre / Protein: 1–6 g/litre / Glucose: low, <1.4 mmol/litre	Acid and alcohol-fast bacilli / Ziehl–Nielsen staining and fluorescence microscopy	See pages 298 – 301
Leptospira ictero-haemorrhagiae (Weil's disease)	Follows exposure to rat urine (sewers) / Associated hepatitis and nephritis / High peripheral WBC: $10-20 \times 10^9$/litre	Lymphocytes: $0.2-0.3 \times 10^9$/litre / Protein: raised by 0.5–1.5 g/litre / Glucose: normal	Serum antibody: rising titre	Penicillin
Lyme disease	Associated with cranial nerve lesions (unilateral or bilateral seventh nerve and assymetrical aethalgia and erythema chronicum migrans	Immunofluorescent antibody tested		Penicillin
Poliovirus	Meningitis (common) / Asymmetrical paralysis (rare) / Polio incidence increasing with decrease in immunisation	Lymphocytes: $0.05-0.5 \times 10^9$/litre / Protein: 0.5–1 g/litre / Glucose: normal	Positive throat swab / Positive stool culture / Serum antibody: rising titre	None

NB Other rare causes: herpes simplex virus; arbovirus; Staphylococcus, Listeria, Pseudomonas, Cryptococcu in immunosuppressed; E. coli, streptococci and Listeria in neonates

Pneumococcal meningitis

Infection may be secondary to pneumococcal pneumonia or it may spread from infected sinuses or ears or through fractures of the base of the skull. It is commoner in paediatric and geriatic practice, and after splenectomy. Symptoms develop rapidly, sometimes within hours, and fever, headache, nausea and vomiting may quickly proceed to coma.

Lumbar puncture

The CSF is purulent with a raised protein, high polymorph count and low sugar. Gram-positive diplococci are present. Blood culture is often positive (as it is in pneumococcal pneumonia).

Treatment

Drug of choice. Benzylpenicillin as for meningococcal meningitis. The dose can be reduced after about 3–4 days provided the fever has fallen and there is clinical improvement. Treatment should continue for 10 days.

Second-line treatment. Cefotaxime or chloramphenicol as for meningococcal meningitis.

Pneumococcal meningitis is extremely serious and especially so if the patient is in coma before therapy is started. The overall mortality is high (20–30%).

Haemophilus influenzae meningitis

This usually occurs in children under 5 years old because after that age they develop specific antibodies. It may be insidious in onset with a longer incubation period than in the meningitides described above (5 days). It usually follows an influenzal-type illness and presents with fever, nausea and vomiting.

Lumbar puncture

The CSF is purulent with a high protein and polymorph count and low sugar. Gram-negative bacilli can be seen, and grown on culture.

Treatment

Drugs of choice. Cefotaxime 1–2 g, 8 hourly, chloramphenicol 3–5 g daily (children 50–100 mg/kg/day for 10 days though a lower dose is required in the neonate) is an alternative.

The overall mortality is 5–10%.

Intrathecal penicillin therapy

There is little evidence to support the use of intrathecal benzylpenicillin therapy through the lumbar puncture needle on finding a purulent CSF. Some physicians consider daily intrathecal and intraventricular therapy of value in pneumococcal meningitis if the patient is unconscious on admission, as the mortality is so high (50%). There is no good evidence that this improves the outlook.

Acute bacterial meningitis of unknown cause

This problem occurs when a purulent CSF is obtained from a patient with meningitis but no organisms are seen with Gram staining. This is most frequently due to pre-admission antibiotic therapy. There is no time to wait for the results of culture and antibiotics should be started immediately. In adults there are a number of recommended courses of action, any of which should treat effectively the common organisms found (i.e. pneumococcus, meningococcus, *Haemophilus influenzae*), i.e.:

- Cefotaxime is the drug of choice
- Chloramphenicol with penicillin is an alternative

The use of chloramphenicol with penicillin, although theoretically inadvisable (bacteriostatic drug with a bactericidal one respectively), is used in some centres with considerable success.

Tuberculous meningitis (see also Tuberculosis, page 298)

This may present as acute meningitis more commonly as an insidious illness with fever, weight loss, and progressive signs of confusion and cerebral irritation leading to mental deterioration and finally coma. The CSF looks opalescent and by investigation resembles viral meningitis but the glucose is very low.

Three or four drugs (rifampicin, isoniazid with pyridoxine, ethionamide and pyrazinamide) should be given initially and the dose of INAH doubled. If streptomycin is used, blood levels must be monitored to prevent ototoxicity. (There is no place for intrathecal streptomycin.)

INTRACRANIAL ABSCESS

The primary source of infection is usually from chronic middle ear infection, the paranasal sinuses, or the lungs (pneumococcus). The clinical presentation is usually that of a space-occupying lesion (headache, nausea, vomiting and papilloedema with or wihout focal signs) plus the evidence of the primary infection. A CT scan or, less satisfactorily, an isotope scan is essential and, if not locally available, the patient should be transferred. Lumbar puncture is potentially dangerous because of the risk of cloning. The CSF shows a normal or raised white cell count and the higher this is, the worse the prognosis tends to be. High-dose dexamethasone, despite the risks with infection, is often given to reduce the surrounding cerebral oedema. Burr holes may be necessary to make the diagnosis, and, if confirmed, the pus may be aspirated through them and antibiotics instilled. The infection is usually due to *Staph. aureus* or anaerobes and systemic antibiotics are given as determined by the sensitivities. Sometimes excision of the abscess cavity is performed later. Even with modern management the mortality rate is 30%. Of those who survive, a third develop epilepsy, and many physicians give anticonvulsants to all survivors.

ACUTE POSTINFECTIVE POLYNEUROPATHY
(Guillain–Barré syndrome)

Clinical features

Symptoms begin 7–10 days after an infectious illness, usually of the upper respiratory tract. Motor nerves are affected more than sensory. Typically paraesthesiae, followed by numbness begins in the toes and is rapidly (hours) followed by flaccid paralysis of the lower limbs which ascends to involve the arms and sometimes the facial muscles, the muscles of the palate and pharynx (causing dysphagia) and the external ocular muscles. Less commonly, the disease affects the upper limbs or the cranial nerves alone, or proximal more than distal muscles, and sensory symptoms are not always present. Sphincters are less affected than in transverse myelitis and there is no clear sensory level. The paralysis is of lower motor neurone type with flaccidity and early loss of reflexes. Maximal disability occurs at 3–4 weeks. The major complications are respiratory failure from weakness of the respiratory muscles, autonomic involvement, pulmonary embolism and cardiac dysrhythmias which may be fatal.

The Miller–Fisher syndrome is a variant with acute onset of external ophthalmoplegia, ataxia and areflexia.

Investigation

The diagnosis is made on lumbar puncture and the CSF characteristically shows a very high protein 300–1000 mg/dl (3–10 g/litre) with no, or very few, white cells.

Differential diagnosis

Poliomyelitis is excluded by:

A known history of complete immunisation.
The presence of sensory symptoms.
The symmetrical pattern of paralysis.
The CSF findings (in polio the protein is lower and the WBCs raised).

Management

Careful nursing with physiotherapy to maintain morale and prevent sores and chest infection and contractures are required in all cases. Careful fluid balance and nutrition may be necessary if dysphagia occurs. Vital capacity must be monitored frequently. If paralysis ascends to involve the respiratory muscles early artificial ventilation is necessary. Shoulder adduction (6,7,8) in a good clinical test of intercostal muscle function. Monitor minute volume, peak flow rate and arterial blood gases. Early tracheostomy is required in all but a very few patients with respiratory failure as muscle activity may take from weeks to months to recover. When recovery occurs it is usually complete, but the mortality is 5–10%. Steroids are contraindicated. Anticoagulants may avoid deep venous thrombosis (DVT) and death from pulmonary embolism, though calf pressure devices may be as satisfactory and also relieve symptoms.

Some centres have used plasmapheresis in severe cases with variable results.

POLIOMYELITIS

Poliovirus is one of the enteroviruses (with echo and Coxsackle virus) and a picorna (pico = small: rna = RNA) virus. The incidence in the UK has fallen dramatically since immunisation began in 1957, but polio remains endemic in the tropics.

Immunisation

Sabin vaccine is live attenuated polio virus types 1, 2 and 3 given as a drop orally.

Clinical features

In areas without an immunisation scheme infection with polio virus is probably quite common, but the serious features of acute meningitis and muscle paralysis are rare.

About 90–95% of infected patients have mild upper respiratory or gastrointestinal symptoms which settle completely. The rest have a more severe early infection with fever, sore throat, diarrhoea or constipation and muscle pains. This *minor illness* usually settles but 1–2% of patients go on to develop a *major illness* 5–10 days later with features of acute viral meningitis. A small number of patients who have acute poliovirus meningitis develop flaccid lower motor neurone muscle paralysis with loss of reflexes as a result of damage to the anterior horn cells. This may be preceded by muscular pain. The legs are most commonly affected and paralysis may spread to involve the arms and the medulla oblongata and lower pons, causing a bulbar palsy.

Respiratory failure is due to paralysis of the respiratory muscles and may be further complicated by aspiration pneumonia following the dysphagia and inability to cough caused by bulbar palsy. There are no sensory neurological changes.

Diagnosis

The cerebrospinal fluid is the same as other forms of virus meningitis (see page 142) with raised protein (50–100 g/dl), increased cells, initially polymorphs, followed by lymphocytes 50–400/mm^3. The sugar is normal.

The virus can be grown from throat, stool and CSF and paired sera will show a rising titre.

Paralytic poliomyelitis must be distinguished from the Guillain–Barré syndrome (page 144).

Management

Patients should be isolated and contacts immunised. Artificial ventilation is required for respiratory failure—the most common cause of death. Careful nursing is necessary in all paralysed patients to prevent sores, combined with monitoring of fluid and electrolyte balance. After the fever has settled, physiotherapy and progressive rehabilitation are started.

Full muscle recovery is rare if limbs are paralysed. Patients with isolated bulbar palsy usually recover completely but those with paralysis of the respiratory muscles rarely do, and may require continued artificial ventilation.

SYPHILIS OF THE NERVOUS SYSTEM

Tertiary syphilis of the central nervous system never develops in a syphilitic patient who has received early and correct treatment. All forms are now rarely seen in the developed world except as chronic cases with residual symptoms and signs; but it remains common world-wide. Tertiary syphilis may be divided into four groups:

- Meningovascular disease occurring 3–4 years after primary infection
- Tabes dorsalis—10–35 years after primary infection
- General paralysis of the insane—10–15 years after primary infection
- Localised gummata

The first three produce symptoms by a combination of primary neuronal degeneration and/or arterial lesions.

Meningovascular syphilis

This affects both the cerebrum and the spine ('*meningo*': producing fibrosis of the meninges and nipping of nerves; '*vascular*': producing endarteritis and ischaemic necrosis). Headache is a common presenting symptom.

Cerebrum. Syphilitic leptomeningitis produces fibrosis and thickening of the meninges with nipping and paralysis of cranial nerves. The second, third and fourth nerves are most frequently involved.
Vascular endarteritis. Produces ischaemic necrosis. Hemiplegia may result. Syphilitic endarteritis is one cause of isolated cranial nerve lesions.
Spinal meningovascular syphilis. Meningeal thickening involves posterior spinal roots to produce pain and anterior roots to cause muscle wasting.
Endarteritis. May produce ischaemic necrosis, and transverse myelitis and paraplegia.

Tabes dorsalis

The signs result from degeneration of the dorsal columns and nerve roots.

Clinical presentation

Lightning pains due to dorsal nerve root involvement characterise the disease. There are severe paroxysmal stabbing pains ('crises') which occur in the limbs, chest or abdomen. Paraesthesiae may also occur. Ataxia follows degeneration of the dorsal columns of the spinal cord. The gain is wide-based and stamping because position sense is lost.

Examination

The facies is characteristic. Ptosis is present and the forehead wrinkled due to overactivity of the frontalis muscle. Argyll Robertson pupils are small, irregular pupils which do not react to light, but constrict with accommodation. There may be optic atrophy. Cutaneous sensation is diminished typically over the nose (tabetic mask), sternum, ulnar border of the arm and outer borders of the legs and feet. Vibration and position sense are lost early in the disease. Deep pain sensation (pressure on testicles or Achilles tendon) may also be lost. Charcot's neuropathic joints are grossly disorganised from painless arthritis (also rarely seen in diabetes mellitus and syringomyelia when there is loss of pain sensation). Absence of visceral sensation results in overfilling of the bladder. The reflexes are diminished or absent in the legs. The plantar responses are flexor in pure tabes dorsalis. Romberg's sign (increased unsteadiness on closing the eyes) is present and is evidence of loss of position sense.

General paralysis of the insane (GPI)

A late manifestation of systemic syphilis. Pathologically the meninges are thickened, particularly in the parietal and frontal regions. Primary cortical degeneration produces a small brain with dilated and enlarged ventricles. The dorsal columns degenerate.

Clinical presentation

The pathological changes are associated with marked mental impairment. This may produce loss of memory and concentration with associated anxiety and/or depression. Later, insight is lost and the patient may become euphoric with delusions of grandeur and loss of emotional response. Epilepsy occurs in 50% of cases.

Examination

Euphoria may be present. The face is 'vacant' and memory lost. Argyll Robertson pupils are present. The tongue demonstrates a 'trombone' tremor. Dorsal column involvement produces limb ataxia from loss of position sensation. Upper motor neurone lesions occur in the legs with increased reflexes and up-going plantar responses.

NB In tabo-paresis there is a combination of the lower limb upper motor neurone signs of GPI and the signs of dorsal root degeneration from tabes dorsalis. This produces a combination of absent knee reflexes with up-going plantar responses.

FTAA and TPHA tests

The TPHA and FTAA tests are the most specific tests available for diagnosis. They may remain positive for years after adequate treatment.

Management

Penicillin by injection is the drug of choice for active syphilitic infection. Improvement, stabilisation or deterioration may occur in any one case despite adequate penicillin therapy.

The Herxheimer reaction is an acute hypersensitivity reaction and results from toxins produced by spirochaetes killed on the first contact with penicillin. Death has been reported and some authorities give steroids during the first days of penicillin therapy.

DISORDERS OF SPINAL CORD

Syringomyelia

A longitudinal cyst in the cervical cord and/or brain-stem (syringobulbia) occurs just anterior to the central canal and spreads, usually asymmetrically, to each side. It may be due to outflow obstruction of the fourth ventricle from congenital anomaly such as the Arnold–Chiari malformation (also associated with spina bifida). It starts in young adults and is usually very slowly progressive over 20–30 years. It is very rare.

Damage to the cord (figure 1, page 5) occurs:

At the root level of the lesion
• in the decussating fibres of the lateral spinothalamic tracts (pain and temperature) since they cross anteriorly
NB   Fibres of the posterior column enter posteriorly and are not involved—hence the dissociated sensory loss
• the cells in the anterior horn where the lower motor neurones start
Distant from the lesion in the upper motor neurones in the pyramidal tracts.

The classical case of syringomyelia therefore presents with
• painless injury to the hands (sensory C6–8)
• weakness and wasting in the small muscles of the hands (T1)
Examination may reveal more extensive dissociated sensory loss in the cervical segments, and upper motor neurone signs in the legs. These are usually asymmetrical. All signs and symptoms are ipsilateral to the lesion. Charcot's joints may occur in the upper limbs. In treatment, surgical decompression and aspiration of cysts should be considered.

Syringobulbia

With progressively more cephalad lesions, the descending root of the trigeminal nerve (pain and temperature) may be involved from the first division downwards, and a Horner's syndrome from involvement of the cervical sympathetic tract. The motor nuclei of the lower cranial nerves may be involved in syringobulbia (true bulbar palsy) and there may be a rotary nystagmus from involvement of vestibular and cerebellar connections.

Subacute combined degeneration of the cord (SACD)

The neurological consequences of B_{12} deficiency include SACD, signs of peripheral neuropathy and, very rarely, dementia and optic atrophy.

'Combined degeneration' refers to the combined demyelination of both pyramidal (lateral columns) and posterior (dorsal) columns, the signs and symptoms being predominantly in the legs. It is now rare.

Clinical presentation

Sensory peripheral neuropathy with numbness and paraesthesia in the feet are the usual presenting symptoms. Less commonly the disease presents as a spastic paraparesis. The signs are of:

- posterior column loss (vibration and position senses, with positive Romber-gism)
- upper motor neurone lesion (weakness, hypertonia and hyperreflexia, with absent abdominal reflexes and up-going toes)
- peripheral neuropathy (absence of all the jerks, reduced touch sense, and deep tenderness of the calves)

Investigation

There rarely may be no anaemia or macrocytosis. The following are indicated:
Serum B_{12} and folate levels.
Marrow histology for megaloblastic change.
Parietal cell and intrinsic factor antibodies.

These and the Schilling test are the only tests of value if the patient has been given vitamin B_{12} injections.

Management

Vitamin B_{12} (hydroxocobalamin 1 mg daily for 1 week, and then 1 mg monthly for life).

Prognosis

Neurological symptoms and signs usually improve to some degree. However, they may remain unchanged or, rarely, continue to progress. Sensory abnormalities resolve more completely than motor, the peripheral neuropathy more than the myelopathy.

Peroneal muscular atrophy (Charcot–Marie–Tooth)

This condition is often confused with the muscle dystrophies. It is rare and genetic counselling is advisable.

Pathology

It may be transmitted as an autosomal dominant, or in some families is recessive and sex-linked. It may be classified into two groups of 'hereditary motor and sensory neuropathy' (HMSA) affecting the peripheral nerves—Type I with thickened peripheral nerves due to repeated demyelination and remyelination (ulnar at elbow, and common peroneal at the neck of the fibula), and Type II due to axonal degeneration, without thickening.

Clinical presentation

Classically it presents about the age of 20 years with wasting and weakness of all the distal lower limb muscles and pes cavus. Later, the upper limbs may be affected. The wasting stops at mid-thigh, producing an 'inverted champagne bottle' appearance, and at the elbows. Fasciculation and sensory loss are sometimes present, and reflexes depressed. The disease usually arrests spontaneously and life expectancy is normal. Contractions may produce talipes equinovarus.

Cord compression

Aetiology

Disorders of vertebrae (extradural). These constitute 45% of cases:
- cervical spondylosis
- collapsed vertebral body (usually secondary to carcinoma, myeloma or, rarely, osteoporosis)
- prolapsed intervertebral disc
- rarely, tuberculosis, abscesses, Paget's disease, reticuloses, angiomata, cervical and lumbar stenosis

Meningeal disorders (intradural). Also constitute 45% of cases:
- neurofibroma (dumb-bell tumours)
- meningioma (usually thoracic and more common in women)

Disorders of spinal cord (intramedullary). 5–10% of cases:
- gliomas
- ependymomas

Clinical presentation

Patients present with a spastic paraparesis: there is upper motor neurone weakness in the legs, loss of sphincter control (an ominous sign) and loss of abdominal reflexes if the lesion is in or above the thoracic cord. The level of the sensory loss indicates the level of the neurological lesion which may, however, be up to two roots higher. Remember that compared with the vertebral column, the cord is about 1 segment short in the lower cervical region, 2 segments short in the upper thoracic region, and 3–5 segments short in the lower thoracic region. The sacral segments and end of the cord lie opposite the L1 vertebra. Remember, also that the cervical spine has 7 vertebrae and the cervical spinal cord 8 segments.

It is important to consider the possibility of cord compression in all cases of spastic paresis. Cord compression is a neurosurgical emergency, particularly if of recent onset and rapid progression. Decompression must be performed as early as possible if recovery is to occur.

NB The tumours which commonly metastasise to bone arise in: bronchus, breast, prostate, thyroid, and kidney.

Investigation

X-ray of the spine and CT scan or NMR if available to show the cord.
X-ray of the chest for carcinoma of the bronchus.
Lumbar puncture for spinal block and raised protein.
Myelography to delineate the level and character of obstructing tissues—this investigation may increase the severity of transverse myelitis and should therefore be performed only after expert advice—it is now rarely necessary.

Differential diagnosis

Other causes of spastic paraparesis are:

Disseminated sclerosis. Demyelination may cause isolated slow progressive paraparesis in the middle-aged.
SACD of the cord.
Parasagittal cranial meningioma.
Transverse myelitis.
Anterior spinal artery thrombosis.
Motor neurone disease.

Cervical spondylosis

Over 70% of the adult population of this country have X-ray changes of osteoarthritis of the joints of the cervical spine. The most frequent and obvious abnormality is the presence of osteophytes. These radiological changes are unrelated to the presence or severity of symptoms.

Clinical features

Most patients are symptom free. Pain in the neck, associated with and precipitated by movements of the neck is the commonest symptom. Occasionally compression of the cervical nerve roots causes root pain, paraesthesiae, numbness and sometimes segmental weakness with muscle wasting (even with fasciculation). Rarely narrowing of the cervical canal with compression of the spinal cord or occlusion of the spinal cord vessels (spinal stenosis) produces brisk reflexes in the arms and upper motor neurone damage affecting the legs.
NB Lumbar spinal canal stenosis may produce weakness of the legs and sometimes pain in the calves on walking (intermittent claudication). It must be distinguished from femoral artery stenosis, the commonest cause of intermittent claudication (or limping).

DISORDERS OF MUSCLES

Mixed connective tissue disease (MCTD) (see also page 166)

A rare overlap disorder presenting with progressive weakness in the proximal limb muscles, usually more marked in the lower limbs. The disease merges with dermatomyositis and scleroderma in which skin manifestations are an obvious feature, with the other collagen disorders such as polymyositis in which muscle weakness may be a marked or dominant feature, and systemic lupus erythematosus (SLE).

Polymyositis and allied disorders

Clinical presentation

The disorder presents at any age, but more commonly in patients over 30 with muscle pain and tenderness with progressive weakness and diplegia (50% of cases). Proximal muscles are affected more than distal ones, and patients may first notice difficulty climbing or standing from a sitting position, and difficulty lifting objects above their heads. Neck muscles are frequently involved (60%) but the facial and ocular muscles rarely (cf. myasthenia gravis). Dysphagia is common (50%) and involvement of the respiratory muscles may be severe and endanger life. Arthralgia occurs in about 25% of cases. Raynaud's phenomenon is common in the young (30%) and may proceed to scleroderma. Skin rashes are common (60%) and range from diffuse erythema to the manifestations of dermatomyositis (page 164).

Prognosis

This is variable but generally worse in older patients. The disease may remit spontaneously, particularly in the young (under 30), but may recur and/or progress to a more diffuse systemic collagen disorder (30–50 years). In patients over 50 the prognosis depends on the underlying carcinoma if present. The overall mortality of untreated cases is about 50%.

Treatment

Corticosteroids (prednisolone 40–60 mg daily) are given initially, and the dose reduced gradually depending upon the patient's clinical state and the serum creatine phosphokinase level. Azathioprine is sometimes given as well and allows a reduction in steroid dosage. This is high during active disease but falls rapidly if therapy is successful. Steroid therapy is usually needed for 1–3 years before being gradually withdrawn. Physiotherapy is usually very helpful.

Differential diagnosis

The differentiation is from other causes of proximal myopathy (page 26). *Trichinella spiralis* infection of muscles may produce acute myositis.

NB Polymyalgia rheumatica usually presents with pain and stiffness. Wasting is not a characteristic feature (page 166). All these conditions are relatively rare.

Investigation

Muscle biopsy

This shows muscle fibre necrosis and inflammatory cell infiltration

Serum aldolase and creatine phosphokinase

These enzymes are greatly elevated in the muscular dystrophies during the most active stage of muscle degeneration (in the second and third decades of life). There may be high titres to nuclear antigens, and the antinuclear factor (ANF) may be positive. In polymyositis, the level of the enzymes is markedly elevated, gives a measure of active muscle destruction and should decline rapidly on corticosteroids coincident with improvement in muscle strength.

Electromyography

In the muscular dystrophies, evidence of decrease in active muscle is shown by the presence of short duration, low amplitude polyphasic action potentials.

Polymyositis produces a similar picture but also with evidence of spontaneous fibrillation, possibly evidence of muscular irritability. Spontaneous fibrillation is characteristic of degenerated muscle undergoing active degeneration, and is associated with evidence of a decrease in the number of motor units on voluntary movement. Electromyograph (EMG) findings often do not fit neatly into the above patterns as the distribution of muscle involvement is patchy and as the EMG recording depends upon the particular region of muscle sampled.

Myasthenia gravis

A very rare disorder of muscle weakness resulting from failure of neuromuscular transmission. There is a reduction in the number of functioning postsynaptic acetylcholine receptors (AChR) and a high titre of specific anti-AChR antibodies has been shown in most cases. Thymoma is associated in 10% of cases and thymus abnormalities in 75%. Excessive muscular fatiguability may also occur in polymyositis and SLE, and there is an increased incidence of myasthenia gravis in thyrotoxicosis. The Lambert–Eaton myasthenic syndrome associated with carcinoma is clinically different (see below).

Clinical presentation

Painless muscular weakness is produced by repetitive or sustained contraction. It is usually most marked in the face and eyes producing a symmetrical ptosis and diplopia. Weakness of speech and swallowing may occur. The proximal muscles are more often affected than the distal, and the upper limb muscles more than the lower. There is no wasting and tendon reflexes are preserved.

Prognosis

The disorder may never progress beyond ophthalmoplegia and periods of remission up to 3 years occur. Death may be rapid if the respiratory muscles are involved. Thymectomy usually improves the outlook unless a thymoma is present.

Diagnosis and treatment

Edrophonium (Tensilon) 10 mg i.v. with cardiac monitor (in case of bradycardia/asystole) reduces the weakness of affected muscles for 3–4 min. The anterior mediastinum should be searched with chest X-rays or CT scan for thymoma. Acetylcholine receptor IgG antibodies are present in 90% of cases. Long-term therapy is achieved with longer-acting anticholinesterases orally such as neo-stigmine or pyridostigmine (Mestinon), preferably by increasing the dose slowly until measured muscular strength is optimal. Overdose may give depolarisation block with weakness. Thymectomy at any age appears to increase the percentage of patients in remission. An alternate day regime of steroids (between 10 and 80 mg alternate days) is of proven value and immunotherapy with azathioprine may be useful and allow a reduction in steroid dosage. Plasma-pheresis has been used in intractable cases but is short-lasting (days–months). The differential diagnosis is from other causes of ptosis (page 4) muscular dystrophies involving the face, familial hypokalaemic paralysis and the

Lambert–Eaton syndrome. In this, a disorder of acetylcholine release, the myasthenia is associated with a carcinoma, usually oat cell, of the bronchus. It differs from classical myasthenia gravis in that the eyes are less frequently affected, that proximal limb muscle weakness is common and their strength initially *increased* by repeated movement, and that there is no response to edrophonium. Oral 3,4 diaminopyridine may help.

Myotonia

Myotonia is the inability of muscles to relax normally after contraction. This produces a 'reluctant' release of handshake, and percussion contraction for instance of the thenar muscles.

Dystrophia myotonica

An autosomal dominant (chromosome 9) disorder producing progressively more severe symptoms and signs with succeeding generations, i.e. 'anticipation'. It is rare.

Clinical presentation

Both males and females are affected with usual onset 15–40 years. UK incidence is 5/100 000. The 'classical' case demonstrates:

Abnormal facies—with frontal balding, ptosis, a smooth expressionless forehead, cataracts and a 'lateral' smile or 'sneer'.
Wasting of the facial muscles, sternomastoids, shoulder girdle and quadriceps. The forearms and legs are involved and reflexes lost. There is no fasciculation.
Myotonia which increases with cold, fatigue and excitement and may reduce with repeated activity.
Testicular or ovarian atrophy with impotence and sterility.
Mental deficiency.

NB The heart may be involved (e.g. heart block) and diabetes mellitus may develop. Phenytoin may reduce myotonia.

Myotonia congenita

This is a hereditary disorder, transmitted as a Mendelian dominant which affects both sexes equally, and first presents in childhood. There is no muscle wasting and no long-term effects. It is very rare. The myotonias should not be confused with two disorders of children:

Amyotonia congenita

A congenital disorder producing weakness and hypotonia which is first noticed in children at the head-lifting stage. The muscle disturbance becomes less severe as the children grow older although contractures may produce scoliosis.

Progressive spinomuscular atrophy (Werdnig–Hoffmann)

A hereditary disorder involving progressive degeneration of the anterior spinal horn cells starting in the first year of life and producing weakness, muscle wasting and fasciculation, and death within 6 months.

Muscular dystrophies

Each family produces its own pattern of disease but some forms are more common than others. They are all rare. Genetic counselling is advised. There is no effective treatment. Chromosome studies may define the carrier state and diagnosis may be made in the male fetus in the first trimester.

Pseudohypertrophic (Duchenne)

A sex-linked recessive disorder affecting males with a prevalence of $3:100\,000$ and incidence of $25:100\,000$ male births. The age of onset is 5–10 years with symptoms of difficulty in climbing stairs, or even walking, and the use of Gowers' manoeuvre to rise from the floor. On examination the posture is lordotic and the gait 'waddling' due to weakness of the muscles of the pelvic girdle and proximal lower limb. The calves are hypertrophied but weak and the creatine phosphokinase level is raised. The electromyogram and muscle biospy are characteristic. In later stages muscle contracture of the legs may produce talipes equinovarus and muscle weakness may spread to the upper limbs, though not to the face. The child dies in the early teens, usually from chest infection or cardiomyopathy. Becker's dystrophy is a mild form.

Facio-scapulo-humeral (Landouzy–Déjérine)

Transmitted as an autosomal dominant and affects both sexes equally. The onset is at puberty with progressive wasting in the upper limb-girdle and face. The disorder may abort spontaneously or progress to the muscles of the trunk and lower limbs. Individuals usually live to a normal age.

Limb-girdle (*Erb*)

Transmitted as an autosomal recessive and affects both sexes equally. It presents at 20–40 years. It involves the muscles of the shoulders and pelvic girdles and is slowly progressive with death usually in middle age.

Other forms may affect the muscles of the face and eyes (oculo-muscular dystrophy) or the distal limb muscles (Gowers' muscular dystrophy). They are very rare.

PSYCHIATRY

Depression and anxiety are the most frequent psychiatric disorders seen in general practice and general medical out-patients. Confusional states and dementia are common in the elderly. A working classification is shown in Table 17.

Depression

Moderate depression, like moderate anxiety, is a normal part of human existence. It it interferes with day to day life, it should be regarded as an 'illness'.

Reactive depression is an excessive reaction to an unpleasant experience. The patient is tired and tearful, lacks concentration and drive, and has reduced ability to cope and to experience pleasure. Somatic symptoms include headache and gastrointestinal problems. The prognosis depends on the patient's personality and the persistence of the precipitating factors.

Table 17. Classification of common psychiatric disorders. After Willis (1989).

Affective (mood) disorders	Anxiety, depression and manic states (common)
Organic disorders	Dementia and confusional states (relatively common, especially in the elderly)
Schizophrenia	Simple (relatively common)
	Hebephrenic (disorders of the content of thought and ideas)
	Catatonic (catatonia denotes the assumption of abnormal postures)
	Paranoid (persecution complexes)
Personality disorders	Obsessional personality and phobias
	Psychopathic personality
Addiction	Drugs and alcohol (common)
Mental subnormality	(Common)
Hysteria	(Rare)

Endogeneous depression is part of an inherited manic-depressive tendency. The mood may be more passive than depressed, with feelings of guilt and unworthiness and with anorexia, weight loss, constipation and early morning wakening. The patient may develop agitated depression (with anxiety, restlessness and rapid speech) or retarded depression (with physical and mental slowing). Occasionally paranoid delusions may mimic schizophrenia, and lack of concentration with apathy may mimic dementia especially in the elderly.

The boundaries between the clinical features of endogenous and exogenous depression are frequently blurred and not universally accepted.

Depression may follow viral infections and some drugs. It may be confused with myxoedema or Parkinson's disease. Suicide is a special risk in both forms of depression: casual hints may be given and must be taken seriously.

Management

In general medical practice, sympathetic support is often sufficient to allow time for spontaneous recovery, particularly after acute grief. It is important to obtain the support of family and friends.

Drug therapy

In severe endogenous depression, treatment should be started immediately since antidepressant drugs take at least 1–4 weeks to work and may be ineffective for some patients. Of the tricyclic drugs, imipramine (Tofranil) 25–50 mg tds is slower acting than amitriptyline (Tryptizol) (25–50 mg tds) but has fewer side-effects. Side-effects of imipramine and amitriptyline result from atropine-like effects and include dry mouth, blurred vision, postural hypotension and tachycardia, and urinary retention. Amitriptyline is also relatively contraindicated in the presence of ischaemic heart disease since it may produce arrhythmias. Newer antidepressive drugs may have fewer cardiac side-effects, e.g. mianserin (Bolvidon, Norval) 30–90 mg/day. Amitriptyline and mianserin are sedative and best given in a single dose at night to help with sleep. Flupenthixol (Fluanxol) 0.5–3.0 mg/day is not sedative.

Monoamine oxidase inhibitors (MAOI) may be less effective and can certainly produce more serious side-effects. They inhibit deaminating enzymes which normally inactivate pressor amines. Hence acute hypertensive encephalopathy and cerebrovascular accidents may result from the combination of MAOI with amphetamine or ephedrine and tyramine-containing foods (Marmite, cheese, yoghurt). They should be reserved for those patients who have not responded to the other antidepressants.

In severe cases, and especially in the presence of suicidal tendencies, or if the above regime is ineffective within 3–4 months, patients should be referred to a psychiatric unit. Electroconvulsive therapy (ECT) is still widely used for endogenous depression.

Mania

Periods of mania may alternate with periods of depression (manic-depressive psychosis). Patients with mania and hypomania show elevation of mood, flight of ideas and talk loudly, forcefully and rapidly. Lithium, sedation and sometimes ECT may be necessary.

Anxiety

The essential feature is an irrational degree of anxiety and worry accompanied by the somatic manifestations of fear, for example sweating, tremor and tachycardia. Fear may amount to panic. The somatic symptoms and signs resemble those seen in thyrotoxicosis and in both conditions there is a disturbance of the autonomic nervous sytem. Anxiety may be associated with depression.

Specific fears are called phobic states. Simple phobias involving for instance spiders, darkness, heights or thunder seldom cause severe problems. Agoraphobia (agora—an open meeting place) involves anxiety about public places such as shops and the possibility of losing control. Social phobias involve anxiety about meeting other people usually at social gatherings.

Management

Mild anxiety is usually self-limiting and requires sympathetic support with or without sedation. Diazepam (Valium 5–10 mg tds) or chlordiazepoxide (Librium 10–20 mg tds) are commonly used. Long-term dependence on benzodiazequines can be a worse and more prolonged affliction than the disease. Anxiety which fails to respond to simple therapy and which is associated with phobias should be referred to a psychiatrist.

Hysteria

The word has many meanings but the most useful concept is of the patient who produces symptoms and signs which act directly to reduce the emotional impact of the cause of his distress. The diagnostic problem shades on one side into malingering, where the patient is aware of what is happening, and, on the other side into the possibility of organic disease where the absence of an identified cause for a symptom or sign does not mean that one does not exist. In conversion hysteria almost any motor or sensory symptom may be produced including aphonia, tic, hyperventilation and blindness. Gross paralysis or sensory loss is unusual. In dissociative hysteria there is altered awareness with fugues, amnesia and trances. Dermatitis artefacta, factitious pyrexia and Munchausen's syndrome are related. Bland indifference to gross disability is common ('belle indifference'). Hysteria is unlikely if there is no obvious 'gain'.

Management

The patient should be observed for a period of time during which the inconstancy of signs and the underlying emotional cause may become apparent. Expert psychiatric advice is often required and behaviour therapy often used.

Acute confusional states

These occur during medical or surgical illness and involve clouding of consciousness with loss of contact between the patient and its environment. There is failure of recent memory, disorientation, and emotional liability. Hallucinations may occur. Confusional states occur relatively frequently in the elderly. Acute confusional states occur in:

Small cerebrovascular accidents.
'All the failures', i.e. cardiac, respiratory (often hypoxia), renal and liver.
Severe acute infections including meningitis, pneumonia and malaria, particularly with high fever.
Drug overdosage, e.g. alcohol, phenobarbitone, salicylates, amitriptyline, LSD, cannabis.
Hypoglycaemia and hyperglycaemia.
Other endocrine disorders, e.g. thyrotoxicosis, myxoedema, Cushing's syndrome and corticosteroid therapy.
Hypercalcaemia, commonly resulting from multiple secondary tumours in bone.
Alcoholics and the elderly may develop an acute encephalopathy due to thiamine deficiency (Wernicke) with confabulation (Korsakoff's psychosis).
Cerebral malaria in travellers.

Treatment

This will depend on the diagnosis. For sedation, chlorpromazine (50–100 mg) intramuscularly can be used. Thioridazine (Melleril) 25 mg tds is a suitable tranquilliser especially in the elderly.

Dementia

Dementia means 'loss of mind'. The earliest feature is loss of memory for recent events. There is a global disruption of personality with the gradual development of abnormal behaviour, loss of intellect, mood changes often without insight, blunting of emotions, and failure to learn (page 14). Eventually there is a reduction in self-care, restless wandering, paranoia and incontinence. In patients under 60 years of age it is usually termed pre-senile dementia, though this distinction is not important. There are two common causes:

1   Alzheimer's disease (senile dementia of Alzheimer type—SDAT) is characterised by a smoothly progressive dementia usually without focal neurological deficits, or epilepsy. It affects 10–15% of people over 65 years of age. Death occurs 5–15 years after onset.

2   Multi-infarct dementia is characterised by a stepwise intermittent progression and is associated with other evidence of arteriovascular disease, plus one or more focal neurological deficits, frequently a shuffling gait and some evidence of a pseudobulbar palsy (page 14) including emotional lability.

In the differential diagnosis, the treatable disorders must be excluded first:

• The pseudodementia of depression
• Overmedication, usually with sedatives often chronically. Remember that the patient may not be taking his medication as prescribed, or may be using another patient's drugs
• Subdural haematoma. This is commoner in the elderly, alcoholics and cirrhotics
• Normal pressure hydrocephalus, where the dementia is associated with fluctuating confusion, ataxia, apraxia and urinary incontinence. A CT scan shows enlarged ventricles without cerebral atrophy. Ventricular shunting can result in great improvement
• Cerebral tumour. Meningiomata may grow very slowly (page 134)
• Hypothyroidism. ('myxoedema madness') (page 183).

The remaining causes are either less amenable to treatment or very uncommon:

• Cerebrovascular disease
• Huntington's chorea (page 134)
• Traumatic
• Epilepsy
• Carbon monoxide poisoning
• Herpes simplex encephalitis
• Secondary malignancy, especially from bronchus, or involvement with haematological malignancies
• Vitamin B_{12} deficiency
• Cerebral syphilis (page 146)
• Multiple sclerosis (page 127)
• AIDS (page 384)
• Creutzfeldt–Jakob disease

NB   Primary dementia is a diagnosis made only by exclusion (in the absence of brain biopsy) and all 'pre-senile dementias' should be investigated.

Investigation

Full blood count, ESR, urea and electrolytes, liver function tests including γ-glutamyl transferase.

Chest X-ray for bronchial carcinoma.

A CT scan of the head to demonstrate cortical thinning (dilated ventricles and widened sulci), subdural haematoma or tumour.

If CT scan not available, skull X-ray for shift of pineal, calcification in tumours, erosion of posterior clinoids in the presence of raised intracranial pressure.

Thyroid function studies.

Serum B_{12}.

Serological tests for syphilis (TPHA and FTAA).

It may be necessary to proceed to:

Examination of CSF.

Brain isotope scan.

EEG.

Schizophrenia

The general physician is unlikely to have patients with this disorder referred to him in the first instance, but certain features should make him suspicious. It affects about 0.5% of the general population but the 'schizoid personality' is said to occur about four times more frequently. The essential features of the illness are due to a lack of contact with reality and involve disturbances of thought, mood and conduct. Hallucinations occur and delusions are common especially delusions of persecution (paranoia). Patients have little or no insight. There is evidence of a familial factor and the schizoid personality occurs more commonly in relatives of the frankly schizophrenic than in the general population. Such persons show withdrawal from life, shyness, suspicion and have bizarre ideas and theories. They may become alcoholic or commit suicide.

Schneider's first-rank delusion symptoms are the most useful diagnostically.

Transmission of thoughts to others (thought broadcasting).

Transmission of thoughts from others (thought withdrawal).

Implantation of thoughts from outside agents (thought insertion).

Feelings of passivity (external control).

Voices discussing, repeating or anticipating thoughts (including 'running commentary').

Actions controlled by outside agents: 'delusional perception' (i.e. persecution perceived from normal events).

Negative symptoms include apathy, mental slowness, and social withdrawal. When symptoms are chronic the prognosis is poor.

Drug management

Treatment by the phenothiazines has greatly improved the prognosis. Chlorpromazine (Largactil) and fluphenazine (Modecate), a long-acting phenothiazine, are the most widely used phenothiazines. They may give rise to a Parkinsonian syndrome, rashes, including light sensitivity, mild jaundice, and they can depress the bone marrow.

Schizophrenia is best managed by experienced psychiatrists.

Connective tissue and rheumatic diseases

Musculoskeletal strains are very common and the cause of most referrals in general practice (sports injuries and low back pain). Osteoarthritis affects almost everyone who lives past middle age.

The connective tissue disorders have usurped syphilis as the 'great imitator' and must often be considered in differential diagnoses even though they remain uncommon diseases. SLE and polyarteritis nodosa (PN) (page 163) in particular should come to mind in the clinical situations of :

- pyrexia of unknown origin (PUO), malaise, and weight loss
- multisystem disease
- renal disorders

The connective tissue diseases are non-organ-specific autoimmune disorders where the lesions affect chiefly skin, glomeruli, joints, serous membranes and blood vessels. The following named diseases describe the commoner clinical pictures though any individual patient may exhibit other features from the total spectrum of the connective tissue disorders:

SYSTEMIC LUPUS ERYTHEMATOSUS (SLE)

SLE most commonly presents in women aged 20–40 years (90%) and is exacerbated by sunlight and infection. Hydralazine usually in high prolonged dosage may give a similar picture as may procainamide, but renal involvement is rare. SLE prevalence in the UK is about 1 :10 000 with a sex ratio of 8 : 1. The American Rheumatism Association criteria tend to exclude milder cases.

Clinical presentation

The commonest early features are fever (75% of cases), arthralgia and general ill health, with weight loss. It can mimic rheumatoid arthritis, subacute bacterial endocarditis and may produce the nephrotic syndrome. The typical 'butterfly' rash on the face may not be present. One or more of the following systems may be involved.

Joints (90% of cases). A migratory, usually symmetrical polyarthralgia, not unlike rheumatoid arthritis but very rarely erosive or deforming, and affecting the finger, wrists, elbows, shoulders, knees and ankles.

Skin (80%). Non-specific erythema, photosensitivity, alopecia and malar (butterfly) rash (60%) are the commonest features. Oral and nasal mucosal ulceration is not uncommon (30%). Nailfold infarcts may occur (10%). Follicles are blocked and telangiectases present. It may involve the ears, neck, chest and upper limbs. Raynaud's phenomenon is present in 10%.

Kidneys (60%). Renal involvement is common and associated with a poor prognosis. Antigen–antibody complexes have been demonstrated by immuno-fluorescence in the arterioles of the glomerular tuft. The clinical presentation is usually of the nephrotic syndrome but asymptomatic proteinuria, an acute nephritic syndrome and chronic renal failure with hypertension may occur. Renal involvement is associated in 50% with hypertension.

Nervous system (60%). Direct involvement is uncommon and symptoms mostly result from arteritis and ischaemia. This may produce cranial or peripheral nerve lesions—single or multiple, motor or sensory or a peripheral neuropathy (10%), usually sensory. Central nervous system manifestations are associated with a poorer prognosis. They include phobias and depression. Confusion and hallu-cination are perhaps more commonly secondary to the corticosteroids used in therapy. Rarely epilepsy is the first presenting feature.

Lungs (50%). Pleurisy with effusion is relatively common. Patchy consolidation and plate-like areas of collapse, and/or diffuse reticulo-nodular shadowing on chest X-ray may be seen.

Cardiovascular system (40%). Pericarditis is sometimes the first indication of SLE. Raynaud's phenomenon (10%) (page 343), cardiac failure of cardiomyo-pathy and non-bacterial endocarditis of mitral (Libman–Sacks) and aortic valves all may occur.

Blood. The sedimentation rate in the acute phase is greatly raised (90%) and it is this which often leads to first suspicion of the disease. Thrombocytopenia (30%) with purpura may be the first indication of SLE. Anaemia (partly haemolytic with reticulocytosis and hyperbilirubinaemia) and leucopenia may occur. There may be splenomegaly.

Lymphatic system. Generalised lymphadenopathy (50%) with or without hepatosplenomegaly (15%) may occur.

Investigation

The antinuclear factor (ANF) is positive in over 95% of cases. The presence of antibodies against double-stranded DNA is diagnostic and found in 73% of those with active disease. Low serum complement, particularly the C3 and C4 fractions, occurs especially in lupus nephritis.

With renal disease, the diagnosis may be made on renal biopsy. Initially a focal nephritis may be seen. Later there is diffuse thickening of the basement membrane of the glomerulus producing the 'wire loop' appearance.

Management

Antibiotics for intercurrent infection, analgesics (aspirin) for joint pain, and blood transfusion is indicated for anaemia.

Steroids in high dosage (prednisolone 40–60 mg daily) for the acute phase. The dosage is slowly reduced depending upon symptoms and severity of involvement of vital organs. Activity is in part reflected by changes in the erythrocyte sedimentation rate (ESR). The CRP is normal except when there is bacterial infection. Immunosuppressive therapy with azathioprine is used in very active cases and may also enable a reduction in steroid dosage particularly when side-effects are troublesome.

Chloroquine has been used usually when skin disease predominates in subacute or chronic forms of the disease. It can cause lens opacities which are not serious clinically (and resolve on stopping it) and retinal degeneration which is rare but irreversible.

Plasmaphaeresis to remove 'antibodies' is used in some centres to treat severe non-responsive generalised vasculitis but its place in routine therapy is yet to be determined.

Prognosis

The history is of episodic relapses and remissions lasting months to years. Five-year survival is over 95% unless there is renal or cerebral involvement, when the percentage survival drops by about 10%. Death usually results from renal failure.

POLYARTERITIS NODOSA (PN)

This is a rare disease which presents in a wide variety of ways. It is commonest in young men (20–50 years). There is fibrinoid necrosis of the media of small- and medium-sized arteries with polymorph infiltration (eosinophils may predominate). The lumen is narrowed and may thrombose giving rise to ischaemic lesions. Healing by fibrosis leads to the formation of small aneurysms (hence the name 'nodosa').

Clinical presentation

Ill-defined malaise, fever, weight loss, arthralgia.

Hypertension (sometimes malignant) occurs almost invariably at some stage, and in 50% at presentation.

Renal disease (80% of cases) with an acute nephritic syndrome, nephrotic syndrome, or progressive renal failure.

Heart (70%). Angina, myocardial infarction, pericarditis.

Gastrointestinal tract (50%). Abdominal pain.

Lungs (40%). Asthma of late onset with diffuse transient patchy lung infiltration and pulmonary eosinophilia—Churg–Strauss syndrome (page 285). The differential diagnosis includes allergic aspergillosis and Loeffler's syndrome.

Nervous system (50%). Mononeuritis multiplex or polyneuritis. Occasionally subarachnoid haemorrhage.

Skin (25%). Tender subcutaneous nodules, arteritic lesions around the nail bed and splinter haemorrhages may mimic bacterial endocarditis (particularly if combined with fever).

Joints (10%). A non-deforming polyarthritis mainly of the lower limbs.

Investigation

There is usually anaemia, and leucocytosis with eosinophilia. Albuminuria, microscopic haematuria and a raised ESR are common. Diagnosis is occasionally confirmed from biopsies of tender muscles, but more reliably from renal biopsy which demonstrates changes of segmental fibrinoid necrosis of the walls of medium-sized arteries and arterioles with cellular infiltration. This causes multiple cortical infarcts. Visceral angiography may demonstrate small aneurysms.

Management

Symptomatic therapy and steroids with immunosuppressive agents as for SLE.

Prognosis

The overall 5-year survival is 40%. The disease may progress rapidly to produce death within weeks or continue for 10 years or more. Renal failure is the most common cause of death, although in a few patients evidence of renal disease may disappear with steroid therapy and not return even after withdrawal.

DERMATOMYOSITIS

Mainly affects women of 40–50 years. About 20% of all cases are associated with underlying malignancy (bronchus, breast, stomach, ovary) and in men presenting over the age of 50 years, over 60% have carcinoma, usually of the bronchus. An acute form occurs in children and is often fatal.

Clinical presentation

The onset may be acute or chronic. Skin and muscle changes occur in any order, or together, sometimes with 2–3 months separating their appearance. General ill health and fever are common.

Skin involvement (60%)

Classically purple 'heliotrope' (a lilac-blue flower) colour occurs around the eyes. The remainder of the face may be involved.
Violet, oedematous lesions over the small joints of the hands with telangiectasia.
Arteritic lesions around the nails.
There may be generalised telangiectasia, especially of face, chest and arms.

Muscle involvement

Tenderness and weakness of muscles occurs, commonly of the shoulder and proximal muscles of the upper limb, and if this predominates the disease closely resembles polymyositis (page 151). Dysphagia is common. Muscle wasting and fibrosis with fixed joint deformity may occur in chronic disease.

Other systems

Lungs with plate-like areas of collapse and diffuse fibrosis.
Heart with cardiomyopathy and cardiac failure.
Sicca syndrome.

Investigation

Investigation of myositis (page 151). As for SLE unless an underlying carcinoma is present.

Management

Steroids are given in high doses (e.g. prednisolone 60–80 mg per day) in the acute stages but are relatively ineffective in the chronic cases. Immunosuppression with azathioprine if there is an inadequate response within 2 months.

Prognosis

Depends upon the underlying neoplasm if present. The disease may progress rapidly but exacerbations and remissions are the rule and continue for 10–20 years until respiratory or cardiac failure occurs.

POLYMYOSITIS

See page 151.

SCLERODERMA (systemic sclerosis)

A disease mainly of middle-aged women. Collagen fibres initially swell and later become sclerotic. Blood vessels show arteritis and thickening. There is progressive fibrosis with atrophy of the skin structures.

Clinical presentation

The following systems may be involved:

General. Lassitude, fever and weight loss.

Skin (75%). Raynaud's phenomenon with sclerodactyly and telangiectasia. In the early stages there is non-pitting oedema of the skin of the hands and feet, later involving the face, neck and trunk. The skin becomes smooth, waxy and tight and finally thin, atrophic and pigmented in 50%. Skin ulcers develop in 40%. Vitiligo may occur. Changes are maximal over the hands, ankles and face, producing a typical mask-like face. Subcutaneous calcification may be present (10%). The sicca syndrome develops in 5%. (Morphoea is a localised indurated sclerodermatous lesion usually on the trunk, neck or extremities. It is benign and only rarely proceeds to systemic sclerosis.)

Lungs. Diffuse interstitial fibrosis progressing to respiratory failure occurs later. Overspill pneumonitis.

Locomotor system. Polymyositis. Polyarthralgia, later proceeds to a rheumatoid picture.

Heart. Pericardial effusion, cardiomyopathy and heart failure are rare.

Oesophagus and intestine. Dysphagia (65%). Steatorrhoea and malabsorption are rare. Barium studies may reveal deformity and diminished peristalsis in the oesophagus and dilatation of the second part of the duodenum.

Kidney. Progressive renal failure (20%), with or without hypertension, is a late but often fatal development.

CREST syndrome. This is a syndrome which includes calcinosis cutis, Raynaud's phenomenon, oesophageal immobility, sclerodactyly and telangiectasia. The outlook is better than in systemic sclerosis, but some progress to the complete syndrome.

Investigation

There is no specific test. The antinuclear factor is positive in 80%, the ESR raised in 50%, the latex fixation positive in 30% and LE cells present in 10%. Anticentromere antibodies are present in CREST.

Management

Symptomatic treatment is commonly all that is required. Antacids and sleeping upright may assist in preventing reflux oesophagitis. Physiotherapy may help stiff fingers and joints and maintain muscle activity. Electrically heated gloves may reduce the symptoms of Raynaud's phenomenon. Non-steroidal anti-inflammatory drops are given for arthralgia. D-penicillamine may help soften the skin. Steroids are sometimes tried in an attempt to suppress systemic symptoms but are usually completely ineffective.

Prognosis

Morphoea is usually benign. Systemic sclerosis is a slow progressive disease. The course is very variable and largely determined by the presence or absence of visceral involvement (renal, cardiac or pulmonary). Oesophageal involvement and calcinosis are not adverse features. Death occurs from lung or cardiac complications. Severe renal involvement is uncommon but is rapidly fatal in association with severe hypertension. The 5-year survival is 75%.

NB Most patients with Raynaud's phenomenon neither have, nor develop, systemic sclerosis.

MIXED CONNECTIVE TISSUE DISEASE (MCTD)

This term is used to describe patients with features of connective tissue disease which do not fall into one of the well-defined syndromes (overlap syndrome). There may be some features from each of the syndromes of SLE, polymyositis and sclerodoma (or 'sclerodermatomyositis'). What may define it as a special entity is the presence of antibodies to ribonucleoprotein (RNP) and absence of DNA antibodies. Steroids may help with the non-sclerodermatous features.

POLYMYALGIA RHEUMATICA

Clinical presentation

Occurs in patients usually over 60 years old and more commonly in women. It presents with muscle pain, stiffness and occasionally tenderness usually in the shoulder girdle and neck, but sometimes in the pelvic region, and is worse on waking. There is little if any weakness or wasting. Joint swelling or pain may occur. The associated findings are headache, lassitude, depression and weight loss. It may be associated with temporal arteritis. The ESR may be very high (>70 mm/h) but is rarely <30.

Management

Steroids (10–20 mg prednisolone daily) are required urgently to relieve symptoms and prevent blindness in patients with associated temporal arteritis. The response is characteristically rapid and good. The dose is reduced often to a very low level, whilst monitoring symptoms and the ESR, which should be kept within normal limits. Treatment should be continued for several years.

Prognosis

A self-limiting disease which usually recovers within 1–8 years.

TEMPORAL ARTERITIS (giant cell arteritis, cranial arteritis)

Clinical presentation

A disease in patients usually over the age of 60 who develop severe headache, with burning and tenderness over the scalp and tenderness over the temporal arteries, sometimes (25%) with visual blurring and even jaw claudication. Systemic manifestations are common with fever, weakness, weight loss, arthralgia and a myalgia identical to that seen in polymyalgia rheumatica in 50%. The ophthalmic arteries may be involved and blindness of one or both eyes results in 30% of untreated patients. Personality changes may occur from involvement of the cerebral vessels. The coronary arteries or other vessels may be involved.

Investigation

The ESR is markedly raised (often above 90 mm/h). The alkaline phosphatase level may also be raised. Diagnosis is confirmed on temporal artery biopsy which shows patchy involvement of the arterial wall with areas of necrosis, large mononuclear cell infiltration and giant cells.

Management

Steroids in high doses (prednisolone 40–60 mg daily) are given urgently to suppress symptoms (this usually occurs within 2 days) and to prevent blindness. Blindness may occur but some may rarely recover vision to some degree if steroids are given rapidly after it occurs. Treatment is given for 3 years or more, gradually reducing the dosage while monitoring symptoms and the ESR.

NB *Polymyalgia arteritica*. This term has been coined to include both polymyalgia rheumatica and giant cell arteritis, since the underlying pathology appears similar though the presentation is different. There is a risk of sudden blindness in both conditions and treatment with high-dose steroids is essential and urgent in both.

ORGAN-SPECIFIC AUTOIMMUNE DISEASE

This refers to a group of disorders characterised by the presence of antibodies to a specific organ which may fail in function. The disorders are more common in women, are familial, and may result from a genetically determined defect of immune mechanisms. Patients with involvement of one organ have an increased incidence of involvement of one or more of the others.

The following disorders characterise this type of disease: Hashimoto's thyroiditis. Addison's (adrenal) disease, idiopathic hypoparathyroidism, premature ovarian failure, pernicious anaemia, alopecia, vitiligo (both skin-markers of organ-specific autoimmune disease), rheumatoid arthritis.

RHEUMATOID ARTHRITIS (RA)

Women are more frequently affected than men (3 : 1). It is usually insidious in onset but may be an acute or a chronic relapsing disease marked by ill health and chronic joint deformity. The dominant clinical feature is a chronic synovitis. However, the name 'rheumatoid disease' may be more appropriate since tissues other than the joints are frequently affected. The overall picture is of a systemic connective tissue disease with the brunt of the disease falling upon the joints. The extra-articular manifestations are very important in determining both the morbidity and mortality of the disease. There is often a family history.

Clinical features

Musculoskeletal

The small joints of the hands and feet are the most commonly affected, usually symmetrically, but other large synovial joints (hips, knees, elbows) are often also involved. The onset may be gradual with progressive pain, early morning stiffness and swelling of joints. The acute onset is associated with fever and general constitutional illness. Examination may show:
• Tenderness and diminished movement of involved joints with characteristic fusiform soft tissue swelling of the metacarpophalangeal and interphalangeal joints of the hands. (The metatarsophalangeal joints of the feet may also be tender on pressure). The wrists are commonly involved. The terminal interphalangeal joints of the fingers are spared (except in psoriatic arthropathy, page 173). The chronic disease may produce fixed deformities and ulnar deviation at the metacarpophalangeal joints.
• Wasting of the small muscles of the hand is common and results from a combination of disuse atrophy, vasculitis and peripheral neuropathy. Wasting may occur in the muscle around any affected joint
• Inflammation of the soft tissues surrounding inflamed joints causes swelling, tenosynovitis (Achilles tendinitis, olecranon bursitis) and even tendon rupture. Localised subcutaneous nodules are present in 25%

Joints less commonly involved are the ankles which have relatively little synovial tissue, the costovertebral joints producing diminished chest expansion, temporomandibular joints, the cricoarytenoid joints (which causes hoarseness and, rarely, acute respiratory obstruction) and the cervical spine. Laxity of the atlanto-axial joint ligaments with some erosion of the odontoid peg may result in acute or chronic cord compression and death. Atlanto-axial subluxation is present in 25% of patients though only 7% have neurological signs. It may be necessary to X-ray the cervical spine in severe cases of rheumatoid arthritis prior to intubation for general anaesthesia.

NB Acute septic arthritis may occur in rheumatoid joints. Acute solitary effusions should be aspirated and examined microscopically and bacteriologically.

Lung

Lung involvement is clinically uncommon but lung function tests will show changes in nearly half of all patients with rheumatoid arthritis. They tend to be commoner in men than in women. It may occur before the arthritis and usually in sero-positive disease. It presents as:

• Isolated unilateral pleural effusion (must be differentiated from primary tuberculosis)
• Rheumatoid nodules, single or multiple, which may be present throughout the lung parenchyma. They are commonly sub-pleural
• Diffuse fibronodular infiltration or fibrosing alveolitis
• Caplan's syndrome: the presence of large (up to 5 cm) rheumatoid nodules in the lungs of coal miners with silicosis but also occurring in other pneumoconioses. They may calcify, cavitate or coalesce and may precede clinical arthritis. The patients are sero-positive

Cardiac

Pericarditis (with or without effusion) is clinically uncommon though found at post-mortem in about 30%.

Vascular

Arteritic lesions characteristically produce nailfold infarcts and minute 'splinter' necrosis in the digital pulps. (This form of vascular necrosis is characteristic of arteritic lesions seen in the collagen diseases although multiple emboli in infective endocarditis may produce a similar picture.) Necrotising arteritis may affect large vessels and give rise to digital gangrene, infarcted bowel or stroke. Chronic leg ulcers result from skin necrosis secondary to vasculitis—the ulcers are frequently on the lateral aspect of the tibia (cf. varicose ulcers). Raynaud's phenomenon (page 343) may occur.

Neurological

• Peripheral neuropathy: this is usually predominantly sensory. Arteritis of the vessels supplying the nerves may be responsible.
• Neuropathy may also follow therapy with gold and chloroquine

- Mononeuritis multiplex, particularly of digital nerves, ulnar nerves and lateral popliteal nerves
- Entrapment neuropathy, e.g. carpal tunnel syndrome and the ulnar nerve at the elbow
- Spinal cord lesions secondary to cervical disease

Reticuloendothelial

The spleen is enlarged in about 5% of cases but only 1% develop leucopenia. Generalised lymphadenopathy is present in 10%.

Infection

Of all kinds (except urinary tract infections) and in all sites (especially joints) is much commoner and should be looked for in all patients who deteriorate suddenly.

Blood

Normochromic normocytic anaemia is common and its severity relates to that of the disease. Iron deficiency may result from bleeding secondary to salicylate or other non-steroidal anti-inflammatory therapy but this is uncommon and peptic ulceration and colonic neoplasms should be excluded. The height of the ESR reflects the activity of the disease. The CRP is raised even in the absence of infection (see SLE page 161).

Renal

Amyloidosis, though common on biopsy, is seldom clinically important in rheumatoid disease. Proteinuria or nephrotic syndrome may complicate treatment with pencillamine and gold.

Ocular

- keratoconjunctivitis sicca occurs in 15% of patients with RA: see *Sjögren's syndrome* (page 173)
- scleritis presents as pericorneal injection with pain and tenderness in 0.6% of RA. It may lead to uveitis and glaucoma
- scleromalacia perforans is even less common and occurs in long-standing RA: a rheumatoid nodule in the sclera which may perforate.
- iatrogenic: lens opacities and retinal degeneration with chloroquine and cataracts from steroids

Iatrogenic

From gold (proteinuria, nephrotic syndrome, skin rash, marrow suppression); aspirin and most non-steroidal anti-inflammatory drugs—NSAIDs (gastric erosion); penicillamine (nephropathy), steroids (page 192) and chloroquine (cataract, retinopathy, photosensitivity).

Investigation of inflammatory polyarthropathy

There is often a normochromic normocytic anaemia. The ESR is performed to assess the activity of the disease and to monitor therapy. Perform ANF and DNA antibodies to exclude collagen disease. The serum uric acid helps to exclude gout particularly if the distribution is asymmetrical. A chest X-ray helps to exclude the hypertrophic arthropathy of bronchial carcinoma and the arthropathy of acute sarcoid which usually affects the ankles and knees. HLA B27 supports the diagnosis of Reiter's disease and the arthropathy of ulcerative colitis or Crohn's disease.

Rheumatoid factor

This is a circulating immunoglobulin of the IgM class which is an antibody to the patient's own IgG. It fixes complement and aids phagocytosis of immune complexes by neutrophils. It agglutinates sensitised sheep red cells (sheep cell agglutination test—SCAT) and also latex particles which have been coated with denatured γ globulin (latex agglutination tests, e.g. F_2LP test in which the 'F_2' fraction of denatured γ globulin is used to coat the latex particles). High titres correlate with more severe arthritis with a worse prognosis, and with a higher incidence of extra-articular disease (nodules, arteritis, leg ulcers, digital gangrene, neuropathy, Felty's syndrome and fibrosing alveolitis).

Rheumatoid factor is positive in:

50–70% of outpatients with rheumatoid arthritis (100% in patients with nodules and Sjögren's syndrome).
25–35% of patients with collagen disease.
15% of patients with juvenile rheumatoid arthritis (Still's disease).
4% of the general population, rising with age. Its presence does not necessarily indicate that rheumatoid disease will later develop.

Rheumatoid factor is usually negative in ankylosing spondylitis, Reiter's syndrome, psoriatic arthropathy and colitic arthropathy.

Radiology

The joints may be normal in early rheumatoid disease. The characteristic sequence of abnormalities is:
* soft tissue swelling and periarticular osteoporosis
* narrowing of joint space and periarticular erosions
* subluxation and osteoarthritis occur in longstanding disease
* fibrosis or bony ankylosis

Management

The objects of therapy are: (a) symptom control of pain and stiffness, enabling the patient to maintain as near normal existence as possible and (b) disease suppression of synovitis and systemic inflammation in more severe disease. A social assessment of occupation, of family help and home conditions is essential when planning therapy.

The assessment of disease severity depends on both clinical and laboratory findings:

- *Mild disease* is characterised by slight joint swelling and pain, with brief morning, stiffness. Haemoglobin and platelet count are normal and ESR less than, say, 20 mm/h.
- *Active disease* has more severe symptomatology, and the laboratory findings abnormal (Hb<12, platelets >400, ESR>40). The rheumatoid factor is more likely to be positive.

Rest diseased joints in splints especially at night to reduce pain and prevent deformity.

Physiotherapy to maintain full joint movement and strengthen weak muscles. Early attention and advice regarding posture may prevent chronic deformity and degeneration of all involved joints.

There are four groups of drugs which are used in disease of increasing severity:

1 *Analgesic.* Simple, such as paracetamol, or a compound, such as coproxamol or cocodamol.

2 *Non-steroidal anti-inflammatory drugs (NSAIDs).* Standard drugs are ibuprofen, indomethacin and soluble aspirin. If there is gastro-intestinal intolerance, H_2-blockade or the prostaglandin E_1 analogue misoprostol may be added.

3 *Disease-suppressing drugs.* Penicillamine, sulphasalazine, gold, and hydroxy-chloroquine.

4 *Steroids and cytotoxic drugs,* such as cyclophosphamide and methotrexate. Systemic steroids should be considered in patients with progressive rheumatoid arthritis who have not responded to less dangerous therapy and whose life and/or occupation is threatened. They should also be considered if severe systemic involvement occurs and fails to respond to other drugs. They are *rarely needed* in the treatment of rheumatoid arthritis. In view of the serious side-effects of systemic steroid therapy, they must only be given after very careful assessment and probably only by an experienced rheumatologist. Local injection of steroids into joints (or other painful sites) may give relief.

Immunosuppressive therapy may be as effective and less toxic than steroids and may allow a reduction in steroid dosage. Depression should not be missed. **NB** Some patients fail to respond to therapy and should be admitted to hospital for rest and further careful assessment of analgesic therapy.

Surgical management. Synovectomy (especially of the knee joint), realignment and repair of tendons, joint prostheses (hip, knee, fingers) and arthrodesis may be required for severe pain or deformity.

Advice of an expert in rehabilitation may allow a severely disabled patient to continue a tolerable and even happy existence at home.

Prognosis

About 60% of patients suffer minimal or only mild disability and are able to continue a full active life; 30–35% suffer serious disability with varying degrees of restriction of activities; and 5–10% progress relentlessly to serious and almost complete disability. The following features indicate a poor prognosis:

- insidious onset
- persistent activity for over a year
- positive serology in high titre within a year
- early bony erosion and subacutaneous nodules
- weight loss and extra-articular manifestations
- anaemia and high ESR

DISEASES RESEMBLING RHEUMATOID ARTHRITIS

Still's disease

Adult-onset Still's disease, like the juvenile form (page 176) is characterised by a high spiking fever (85%), an evanescent rash (80%) and arthritis (100%), but occurs after the age of 15 years. Other features include splenomegaly (35%), pleurisy (30%), pericarditis (20%), neutrophil leucocytosis (100%), lymphadenopathy (70%), and hepatic abnormalities (85%). Roughly half go into remission off medication. NSAIDs are the treatment of choice e.g. naproxen. Steroids are often needed in the acute phase.

Sjögren's syndrome

It is commoner in women than in men (9:1). The major clinical features (sicca syndrome) result from reduced secretions from the lachrymal and salivary glands which produce dry 'gritty' eyes and corneal ulcers (keratoconjunctivitis sicca) and a dry mouth (xerostomia) with dysphagia. Recurrent respiratory infections occur from diminished bronchial secretions. About 50% are associated with rheumatoid arthritis, 30% are uncomplicated and 20% associated with other autoimmune disease (mostly non-organ specific). Rheumatoid factor is usually present, ANF frequently present (70%), anti-R_o is often present, (40–60%), and LE cells seldom present (15%). In Schirmer's test, filter paper is hooked over the lower eyelid; in normal people at least 15 mm is wet in 5 min and in the sicca syndrome usually far less. Fluorescein demonstrates corneal ulceration. Labial salivary gland biopsy, may show diagnostic histology. Treatment is symptomatic with artificial tears (1% methylcellulose) and the arthritis is treated as uncomplicated rheumatoid arthritis.

Felty's syndrome

Some patients with severe rheumatoid arthritis have enlarged lymph nodes, splenomegaly, and hypersplenism (anaemia, leucopenia and thrombocytopenia). Removal of the spleen often reverses blood abnormalities but the underlying rheumatoid process is not affected and operation is seldom indicated. Leg ulcers are common due to vasculitis. The ANF is usually positive.

Psoriatic arthritis

An arthritis similar to but distinct from rheumatoid arthritis may complicate psoriasis (page 344). The clinical picture resembles rheumatoid arthritis and may be clinically indistinguishable from it in 30% but:

- psoriasis is present
- joint involvement is usually asymmetrical and deforming and involves the

terminal interphalangeal joints which may be the only affected joints (50%)
- pitting occurs in the nails (80%)
- subcutaneous nodules do not occur
- sacroiliitis is more common (30%)
- tests for rheumatoid factor are negative

ANKYLOSING SPONDYLITIS (sacroiliitis)

Clinical features

A disease mainly of young adult males (20–40) (cf. rheumatoid arthritis) with a 6% familial incidence. Joint involvement affects the sacroiliac joints causing low back pain with morning stiffness. The disease may involve the spine, producing pain and stiffness initially of the lumbosacral region and eventually of the thoracic and cervical spine. The hips are involved in 50% of patients. Examination reveals decreased spinal movements and loss of the normal lumbosacral curvature. 'Springing' the pelvis (i.e. pressing the iliac crests towards each other) causes sacroiliac pain.

Peripheral joints are involved in 25%, especially the knees and ankles. The ribs fuse to the vertebrae. Up to 15% may present with a peripheral arthropathy. The arthropathy differs from rheumatoid arthritis in that it is asymmetrical and affects large joints more than small joints.

Other features of ankylosing spondylitis are:
- general ill health
- uveitis (in 25–30% of cases and up to 40% in longstanding cases)
- ulcerative colitis—more common in patients with ankylosing spondylitis and vice versa
- aortic regurgitation due to aortitis
- respiratory failure may result from the fixed rib cage with kyphoscoliosis, and from fibrosing alveolitis

Investigation

Tests for rheumatoid factor are usually negative. The ESR is raised in 80%. HLA B27 is present in 96% (compared with 7% in the general population, and 50% of asymptomatic relatives).

Radiology

The sacroiliac joints are irregular with sclerosis of the articular margins. Bony ankylosis occurs late. The intervertebral ligaments calcify and finally ossify to produce a 'bamboo' spine.

Differential diagnoses

Osteoarthritis of the spine.
Prolapsed intervertebral disc.
Tuberculosis which may affect only one sacroiliac joint.

and rarely:

Psoriatic arthritis.
Reiter's disease.
The sacroiliitis of ulcerative colitis.

All these may be variants of ankylosing spondylitis.

Management

Bedrest is contraindicated because it increases stiffness and ankylosis.
Careful posture with spinal muscle exercises is essential to prevent chronic deformity. Sleeping on a firm bed without pillows should help prevent fixed spinal flexion.
Analgesics. Phenylbutazone (Butazolidine) 200–300 mg/day is particularly effective but must now be reserved for specialist use.
Indomethacin or other NSAIDs may be given as an alternative.
Radiotherapy although effective in reducing pain is inadvisable except in those with intractable pain as there is an increased risk of leukaemia (0.3%).
Sulphasalazine (500 mg starting dose to maintenance dose of 2–3 g/day) as in rheumatoid arthritis, offers symptomatic improvement more of peripheral joints than sacroiliitis in 2–3 months, probably by altering the immune process.

Prognosis

Many mild cases may never present to a physician. With expert care 70–80% will maintain complete or almost complete activity. More severe cases develop moderate to severe bony ankylosis of the spine to produce fixation of mobility and rounded kyphosis of the cervical and thoracic spine. This may impair ventilation. In severe cases extreme rigidity of the spine may occur within 3–5 years. The disease may remit at any stage but recurrent episodes may occur.

REITER'S SYNDROME

A disease usually of young men presenting with urethritis, arthritis and conjunctivitis (only 30%). There is usually a history of sexual intercourse 2–4 weeks previously. It occurs in <1% of patients with non-specific urethritis. The disease may, less commonly in the UK, follow bacillary (shigella) dysentery.

Clinical features

Arthritis: typically acute or subacute and usually polyarticular and asymmetrical affecting large joints of the lower limbs.
Sacroiliitis occurs in 30%. Plantar fasciitis, calcaneal spurs and Achilles tendinitis may occur (20%).
Conjunctivitis is common in the acute disease. Iritis is associated with chronic recurrent disease, particularly when associated with sacroiliitis.
Skin lesions: mouth ulcers are common. Urethritis and prostatitis are associated with superficial skin ulceration around the penile meatus (circinate balanitis).
Pustular hyperkeratotic lesions of the soles of the feet and less frequently the palms of the hands (keratoderma blennorrhagica) may occur (15%).
Cardiovascular lesions may occur.

Tests for rheumatoid factor are by definition negative.
HLA B27 is present in 70%.

Differential diagnosis

Gonococcal arthritis (the gonococcus is present in up to half the cases and is detected in urethral discharge or blood culture)
Ankylosing spondylitis
Behçet's disease
Psoriatic and rheumatoid arthritis

Management

The treatment of the acute stage is symptomatic.
Rest and aspirate the inflamed joints.
Indomethacin is the drug of first choice.
The majority of cases settle spontaneously within 4–10 weeks, but the disease may recur in 50%. (The urethritis may respond to tetracycline 2 g/day for 10 days.)

ACUTE GENERALISED ARTHRITIS

Still's disease—juvenile form

A childhood disease usually of acute onset with fever and skin rashes. Joint pain is not an essential feature (absent in 25% at onset) and may be monoarticular (30%) at the onset. Subcutaneous nodules are rare. Eye changes include chronic iridocyclitis (10%), corneal band opacity and complicated cataract. Lymphadenopathy is present in 30%, splenomegaly in 20% and simple pericarditis in 10%. One-third of patients present with a history of insidious polyarthritis as in adult rheumatoid arthritis. Tests of rheumatoid factor are usually negative (85%).

Prognosis

The majority of cases settle spontaneously with minimal or no disability. Bone growth may be retarded. In one-third the disease continues into adult life.

ACUTE RHEUMATIC FEVER

An acute febrile systemic disorder affecting mainly the heart and joints following a streptococcal infection (group A, β-haemolytic), occurring usually between the ages of 5 and 15 years. The disease is now very rare in the UK.

Diagnosis

In the text below, double asterisks denote major criteria, single asterisks minor criteria. The diagnosis is made if there are one major and two minor, or two major with evidence of previous streptococcal infection.

Symptoms

The disease usually presents with flitting **polyarthropathy or **carditis (40%), the former being more common in adults and the latter in children. Both may be present at the same time but carditis is uncommon over the age of 20. The involved joints may be exquisitely *tender. There may be a history of streptococcal infection of the throat or skin 10–20 days previously. Rarely, children may present with **chorea.

Examination

General

The dominant features are *fever (90%) and flitting arthropathy of large joints (small joints may be affected in the elderly) which are exquisitely tender. Erythema nodosum and erythema *marginatum (5%) are more common in children. Symmetrical subcutaneous **nodules (10%) lying over bony prominences and extensor surfaces occur virtually only in children and their presence probably correlates with severe carditis.

Sign of carditis

Myocarditis: tachycardia, cardiomegaly, heart failure. Endocarditis: any valve may be involved and cause transient murmurs. A transient mitral diastolic murmur (Carey–Coombs) is the most common. Mitral systolic and aortic murmurs also occur.
Pericarditis: friction rub or small effusion.

Investigation

The *ESR is raised. *ASO titre may be raised or rising (more than 200 units/ml) and *haemolytic streptococci may be isolated from the throat. The *WBC is raised and a hypochromic normocytic anaemia, unresponsive to iron therapy, may develop. The ECG may show *first degree heart block. Almost any rhythm disorder may occur. Chest X-ray may demonstrate progressive cardiac enlargement.

Management

Bed rest
Immobilise inflamed joints.
Acetylsalicylic acid. The oral dose is 6–12 g/day to achieve blood levels of 2.1–2.4 mmol/litre (30–35 mg/100 ml). Side effects of nausea, tinnitus and blurring of vision may limit the dosage. The symptomatic response to salicylates is characteristic. Steroids are frequently used with salicylates but there is no evidence that either improves the prognosis.
Penicillin G is given during the acute stages and oral penicillin (125–250 mg bd) continued in those with cardiac involvement for at least 5 years and preferably until 20 years of age to prevent recurrence. Erythromycin is used for patients sensitive to penicillin.
NB Sodium salicylate is best avoided because of the sodium load and because it is a less effective analgesic.

POSTINFECTIOUS ARTHRALGIA

Low-grade polyarthralgia may follow some infections e.g. glandular fever, German measles, *Mycoplasma pneumoniae* and viral hepatitis, meningococcal septicaemia and persist for months or years. The asociation of this with erythema chronicum migrans occurs in Lyme disease following tickborne infection with the spirochaete *Borrelia burgdorferi* (this may present as viral meningitis with isolated cranial nerve lesions. Diagnosis is by an immunofluorescent antibody test. Penicillin or cefotaxime are the antibiotics of choice.)

OSTEOARTHRITIS

A common degenerative disorder of the joint surface. It is related to age, obesity, previous joint injury and deformity.

Incidence

It is radiologically universal after the age of 55 years and present in distal interphalangeal joints of the hands (50%), the carpometacarpal joints of the thumb (30%), cervical spine (40%), lumbar spine (40%), knees (30%) and hips (20%).

Clinical features

There is pain worse with movement and towards the end of the day. There is also stiffness, immobility, deformity and occasionally nerve root involvement. The joints may be red, warm and tender and even produce an effusion (beware of an infected effusion). Joint involvement is asymmetrical. The stiffness tends to wear off in 10–15 min of exercise (cf. rheumatoid arthritis in 1–2 h).

Investigation

Joint X-rays show a loss of joint space, osteophytes and sclerosis of subchondral bone sometimes with cyst formation. Synovial aspirates produce <100 WBC/mm^3 and these are chiefly monocytes.

Management

Effective analgesia with or without anti-inflammatory agents including paracetamol and the NSAIDs. Obese patients should lose weight if the arthritis affects weight-bearing joints.

A walking stick and special orthopaedic shoes may be very effective in relieving symptoms. Orthopaedic surgery can offer arthrodesis, arthroplasty, and joint replacement (hips, knees, fingers and perhaps elbows).

Endocrine disease

Diabetes mellitus (page 198) and disorders of the thyroid gland are the only common forms of endocrine disease.

THYROID

Enlargement of the thyroid of varying degrees is frequent, especially in women, and large non-toxic goitres are not uncommon. Both hypothyroidism and hyperthyroidism are relatively common. Thyroid cancer is rare.

Non-toxic goitre

Aetiology

The enlargement of the gland (visible and palpable) is due to an increased secretion of thyroid stimulating hormone (TSH) secondary to diminished output of thyroid hormones. The causes are:

Simple goitre. Iodine deficiency especially in areas of endemic goitre. Sporadic goitre is probably due to relative iodine deficiency for that patient. Iodine requirement is increased at puberty in girls and during pregnancy. The gland tends to become nodular as age increases.

Goitrogens, e.g. iodides in large doses (in some cough linctuses), antithyroid drugs such as para-aminosalicylic acid (PAS), phenylbutazone, lithium and many others, are rare as causes (except when used therapeutically, e.g. carbimazole).

Inborn errors of thyroid hormone synthesis (dyshormonogenesis). Six types of enzyme defect are known. All are rare. They are autosomal recessive and the commonest is associated with nerve deafness (Pendred's syndrome) and due to impaired organic binding of iodine.

Clinical presentation

A painless swelling of the thyroid is usually noticed by the patient or relatives. If untreated it may develop into a large nodular goitre and give pressure symptoms, especially if there is retrosternal extension.

Differential diagnosis

Autoimmune thyroiditis (Hashimoto's disease).
Toxic goitre.
Cancer of the thyroid.
Solitary nodule—benign (rare) and carcinoma (very rare).

Investigation

Serum T_3, T_4 and TSH if hyperthyroidism is suspected, or T_4 and TSH if hypothyroidism.

Thyroid antibodies for Hashimoto's disease.

X-ray of neck thoracic inlet if pressure symptoms are present.

Ultrasound will distinguish solid or cystic masses and whether single or multiple.

Fine needle aspiration with cytology may be diagnostic but some surgeons prefer excision.

Prophylaxis

Iodised salt, especially during pregnancy. Seafish in the diet.

Treatment

Thyroxine 0.1–0.15 mg daily for long periods to suppress TSH hypersecretion. Surgery for pressure symptoms (rarely necessary) and removal of cold nodules.

Thyrotoxicosis (hyperthyroidism)

Aetiology

The clinical picture results from an excess of thyroid hormones (T_4 and/or T_3). Graves' disease refers to the common form of hyperthyroidism in which eye signs and toxic symptoms accompany diffuse enlargement of the gland (F : M = 5 : 1) with antibodies and occasional pretibial myxoedema. Thyrotoxicosis is an autoimmune disease associated with thyroid stimulating immunoglobulins (TSI), against the TSH receptor site on the thyroid follicular cell membrane. There also appears to be a thyroid growth immunoglobulin (TGI), which may independently determine the size of any goitre. An ophthalmopathic immunoglobulin to eye muscle basement membrane may be causative and independent. There is an association with HLA B8 and DR3. Rarely a single toxic nodule may produce thyrotoxicosis. There is a strong genetic factor. Self-administered thyroxine should not be forgotten as a cause of hyperthyroidism, particularly in doctors and nurses. Iodine in health foods and some cough medicines may precipitate hyperthyroidism.

Clinical presentation

The symptoms and signs, except the eye signs, can be deduced from a knowledge of the pharmacological action of thyroxine (T_4) and triiodothyronine (T_3).

The most helpful symptoms are preference for cold weather, excessive sweating, increased appetite and weight loss, 'nervousness', tiredness and palpitations.

The most helpful signs are goitre, especially with a murmur over it, exophthalmos, lid retraction and lid lag, hot moist palms, tremor and excessive movements, tachycardia or atrial fibrillation.

Atypical presentations

Atrial fibrillation, tachycardia or cardiac failure in middle age or older should always suggest thyrotoxicosis.

Unexplained weight loss in apparently euthyroid patients.
Very rarely. Toxic manic confusion. Severe proximal limb girdle myopathy. Diarrhoea.

Differential diagnosis

Thyrotoxicosis is often difficult to differentiate from an anxiety state particularly when this is associated with a simple goitre. The palms tend to be moist but cold in anxiety state.

Investigation

Always carry out at least one, and preferably two, tests before starting treatment to confirm and document the diagnosis. Use serum T_3, T_4 (raised) and TSH (suppressed) in borderline cases. CT scan of the orbit demonstrates thickened external ocular muscle. The orbit contains excess mucopolysaccharide (and water).

Treatment

Antithyroid drugs. Carbimazole can be given in a titration regime to block thyroid hormone synthesis and sufficient to produce a euthyroid state. For this, give carbimazole 15 mg three times a day for 3 weeks reducing to 5 mg three times a day or more according to the response and maintained for 12–18 months. Review at 6 months, 1 year and 18 months. When the drugs are stopped, relapse occurs in at least two thirds within 1 or 2 years and either surgery or radioiodine is used (see below).

In the block-replacement regime, enough carbimazole is given to block all thyroid hormone production with 40–60 mg in a single daily dose, plus replacement of normal thyroid requirements with l-thyroxine, 100–150 µg/day. Compliance is improved, thyroid status more stable and relapse possibly less common after treatment is stopped. Side-effects of carbimazole include skin rashes, loss of hair and neutropenia (sore throat is usually the first symptom). Propylthiouracil is a suitable alternative. In pregnancy, carbimazole in the usual doses remains the treatment of choice, with tests of thyroid function kept at the upper end of the normal range. The baby can be breast fed if the patient remains on the drug.

Propranolol 20 mg three times a day may give rapid improvement in cardiac symptoms and sense of well-being. It should not be used alone in thyrotoxic heart failure or as the sole therapy.

Radioactive iodine therapy is given after rendering the more toxic patient euthyroid with drugs, stopping them 4 days before administration, and reintroducing them 4 days afterwards while awaiting the 5-week delay before the effects of radiotherapy become apparent.

One strategy is to give an ablative, or near-ablative dose of radioiodine (about 550 MBq = 15 mCi) followed by standard replacement doses of thyroid hormone. Patients given more conventional doses of radioiodine experience an inexorable cumulative incidence of hypothyroidism of about 4% per year. Between 5% and 15% develop hypothyroidism in the first year.

Patients with a single toxic adenoma or a toxic multinodular goitre can have a large dose of radioiodine with relatively little chance of hypothyroidism, because the unaffected parts of the thyroid have been dormant following suppression of thyroid-stimulating (thyrotrophic) hormone (TSH) by excessive thyroid hormone secretion, and do not take up the radioiodine.

Surgery. This requires adequate pre-operative treatment with carbimazole and later potassium iodide. Subtotal thyroidectomy is advised for (*a*) failure of medical treatment, and drug sensitivity in the young, and (*b*) large multinodular goitres especially with pressure symptoms as they may enlarge with medical therapy, and for cosmetic reasons. One year later about 80% are euthyroid, 15% hypothyroid and 5% have relapsed. Complications include hypothyroidism (eventually 10–15% in those with high antibody titres), recurrence of hyperthyroidism, recurrent laryngeal nerve palsy (rare), hypoparathyroidism (rare).

Treatment of complications

Eye. Lid retraction (sclera visible below the upper lid) usually responds to treatment of the thyrotoxicosis. Exophthalmos (sclera visible above lower lid) results from the swelling of retro-orbital tissues and may not improve and may progress. In malignant exophthalmos there is weakness of the external ocular muscles, often with diplopia, oedema of the conjunctivae and corneal damage from exposure. Treatment is difficult. The strabismus and lid retraction of dysthyroid ophthalmopathy may respond to intramuscular injection of botulinum toxin (neurotoxin A) but the place of this in routine therapy is not yet determined. Local or systemic steroids may be required with tarsorrhaphy in severe cases. Orbital decompression may be required. The condition remits slowly over years with or without treatment.

Atrial fibrillation responds poorly to digoxin and larger doses are often needed until the patient is euthyroid. Cardioversion may then be used. Propranolol or other β-blocker may control severe tachycardia. Heart failure is unusual and responds to antithyroid drugs plus conventional treatment.

Thyrotoxic crisis. This is rare but dangerous. Dexamethasone (2 mg qds) inhibits T_4 conversion to T_3 in the tissues. Oral carbimazole (60–120 mg) is followed by potassium iodide (60 mg daily in divided doses). Beta-blockade (propranolol 80 mg qds) is usually required. Oxygen should be given and particular attention paid to fluid balance since sweating is marked.

Hypothyroidism

This results from a low level of circulating thyroid hormone, either free thyroxine (T_4) or triiodothyronine (T_3). The term 'myxoedema' means that there is a deposition of a mucopolysaccharide beneath the skin producing a non-pitting swelling of the subcutaneous tissues.

Aetiology

Autoimmune thyroiditis. This may present as Hashimoto's disease when a goitre is present, or as 'spontaneous' or 'primary' hypothyroidism if the gland atrophies without producing a goitre. Circulating thyroid antibodies are present.

Destructive therapy for hyperthyroidism or carcinoma by operation or by radioiodine.

Primary thyroid agenesis may produce cretinism in infants.

Ingestion of goitrogens, usually an antithyroid drug (including iodine) in too large doses or for too long.

Secondary to hypopituitarism; this is rare.

Inborn errors of thyroid metabolism (dyshormonogenesis).

There may be a family history of thyroid disease or of autoimmune disease, e.g. 10% have pernicious anaemia.

Clinical presentation

The onset is insidious, difficult to distinguish from depression and the condition may be far advanced before it is recognised. All who have had destructive therapy to the thyroid should be followed up at 6-monthly intervals. Many of the symptoms occur also in euthyroid individuals, e.g. tiredness, loss of hair. Those which have the greatest diagnostic value are intolerance of cold, diminished energy, physical tiredness, slow cerebration, increase in weight, hoarseness of voice, diminished sweating, dry and rough skin, dry and unruly hair, deafness, constipation, muscular pains and paraesthesiae (carpal tunnel syndrome).

The physical signs include a typical facial appearance with periorbital puffiness and pallor, coarse and cold skin, slow movements, hoarse voice, slow pulse and a slowing of the recovery phase of the ankle jerk reflexes. Ischaemic heart disease is common. CNS involvement may produce intellectual impairment and dementia (myxoedema madness) and coma (with hypothermia). Only 5% of patients presenting with hypothermia have hypothyroidism.

Investigation

All suspected cases should be investigated: Serum T_4 is reduced and this stimulates pituitary secretions of TSH (raised in primary hypothyroidism)

Raised serum cholesterol (page 210) is present though not important in the diagnosis

Anaemia (normochromic or macrocytic)

ECG shows slow rate and low voltage with flattened or inverted T waves

Rise in titre of thyroid antibodies

Treatment

Thyroxine is given in doses of 25–50 µg a day, starting with a low dose and raising it every 14 days to achieve normal levels of TSH. The average maintenance daily dose is 150 µg. Free T_4 levels are above the normal range given for the untreated patient. If ischaemic heart disease is present, the lowest dose should be used initially. Patients should be warned that treatment is for life. Osteoporosis is a long term risk of over-treatment.

Autoimmune thyroiditis

This term usually refers to disorders of the thyroid gland in which circulating thyroid antibodies are present in the plasma; in addition lymphoid and plasma cells are found in excess in the thyroid gland. The patients may be hypothyroid, euthyroid or hyperthyroid. Hashimoto's disease refers to the condition in which autoimmune thyroiditis has produced a hard nodular goitre. Destruction of thyroid-hormone-producing tissue causes a rise in TSH which leads to thyroid enlargement. At this stage, the level of the circulating thyroid hormones, although reduced for that person, may be within the 'normal limits' and there is no evidence of hypothyroidism. However, thyroid reserve is diminished, and later the free thyroxine falls further and symptoms of hypothyroidism occur in about 2% per annum. By then the patient has a goitre which is often hard and sometimes nodular. In some patients the development of autoimmune hypothyroidism is associated with progressive fibrosis of the gland without the production of a goitre. These patients present with hypothyroidism without a goitre.

Clinical presentation

Hashimoto's disease presents as a patient with a goitre who is either euthyroid or hypothyroid. The goitre must be distinguished from other types of non-toxic goitre and from carcinoma of the thyroid.

Investigation

Thyroid antibodies may be directed against thyroglobulin or the microsomal fraction of thyroid cells. The former include the highly specific but relatively insensitive precipitin test, and the sensitive but less specific tanned red cell agglutination test. The complement fixation test against microsomal antibodies is not very specific. The gland usually takes up a normal amount of iodine, i.e. the radioiodine uptake is within normal limits but there is faulty utilisation of iodine and the iodine is discharged from the gland by potassium perchlorate in about half the cases. The T_4 is in the lower range of normal or in the hypothyroid range.

Management

Thyroxine in full doses will suppress TSH, cause the gland to diminish in size, and relieve any symptoms of hypothyroidism if present.

Acute thyroiditis

Although relatively uncommon, acute thyroiditis may often follow an upper respiratory tract infection or other microbial infection (e.g. measles, infectious mononucleosis, mumps, coxsackie). There is fever and malaise, usually with some local swelling and tenderness of the gland and sometimes dysphagia. Initially there may be some hyperthyroidism. The serum thyroxine may be normal or raised but the radioiodine uptake is suppressed. The differential diagnosis includes carcinoma (less tender but harder), haemorrhage into a cyst or Hashimoto's thyroiditis. Pyogenic infection in the thyroid causes a more severe illness.

Management

Simple analgesia may suffice. Prednisolone 10 mg tds may be necessary and can usually be tailed off rapidly.

Thyroid cancer (page 40)

All types are rare and some carry a relatively good prognosis. Ionising radiation during childhood is a predisposing factor. The main types and their clinical features are:

Papillary

Commonest type. It occurs in the relatively young and may present with lymph gland enlargement (lateral aberrant thyroid). It is often TSH-dependent and regresses if thyroxine is given. The prognosis is relatively good.

Follicular

Often produces functioning secondaries which are sensitive to radioiodine. It has a relatively good prognosis and is relatively common.

Anaplastic

Usually presents with gland enlargement in the elderly and is highly malignant.

Medullary

Rare. It secretes calcitonin and may produce ectopic corticotrophin and other substances. It may be associated with a phaeochromocytoma (page 196). The prognosis is poor though relatively better than anaplastic cancers. Relatives should be screened.

Thyroid nodules

A thyroid nodule which appears to be single is usually not single. Even if it is, the likelihood of malignancy is low. Ultrasound may distinguish solid from cystic lesions, but this does not distinguish between the presence or absence of thyroid carcinoma. Fine needle biopsy and aspiration of fluid for cytology may miss a carcinoma and single cysts tend to refill.

PITUITARY

The hypothalamus controls the secretion of the anterior and posterior pituitary hormones. Hypothalamic nerve fibres liberate substances which are carried in the portal bloodstream to the pituitary gland and there cause release, synthesis or inhibition of pituitary hormones. At least nine factors have been suggested and three, corticotrophic releasing hormone (CRH), thyrotrophin releasing hormone (TRH) and gonadotrophin releasing hormone (GnRH), have been isolated and their chemical structure determined. The latter causes release of both LH and FSH. Prolactin release is inhibited by dopamine.

The anterior lobe produces at least six types of hormone—growth hormone (GH), follicle stimulating hormone (FSH), luteinising hormone (LH), thyroid stimulating hormone (TSH), adrenocorticotrophic hormone (ACTH), and prolactin (PRL). The posterior lobe secretes two hormones, antidiuretic hormone (ADH) and oxytocin. The gland has a close anatomical and physiological relationship to the hypothalamus. The anatomical relationship to the optic chiasma is important and all patients with suspected pituitary tumours should have their visual fields plotted. X-ray of the pituitary fossa and CT scan will accurately define the pituitary fossa.

The clinical features of pituitary disease differ according to the type of the lesion and the region of the gland which is predominantly affected. All are rare and in examinations will have received some treatment. Failure of secretion is more common than increased secretion. Non-functional (chromophobe) adenoma is the commonest cause of hypopituitarism. It also gives rise to increased intracranial pressure and to local pressure effects. Prolactinomas are the commonest secreting tumours of the pituitary. They cause infertility in women, and impotence with gynaecomastia in men. The commonest tumour in childhood is the craniopharyngioma which often calcifies. Classically eosinophilic tumours (rare) give giantism in the child or acromegaly in the adult; and basophil hyperplasia or adenoma produce Cushing's syndrome. About 10% of Cushing's syndrome is due to a larger, non-functional adenoma. However, acromegaly may be associated with eosinophil, chromophobe or mixed-cell tumours.

Hypopituitarism (Simmond's disease)

The pattern of deficiency depends on the nature of the lesion and its rate of progress. In general, deficiencies of GH, FSH and LH secretions occur early, TSH and ACTH next. Last of all ADH secretion fails if the posterior lobe is involved by surgical intervention or suprasellar disease. Deficiency of each hormone is measured by suitable blood hormone assay and the integrity of the target organs assessed by applying the appropriate physiological stimulus, e.g. ACTH.

Aetiology

Iatrogenic from hypophysectomy or irradiation—adequate replacement therapy prevents symptoms from occurring.

Non-functional (chromophobe) adenoma.

Post-partum pituitary necrosis in the female (Sheehan's syndrome). This is now extremely rare with improved standards of midwifery.

Other tumours (including secondary tumours), granulomas (sarcoid and tuberculosis) and head injury—all rare.

Clinical presentation

In children hypopituitarism produces pituitary infantilism (Peter Pan Dwarfs i.e. small but well formed and in proportion). In adults the presentation depends upon (a) the pattern of deficiency of the various hormones; and (b) associated pressure symptoms. The symptoms and signs can be worked out from a knowledge of the functions of the target organs involved.

Hormone deficiency

Loss of sexual function occurs, both primary with amenorrhoea and loss of libido, and secondary with loss of body hair (male patients may find shaving unnecessary).

Adrenal insufficiency (page 194) from failure of ACTH occurs but there is little change in electrolyte metabolism since aldosterone is still secreted.

Pallor and skin depigmentation occur.

Symptoms of hypothyroidism (page 182) from lack of TSH appear but there is no myxoedema, e.g. the face is not coarsened.

Coma may occur from low cortisol levels, spontaneous hypoglycaemia or hypothermia.

Pressure effects

Compression of the optic chiasma produces bitemporal hemianopia and optic atrophy.

Pressure on the hypothalamus may cause somnolence and weight gain.

NB In the male, hypopituitarism is usually due to a non-functional adenoma or large prolactinoma. In Sheehan's syndrome, there is a history of post-partum haemorrhage, failure of lactation with atrophy of breast tissue, and amenorrhoea in addition to the other effects described.

Investigation

Assessment of pituitary function involves:

- measurement of pituitary hormones (TSH, ACTH, FSH, LH, GH and PRL)
- measurement of target organ secretion (thyroid and adrenal, and sex hormones)
- dynamic tests of hypothalamic pituitary function:
  insulin hypoglycaemia test (page 195)
  tetracosactrin tests (page 195)
  metyrapone test (page 192)
  TRH stimulation test
  LH–RH test

Treatment

The pituitary is removed if there are pressure symptoms, particularly visual loss unless a prolactinoma is present, when bromocriptine usually shrinks the tumour without surgery.

Replacement therapy by:

- cyclical oestrogen–progesterone therapy in women or intramuscular depot testosterone esters every 2–4 weeks (e.g. Sustanon 250) in men
- hydrocortisone 20 mg in the morning and 10 mg at night. Fludrocortisone is not usually required
- thyroxine 0.1–0.3 mg (100–300 μg) daily
- coma is treated as in Addisonian crisis (page 194)

Acromegaly

Excess growth hormone gives acromegaly in the adult (after the epiphyses have fused) and giantism in earlier life. The onset is between 20 and 40 years.

Giantism is almost always the result of the action of excessive secretion of GH before the epiphyses have united. Later in life pituitary failure tends to occur and giants are therefore not usually strong, aggressive or virile.

Aetiology

Excessive secretion of growth hormone from an adenoma of the pituitary, often of eosinophil cells. Growth hormone causes overgrowth of soft tissues including the skin, tongue and viscera and of bones. It has an anti-insulin action.

Clinical presentation

The onset is insidious often with early changes (look at old photographs). Headache occurs early due to stretching of the dura mater. Pressure effects with bitemporal hemianopia are rarer. Excessive secretion of GH causes:

Face. Increase in size of skull, supraorbital ridges, lower jaw (separation of teeth) and the sinuses.
The tongue is enlarged.
Vertebral enlargement, and kyphosis from osteoporosis.
Hands and feet are spade-shaped and carpal tunnel syndrome may be present.
Enlarged heart, liver and thyroid.
Hypertension (15%).
Diabetes mellitus (10%) and reduced glucose tolerance (30%).
Arthropathy (50%).

The following also occur:

Acne, hirsutes, excessive sweating.
Gynaecomastia and galactorrhoea (prolactin excess).
Hypogonadism, oligomenorrhoea.

Investigation

Assay of growth hormone by radioimmunoassay; the levels are raised only in active disease and are not suppressed by glucose in a standard GTT.
Perimetry for bitemporal visual field defects (50%).
X-ray of skull for enlargement of the sella, erosion of the clinoid processes, supraorbital ridges and lower jaw. The floor of the pituitary fossa may appear eroded or double in lateral view tomograms.
CT scan to show suprasellar extension.
X-ray of hands for tufting of the terminal phalanges and increased joint spaces due to hypertrophy of the cartilage. The heel pad is usually thickened. These tests are interesting rather than diagnostic.
The glucose tolerance curve may be diabetic.
Fasting serum phosphate may be raised but is of no diagnostic value.
Chest X-ray and ECG may show left ventricular hypertrophy from hypertension.

Prognosis and treatment

Life expectancy is halved due to cardiorespiratory complications. Successful management means destruction of the tissue producing excess growth hormone. Surgery is indicated for progressive visual deterioration (regular perimetry is obligatory) and some would recommend it for all acromegalics who are fit for surgery. Transsphenoidal hypophysectomy is the treatment of choice. Craniotomy is sometimes used in those with suprasellar extension. Yttrium-90 implants or external irradiation are alternatives to surgical removal in active disease, but may cause further damage to the optic tracts, diabetes insipidus and aseptic bone necrosis, and have much lower cure rates. Cerebrospinal rhinorrhea may result from yttrium implantation. Bromocriptine reduces growth hormone and prolactin levels and may be a useful adjunct to conventional therapy or used as sole therapy. Unlike destructive therapies, diabetes insipidus is not produced. Somatostatin analogues (octreotide) may be used, particularly for young patients, male or female, who wish to retain fertility.

Diabetes insipidus
A very rare disease due to deficiency of ADH (vasopressin).

Aetiology
Idiopathic, often familial and the commonest form

Tumours
Craniopharyngioma or secondary tumour.
Surgery or radiation to pituitary gland.
Head injury—usually mild and short-lived. Rarely complete and permanent with transection of the pituitary stalk with frontal vault fractures.
Granulomas, e.g. sarcoid; or infections, e.g. basal meningitis.

Clinical presentation
Polyuria and polydipsia—5–20 litres urine/24 h.

Investigation
The specific gravity of the urine is very low and fails to increase with water deprivation. Fluids are allowed overnight and stopped in the morning. It is dangerous to lose more than 2–3% of the body weight. In normal people plasma osmolality does not rise above 300 mosmol/kg and urine osmolality rises to 600 mosmol/kg. In diabetes insipidus the former rises and the latter does not, or remains at about plasma level. Vasopressin corrects the abnormality in ADH deficient diabetes insipidus but not in the nephrogenic type.

Differential diagnosis
Psychogenic polydipsia. Thirst dominates the picture. The patient resents the water deprivation test, and surreptitious drinking is common. Renal concentrating power may be moderately reduced due to the prolonged polyuria and consequent low medullary osmolality.

Nephrogenic diabetes insipidus. This refers to a vasopressin (ADH)-resistant polyuria. This is a rare sex-linked recessive inherited disorder with a primary renal tubular defect of water reabsorption. Secondary nephrogenic diabetes insipidus occurs with:

- diabetes mellitus (glycosuria)
- chronic renal failure
- post-obstructive uropathy
- hypercalcaemia
- hypokalaemia
- lithium toxicity

Treatment

Desmopressin (DDAVP or arginine vasopressin) nasal spray 10–20 µg bd has replaced lysine vasopressin in the treatment of ADH deficiency.

Carbamazepine 200–800 mg daily may increase the renal response to ADH. Chlorpropamide (100–300 mg daily) acts similarly but is obsolescent due to the risk of hypoglycaemia.

Thiazide diuretics probably act by reducing glomerular filtration rate and are also used in nephrogenic diabetes insipidus.

Prolactinoma

These tumours cause galactorrhoea in both sexes and gonadal dysfunction—infertility in the female and impotence in the male. Measurement of prolactin levels suggests the diagnosis usually before pressure symptoms occur. The tumours vary in size from pinhead (microadenoma) to very large (rare) and may necrose. Hyperprolactinaemia may be caused by a variety of physiological stimuli such as pregnancy and stress and by certain drugs such as oestrogens and tranquillisers. Bromocriptine (1.25–10 mg or more daily) inhibits prolactin secretion and is usually tried before surgery or radiotherapy. Visual fields need checking periodically because pituitary tumours may press on the optic chiasma to cause a bitemporal field loss. If the patient becomes pregnant, a small tumour may enlarge rapidly.

ADRENAL

Adrenal glands

The medulla secretes adrenaline and noradrenaline. The cortex produces steroid hormones of which the most important are cortisol (hydrocortisone) and aldosterone. The secretion of most of the steroids is controlled by pituitary corticotrophin (ACTH) which itself is released by the hypothalamic hormone—corticotrophin releasing hormone factor (CRF). The secretion of aldosterone is independent of the pituitary and controlled by the renin-aldosterone system. The adrenals also produce androgens and oestrogens. The effects of the three main groups of adrenocortical hormones differ. In summary they are:

Glucocorticoids (e.g. cortisol)

Raise the blood sugar and antagonise insulin. They have a permissive effect on the action of catecholamines on the heart and blood vessels and are essential for the body's response to shock. They suppress the reaction to injury, infection and inflammation. In excess they have a protein catabolic effect, atrophy skin and weaken capillaries. They reduce the circulating eosinophil and lymphocyte counts. They cause sodium retention and potassium depletion and alkalosis when given in large doses or over long period.

Mineralocorcoids (e.g. aldosterone)

Cause sodium retention and potassium depletion, with hypertension, alkalosis and oedema. The synthetic steroids, fludrocortisone and deoxycorticosterone acetate have similar actions.

Sex hormones

Produce effects depending on the dominance of male hormone, e.g. androsterone, or female hormone, e.g. oestrogens and progesterone. Hence they may be virilising or feminising. Androgens antagonise some of the metabolic effects of the glucocorticoids.

Cushing's syndrome

Aetiology

The syndrome is the result of *excess corticosteroids* and by far the commonest cause is *prolonged treatment with relatively large doses*. Most of the synthetic analogues of cortisone produce these side-effects but they are less liable to give rise to sodium retention. Apart from iatrogenic disease, this disorder is very rare.

The other causes are:
- *Basophil* or *chromophobe hyperplasia* or *adenoma* of the pituitary gland, with excess production of corticotrophin (60%). This produces bilateral adrenal hyperplasia and is called pituitary-dependent Cushing's syndrome and is properly called Cushing's disease
- *Primary tumours* of the adrenals, either adenoma (20%) or carcinoma (10%)
- *Secondary* to carcinoma elsewhere—usually an oat cell carcinoma of the bronchus causing the 'ectopic ACTH syndrome'. Other sites are the thymus, pancreas, thyroid or ovary. Pigmentation may occur in this condition

Clinical presentation

The onset is insidious with:

Alteration in appearance with redistribution of body fat, 'mooning' of the face and truncal or 'buffalo' obesity (about 90%). The limbs are often spared but the obesity may be generalised. Growth is retarded in children.

Protein breakdown leads to muscle weakness which may present as a proximal myopathy, wide purple striae (50%) on the abdomen, thighs and buttocks, and easy bruising (30%). The striae of obesity are pink.

Osteoporosis with backache and vertebral collapse (50%).

Disturbance of carbohydrate tolerance which may amount to diabetes (10%).

Electrolyte disturbance with sodium retention, potassium loss and hypokalaemic alkalosis—especially in the ectopic ACTH syndrome, where ACTH levels are very high. Renal stones may occur (20%).

Hypertension, probably related to sodium retention (60%).

Masculinisation due to adrenal androgens—amenorrhoea, hirsutism, deep voice, greasy skin with acne in the female (80%).

Mental disturbance—depression or mania and sometimes exaggeration of previous psychiatric abnormalities.

NB Almost all of these can be produced by large doses of corticosteroids.

Investigation

Estimate of plasma cortisol—looking for absence of normal diurnal variation. Radioimmunoassay of ACTH.

Increase in urinary 24-h urinary free cortisol (or 17-hydroxycorticosteroids, which are normally <1% of total cortisol).

Determine whether it is adrenal- (adenoma or carcinoma) or pituitary-dependent using metyrapone and dexamethasone suppression tests. If CT scan shows bilateral hyperplasia this indicates external ACTH stimulus either from the pituitary or from a carcinoma. Inferior petrosal sinus sampling after CRF stimulation will confirm the diagnosis of Cushing's disease.

Screening of basal function

24-h urinary free cortisol (UFC)— 11-OHCS—is raised in Cushing's syndrome cases but not in simple obesity or polycystic ovary syndrome.

24-h excretion of steroid metabolites, 17-oxogenic steroids. This measures the compounds which can be converted to oxosteroids by oxidation and includes cortisol, its metabolites and some other steroid compounds. Normal 24-h ranges: 25–70 μmol (7–20 mg male) and 20–55 μmol (5–15 mg female). The test is not specific and values are often slightly raised in simple obesity, and up to 25% of patients with Cushing's syndrome may have normal results. It is used when UFC is not available.

Diurnal variation in serum cortisol. The patient should be unstressed at the time of sampling. This level is normally highest at 9 a.m. 200–700 nmol/litre (7–25 g/100 ml) and lowest at midnight. The midnight value is almost always raised in Cushing's syndrome. It is the loss of diurnal variation which is the important observation.

CT scan of adrenal area.

Dynamic tests of adrenocortical–pituitary function

Dexamethasone suppression tests. Short screening test. 1 mg is taken between 11 p.m. and midnight and the 9 a.m. plasma cortisol estimated (normal <200 nmol/litre)

6-day tests. Twenty-four hour urines for 17-oxogenic steroids are collected; 2 days control, 2 days while the patient takes 0.5 mg 6-hourly and 2 days on 2.0 mg 6-hourly. In patients with Cushing's syndrome 17-oxogenic steroids do not fall below 20 μmol/24 h on the low dose. (Many 'normal' patients do not suppress either—40%.) The high dose of dexamethasone may help to differentiate between pituitary-dependent disease (which may suppress completely at this dose) and patients with ectopic ACTH or adrenal tumour. The results of these test are not always reliable.

A useful system is to use 24-h urinary-free cortisol and start dexamethasone test as a screen followed, if indicated, by a high-dose dexamethasone test (as an in-patient). If pituitary-dependent, the diagnosis is confirmed by inferior petrosal sinus sampling.

Management

Hypophysectomy is the treatment of choice for pituitary-dependent Cushing's syndrome. In some centres metyrapone and aminoglutethimide which block adrenal cortisol production are used to control the plasma cortisol and produce regression of symptoms in all patients with Cushing's syndrome of adrenal or pituitary origin before definitive surgical therapy. Others use mitotane (o.p.'-DDD). When bilateral adrenalectomy is performed to treat Cushing's syndrome due to a pituitary basophil or chromophobe adenoma, Nelson's syndrome may result with hyperpigmentation from excess β lipotrophin activity (MSH and ACTH) which is now not suppressed by high blood cortisol.

If the disease is primarily adrenal (yet to be called 'adrenal-dependent Cushing's syndrome'), unilateral or bilateral adrenalectomy is performed and the later is followed by replacement therapy with cortisol 20–40 mg daily and fludrocortisone 0.1 mg daily.

Removal of ectopic ACTH sources is rarely possible (bronchial carcinoma).

Conn's syndrome (primary hyperaldosteronism)

This is a very rare condition caused by a solitary benign adenoma or hyperplasia of the zona glomerulosa producing excess of aldosterone.

Clinical presentation

Hypokalaemia and muscle weakness often in attacks. Polyuria and polydipsia are secondary to the hypokalaemia.

Sodium retention often leading to hypertension but there is usually no oedema. It may mimic hypertension from other causes especially when potassium-losing diuretics are being given, or Cushing's syndrome.

Investigation

The condition is marked by renal potassium wasting i.e. serum potassium reduced often <3 mmol and urinary potassium increased for serum blood level. It is usually associated with a metabolic alkalosis. The serum sodium is usually over 140 mmol.

Stop diuretics for 3 days and if potassium is still <3.2 mmol check the urinary output of potassium: if it is <20 mmol this is appropriate to the blood concentration and is probably normal: if it is >30 mmol further investigation for primary hyperaldosteronism is required.

The serum renin is low and this differentiates it from secondary aldosteronism (which occurs in the nephrotic syndrome, cirrhosis of the liver with ascites and, rarely, in congestive cardiac failure and bronchial carcinoma).

The best screening test is a 24-h urinary aldosterone. If this is raised, take a 7 a.m. plasma specimen from a rested and recumbent patient for renin and aldosterone.

Management

Surgical resection should be considered because some tumours are malignant. Spironolactone is an antagonist to aldosterone and may be given in primary or secondary aldosteronism.

Adrenogenital syndrome

A very rare condition of infancy or childhood due to a congenital enzyme defect (usually of 21-hydroxylase) affecting cortisol synthesis. The resulting decrease in circulating cortisol stimulates overproduction of ACTH, which in turn stimulates the adrenals to produce excess of androgenic steroids. Females show virilisation early in life and are treated with cortisol. Males are less often diagnosed and may die in acute adrenal insufficiency, but if the infant survives, growth is excessive though precocious puberty results in a short final height. Treat with corticosteroids sufficient to suppress excess ACTH.

Adrenal insufficiency (Addison's disease)

Acute

Adrenal crisis. There is apathy, coma and epigastric pain. The blood sugar is low. It occurs after trauma, severe hypotension and sepsis.

Less commonly it may occur in patients previously (within 1–1½ years) or currently being treated with corticosteroids when there is trauma, surgery or acute infection or withdrawal of steroids. It may follow surgical removal of the adrenals for Cushing's syndrome or in the treatment of breast carcinoma unless there is adequate replacement therapy.

NB The Waterhouse–Friderichsen syndrome of severe acute meningococcal septicaemia, associated with purpura, is usually associated with raised levels of circulating corticosteroids despite the massive bilateral adrenal haemorrhage. It appears to be a special form of vascular rather than adrenal collapse. Adrenal haemorrhage is frequently found at postmortem as a non-specific finding.

Chronic

Insidious onset of weakness and fatigue with gastrointestinal symptoms of anorexia, weight loss, nausea, vomiting, intermittent abdominal pain and diarrhoea. Hypotension, often postural, and tachycardia occur late in the disease. Hyperpigmentation occurs in exposed areas, friction areas, hand creases, and buccal mucosa.

Chronic adrenal insufficiency (Addison's disease) is rare (4/100 000 prevalence in UK) and causes include: autoimmune adrenal destruction; adrenal infiltration with secondary carcinoma, Hodgkin's or leukaemic tissue; destruction in tuberculosis, haemochromatosis, amyloidosis and histoplasmosis where prevalent. It may be associated with other organ-specific autoimmune disease, especially Hashimoto's thyroiditis (Schmidt's syndrome).

It may occur secondary to hypopituitarism (page 186) during treatment of adrenal (or renal) tuberculosis and in the adrenogenital syndrome (page 194).

Investigation

Plasma cortisol levels are usually low and show no diurnal variation.

No increase in output after tetracosactrin (Synacthen). Serum electrolytes are usually normal but in impending crisis the sodium may be low, the potassium high and the blood urea raised.

There is a high plasma ACTH.

Screening of basal function

Both 24-h urinary 17-oxogenic steroids and 8 a.m. cortisols may be well in the normal range, even in strongly suspected cases.

A *single basal plasma ACTH assay* shows high levels in primary adrenal disease and undetectable values in pituitary disease.

Dynamic tests

Synacthen (tetracosactrin) tests

- *Short Synacthen test.* Take blood at 0, 30, and 60 min. In normal subjects, the initial level should be >170 nmol/litre (6 μg/dl), and rise by at least 190 nmol/litre (7 μg/dl) to >580 nmol/litre (21 μg/dl). If the response is flat, proceed to a long Synacthen test
- *Five-hour test* to 1 mg of depot tetracosactrin. In normal patients the serum cortisol more than doubles in the first hour
- *Three-day test.* This involves two baseline and three post-stimulation 24-h urine collections for 17-oxogenic steroids. 1 mg depot tetracosactrin i.m. is given daily. Adrenals suppressed by prolonged steroid therapy may show a response to this prolonged stimulus when they may not to a short one

Insulin hypoglycaemia test

This test is potentially lethal, particularly in adrenal failure, and is performed only by experienced hands. A blood glucose of <2 mmol/litre stimulates the hypothalamic pituitary to produce ACTH and growth hormone. Soluble insulin 0.1 to 0.2 units/kg is given intravenously (with an indwelling needle for resuscitation). The lower dose is used in patients with suspected hypofunction (pituitary) and the higher dose for those with suspected hyperfunction. The serum cortisol, glucose, growth hormone and ACTH may be measured half-hourly for 2 h. This is a fuller test of function than that below (and quicker to perform) because it includes 'stress' in the test.

Treatment

Maintenance therapy—hydrocortisone 20 mg a.m. and 10 mg p.m. and fludrocortisone 0.1 mg daily. The doses are adjusted according to response as judging by lying and standing blood pressure, plasma urea and electrolytes and clinically.

In acute crisis—intravenous hydrocortisone 100 mg 6-hourly, intravenous saline and glucose are required. Underlying infection must be treated.

Phaeochromocytoma

This is usually a benign tumour of the adrenal medulla. It can arise from other chromaffin tissues of the sympathetic nervous system, e.g. the para-aortic ganglia, and it may be associated with neurofibromatosis. Medullary thyroid carcinoma (calcitonin-producing) and parathyroid adenoma are associated with it. Very rarely it is malignant.

It is a very rare cause of hypertension (<1 in 200) but it is important to recognise, since it is treatable. It can be familial and bilateral.

Clinical presentation

The clinical features depend on the activity of the tumour and the relative amounts of adrenaline (β- and some α-effects) and noradrenaline (α-effects). Usually α-effects predominate. Some tumours secrete intermittently.

The β-effects include a rise in systolic blood pressure with an increase in heart rate, increase in the cardiac output and dilatation of muscle vessels. The α-effects include a rise in both systolic and diastolic blood pressure with reflex slowing of the heart rate and constriction of blood vessels.

A few patients have normal blood pressure between attacks of paroxysmal hypertension, but most are hypertensive all the time. In a typical attack there is pallor, palpitation, anxiety and sometimes angina, headache, sweating and nausea. The blood pressure may be very high and death may occur from myocardial infarction or a cerebrovascular accident. Hyperglycaemia may occur if adrenaline is secreted.

NB Paroxysmal bradycardia (an α-effect) may occur.

Investigation

Estimation of catecholamines (adrenaline and noradrenaline) in the blood or urine or the urinary metabolite vanillylmandelic acid (VMA) or hydroxy-methyl-mandelic acid (HMMA).

Abdominal CT scan will usually show the tumour. This has superseded aortography, which may precipitate an attack. The patient must be fully α- and β-blocked before any interventional investigation or surgery.

Treatment

The tumour is removed under cover of α- and β-blocking agents given 3–4 days previously to prevent the effects of the release of catecholamines during operation. Plasma volume must be monitored throughout the period of sympathetic blockade and during surgery the central venous pressure should be monitored because changes in pulse and blood pressure are blocked.

In emergencies, α-effects may be antagonised by phentolamine and β-effects by propranolol.

Multiple endocrine adenomatosis (MEA syndrome)

There are two main autosomal dominant syndromes, Type 1 (Wermer) and Type II (Sipple). These are tumours originating from two or more endocrine (or neural) tissues which produce peptide hormones. They are very rare.

MEA Type I refers to benign adenomas of parathyroid, pancreatic islets (hypo- or hyperglycaemia, watery diarrhoea, hypokalaemia, achlorhydria or Z–E syndrome), pituitary (prolactin), adrenal cortex and thyroid (in that order of frequency).

MEA Type II refers to the association of a phaeochromocytoma, commonly bilateral, and occasionally malignant, calcitonin-producing medullary carcinoma of the thyroid and, less commonly, parathyroid adenoma or hyperplasia.

Families tend to run true. Patients with any one of the above tumours should be screened for others within the type and, if these are discovered, all other members of the family too. In Type II there are provocative tests for calcitonin excretion (e.g. pentagastrin). Assays of both calcitonin and catecholamines are used to assess complete removal of tumour and for early recognition of recurrence.

SHORTNESS OF STATURE

The term dwarf is better avoided. The common cause is short parents. Other causes are:

Deficiency of growth hormone—sometimes familial (see *Hypopituitarism* page 186), often associated with delayed or failure of sexual development. Bone age is retarded.

Bone diseases, e.g. achondroplasia and rickets.

Malnutrition including the malabsorption syndrome.

Renal (relatively common), liver or heart failure in early childhood.

Large doses of steroids in childhood.

Cretinism and childhood hypothyroidism.

Metabolic disease

The commonest metabolic diseases are obesity and diabetes mellitus. Osteoporosis is common in the elderly.

DIABETES MELLITUS (see also pages 102–108)

The clinical picture of diabetes is due to diminished availability or effectiveness of insulin.

Primary (idiopathic diabetes)

There are half a million cases diagnosed in the UK and surveys suggest another half a million undiagnosed; i.e. roughly 2% of total population.

Secondary diabetes

This is, in comparison, uncommon and due to
- other causes of glucose intolerance: thiazide diuretics, thyrotoxicosis and pregnancy
- pancreatic destruction: carcinoma of the pancreas, pancreatitis, pancreatectomy, cystic fibrosis, haemochromatosis
- insulin antagonism: steroid therapy, Cushing's syndrome, acromegaly and phaeochromocytoma

Clinical presentation (pages 102–106)

See table 18. Only 36% of identical twins, and about 10% of non-identical twins (and sibs of diabetic subjects) develop diabetes. Genes of the histocompatibility locus antigen (HLA) system on chromosome 6 are associated particularly HLA DR3 and HLA DR4. Up to 60% of the normal population have these, and relative risk of an individual with these developing insulin-dependent diabetes mellitus (IDDM) is only 5 times that of a person without them. Non-genetic factors are thus important and a virus infection at a time of susceptibility peaking between the ages of 10 and 15 years seems likeliest.

NB If glycosuria is discovered as an incidental finding, check the drug history (diuretics and steriods) and for pregnancy.

Diagnosis

This is made on finding random blood glucose of more than 11.0 mmol/litre.

Table 18. Types of diabetes mellitus and other categories of glucose intolerance. From *Weight Concern* (1985). No. 3 (special issue). Diabetics and the Overweight.

Clinical classes	Distinguishing characteristics
Diabetes mellitus (DM) Type I insulin-dependent diabetes mellitus (IDDM)	Patients may be of any age, are usually thin, and usually have abrupt onset of signs and symptoms with insulinopenia before age 40. These patients often have strongly positive urine glucose and ketone tests and are dependent upon insulin to prevent ketoacidosis and to sustain life
Type II Non-insulin-dependent diabetes mellitus (NIDDM) (obese or nonobese)	Patients usually are older than 40 years at diagnosis, obese, and have relatively few classic symptoms. They are not prone to ketoacidosis except during periods of stress. Although not dependent upon exogenous insulin for survival, they may require it for stress-induced hyperglycaemia, and hyperglycaemia that persists in spite of other therapy
Other types of impaired glucose tolerance Impaired glucose tolerance (IGT) (obese or nonobese)	Patients with impaired glucose tolerance have plasma glucose levels that are higher than normal but not diagnostic for diabetes mellitus
Gestational diabetes mellitus (GDM)	Patients with gestational diabetes mellitus have onset or discovery of glucose intolerance during pregnancy

The standard oral glucose tolerance test is rarely required to establish the diagnosis, (75 g of glucose is taken and capillary or venous whole blood taken to be analysed by the oxidase method). Accepted values are as follows (table 19):

Table 19. Diabetes mellitus—diagnostic blood glucose values.

	Diagnostic	
	Capillary	Venous
Fasting	≤7	≤7
2 hours	≤11	≤10

Complications

Vascular

These account for 75% of deaths.
- *Large vessel disease*. Atheroma (page 308) is widespread and early in onset. Ischaemic heart disease produces angina and myocardial infarction (five times more common in middle-aged diabetics than in the general population). Atheromatous occlusion of large vessels is 40 times more common and may produce gangrene of the feet (page 342) (see *Hyperlipidaemia* (page 209)
- *Small vessel disease*. Diabetic microangiopathy is associated with homogeneous thickening of the vascular basement membrane and endothelial proliferation. It produces renal failure (invariably associated with retinopathy) and gangrene of the skin of the feet with wedge-shaped infarcts—arterial pulses are usually present and the skin warm. It carries a poor prognosis for life

Eye

20% of diabetics. Large changes in blood glucose levels can affect refraction reversibly.
Good control of diabetes appears to result in fewer eye complications and to slow its progress when present.
- *Background retinopathy* is evidence of increased capillary permeability. This is characterised by haemorrhages, hard exudates and microaneurysms and, although common, has little effect on vision. Microaneurysms are bulges in capillary walls, usually appearing first on the temporal side of the macula, which leak plasma to produce hard exudates. (Soft 'cotton wool' exudates are small deep retinal infarcts.) Macular oedema may develop, especially in the elderly, noninsulin-dependent diabetes mellitus (NIDDM) patient, and reduce visual acuity
- *Proliferative retinopathy* is evidence of capillary non-perfusion, and presents chiefly in the young-onset diabetic, often 15–20 years after initial diagnosis. There is new vessel formation (mainly near the disc), venous irregularity, cluster haemorrhages and cotton wool spots. Haemorrhage into the vitreous causes sudden blindness and is followed by fibrosis; this contracts leading to retinal

detachment and thrombotic glaucoma. Once it occurs, blindness follows within 5 years in 50%. Argon laser therapy is used for new vessel formation and though destructive may stop progression. Cataracts (20% of diabetic blindness) occur at a younger age in diabetic patients.

Kidney

Renal disease accounts for 30% of diabetic deaths under the age of 40 years. Uraemia and hypertension are common but both treatable conditions, the first by renal dialysis or transplantation, and the second with antihypertensive medication, particularly angiotensin-converting enzyme (ACE) inhibitors. Nephrotic syndrome occurs in under 10%; it is associated with a high mortality often within 3 years of onset.

• *Diffuse glomerular sclerosis.* This occurs in over 70% of diabetics (100% on electron microscopy). Its severity tends to correlate with the degree of renal failure. There is thickening of the basement membrane and hyaline degeneration of afferent and efferent arterioles. Similar changes may occur with arteriosclerosis and glomerulonephritis

• *Nodular glomerular sclerosis.* (Kimmelstiel–Wilson lesion). There are focal homogeneous acellular eosinophilic nodules usually at the periphery of the glomerulus consisting of excess mesangial matrix. There may be localised basement membrane thickening. This lesion is pathognomonic of diabetes; but its severity correlates poorly with the nephrotic syndrome

• *Pyelonephritis.* Glycosuria predisposes to infection; catheterisation should be avoided

• *Renal papillary necrosis* may occur in diabetes in the absence of analgesic abuse. It is caused by infarction of the papillae producing haematuria and renal failure. The papillae may slough and cause obstruction

Neuromuscular

These occur in 30% of cases.

• *Peripheral neuropathy.* This is the commonest neurological complication. Patients present with numbness, night cramps and paraesthesiae in the feet. The neuropathy is predominantly sensory and affects the lower limbs with early loss of vibration sense and absent ankle jerks. Later there is loss of pain sensation resulting in chronic painless ulcers at pressure points (even if good arterial pulses are present)

• *Mononeuritis.* Single nerve palsies may result from occlusion of the nutrient artery to the nerve, commonly the third cranial nerve, ulnar nerve or lateral popliteal nerve. These are often transient. More than one nerve can be involved (page 137)

• *Diabetic amyotrophy.* This usually occurs in middle-aged diabetics who develop painful, asymmetrical weakness and wasting of the quadriceps muscles. Recovery is the rule and appears to be related to good diabetic control

• *Autonomic neuropathy.* This may produce impotence (25% of male patients), nocturnal diarrhoea, postural hypotension (table 20) and occasionally urinary retention with overflow

Table 20. Autonomic function tests.

Parasympathetic:
  Heart rate response to deep breathing
  Heart rate response to standing
  Heart rate response to the Valsalva manoeuvre
Sympathetic:
  Blood pressure response to standing
  Blood pressure response to muscle exercise such as sustained hand grip

NB The autonomic effects of hypoglycaemia, especially pallor, sweating and tachycardia, may be reduced or absent in diabetics with an autonomic neuropathy and in patients on β-blockers.

Skin

- *Insulin sensitivity* may occur in the first month of insulin therapy with the production of tender lumps after each injection. Spontaneous recovery occurs and no change of therapy is indicated
- *Lipoatrophy.* There is painless fat atrophy and hypertrophy at injection sites. The patient should discontinue using these sites for injections because there is unpredictable absorption of insulin from them. The patient should be transferred to human insulin
- *Necrobiosis lipoidica diabeticorum.* This is rare but pathognomonic of diabetes and may precede it. It occurs usually over the shins and is characterised by atrophy of subcutaneous collagen. The lesions are violet rings with yellow masses at the periphery and scarring and atrophy at the centre
- *Photosensitivity* may occur with chlorpropamide

Intercurrent infection

This is common in diabetic patients, particularly of the urinary tract and skin. Tuberculosis and moniliasis (vulvitis and balanitis) are more common in diabetes.

Management

Most diabetics are best managed in diabetic clinics (where there is close liaison between expert physicians, special experienced nursing staff, ophthalmologist, dietician and chiropodist, and continuing education of the diabetic can be best co-ordinated) in combination with mini-clinics in general practice.

Annual review should include an assessment of diabetic control at home from the patient's record of blood glucose estimation and hypoglycaemic symptoms; visual acuity by Snellen's chart; examination of the optic fundi after dilatation of the pupils (with tropicamide) for background retinopathy (exudates and microaneurysms) and for proliferative retinopathy (neovascularisation); blood pressure check; blood urea, creatinine, urine for albuminuria and microalbuminuria; examination of the feet for neuropathy (sensation, ankle jerks), for arteriopathy (arterial pulses and temperature) and for infection and nails and calluses; inspection of injection sites.

NB Regular expert chiropody may prevent serious complications, particularly in the elderly.

Non-insulin-dependent diabetes mellitus (NIDDM)

Reduction of dietary calorie intake to roughly 1200–1500 calories with weight loss may be sufficient to reduce the blood sugar towards normal and to abolish symptoms. If not, give oral hypoglycaemic agents. Start with a sulphonylurea (e.g. glibenclamide 5–20 mg). The biguanide metformin (500–850 mg bd) may later be added. In the elderly, diet alone is usually sufficient.

NB Metformin may cause gastrointestinal side-effects and occasionally produce megaloblastic anaemia, and may predispose to lactic acidosis.

Particular attention must be paid to the care of the feet and toenails, which are frequently infected.

Insulin-dependent diabetes mellitus (IDDM)

The immediate object of therapy is to prevent hypoglycaemic and hyperglycaemic states. Good control decreases the incidence of intercurrent infection, coma, ocular and possibly neurological and renal disability. The other complications appear not to be affected by the standard of control. Hypoglycaemia remains the commonest complication of insulin therapy.

The new patient is instructed about diet, the effects of exercise, insulin therapy, injection technique, urine testing for ketones, and home blood glucose monitoring and recording. Most are controlled on empirical twice-daily insulin injection combining short- and medium-acting preparations (e.g. 12–20 units bd depending on the blood glucose) or basal/bolus with Actrapid tds (usually from a pen device) and evening Ultratard. After pancreatectomy patients usually need 20–30 units per day. Dietary caloric intake, unless excessive, is best chosen by the individual patient with professional dietetic advice, according to his personal needs, and insulin therapy adjusted for the chosen diet. Most patients are now given a low fat, high fibre, controlled calorie diet. Control is probably best monitored by home blood glucose estimations, with periodic HbA_{1c} or fructosamine at the clinic.

Though tight control of diabetes might reduce the long-term complications of retinopathy and, less likely, kidney damage, the incidence of hypoglycaemia, occasionally severe (and dangerously so), is considerably increased.

Diabetic coma

There are two common types:
- hypoglycaemic
- hyperglycaemic ketoacidosis

In clinical practice there is rarely any difficulty in differentiating between these two clinical situations. Should there be any difficulty the problem may be solved by estimating the blood sugar at the bedside with 'stix'. Unfortunately they may be unreliable in hypoglycaemia and if still in doubt 20 ml of 50% intravenous glucose can do no harm (take a blood sample first). Glucagon, 1 mg i.m. may be used if a vein cannot be found.

Hypoglycaemia

The patients are usually known diabetics on insulin or, less commonly, sulphonylurea therapy, and very rarely have insulinoma or, Addison's disease. It is caused by excess antidiabetic therapy, excess exercise, decreased food intake or an alcoholic binge. The rate of onset of symptoms is rapid. Most patients are aware of impending coma and may prevent it by taking sugar (2 lumps = 20 g). Patients present either in pre-coma with agitated, often aggressive confusion, or in coma when marked sweating is usually present.

The differential diagnosis of hypoglycaemia involves the following considerations:

- Excess insulin, which may be exogenous, endogenous (usually from insulinomas) or due to sulphonylurea therapy (frequently chlorpropamide or glibenclamide, because of their long durations of action)
- Post-gastrectomy and functional hypoglycaemia
- After excess alcohol
- Hypopituitarism and hypoadrenalism
- 'Hungry neoplasm', e.g. hepatic carcinoma

Management

Oral glucose in water or, if necessary, intravenous glucose (20–40 ml of 50%) will reverse symptoms within a minute. Glucagon 1 mg i.m. acts as rapidly and can be given by relatives.

NB Hypoglycaemia must be treated rapidly since it may produce irreversible brain damage. Corticosteroids are required in addition to glucose if Addison's disease is present.

The hypoglycaemia of chlorpropamide therapy may require continued glucose administration for 24 h (the drug's effects last up to 48 h).

Rarely, warning symptoms of hypoglycaemia may be absent on human insulin, or in those on β-blockade.

Hyperglycaemic ketoacidotic coma

This appears to be occurring less frequently perhaps due to better education of patients.

Pre-coma is of slow onset, i.e. hours or days. There is often evidence of infection (25–35%) particularly of the renal, respiratory or gastrointestinal tracts. Septicaemia and meningitis are uncommon but important causes. The patient has usually not been eating properly and has stopped taking insulin. In 25–35% there is no obvious precipitating cause and 10–20% are new cases. The patient may be confused, vomiting, hypotensive, severely dehydrated and overbreathing. The breath may smell of ketones.

Management

Venous blood should be taken for glucose, urea and electrolytes (including bicarbonate) haemoglobin and haematocrit. Arterial acid–base studies and blood gases must be performed to quantiate the acid–base disturbance:

1 *Aspiration.* There is usually gastric dilatation, and death can occur from aspiration pneumonia. If the conscious level is depressed, the gastric contents should be aspirated, preferably continuously and initially with the patient's head down.

2 *Fluid.* Start intravenous fluid therapy immediately. No fixed regime can be given and therapy depends upon an assessment of the degree of dehydration. (The average deficit is 6–8 litres—to be replaced in the first 24 h in addition to the daily requirement.) The patients are water, sodium and potassium depleted and acidotic. For moderate to severe cases, in young people, 1 litre of normal (0.9%) saline may be given in the first half-hour and repeated in the following hour and continued at a rate of 0.5–2 litres/h for the first 2 h depending upon the degree of hydration.

3 *Electrolytes.* Nearly all these patients have a low total body potassium with a deficit of 200–400 mmol on admission. Both insulin and bicarbonate will tend to exacerbate the dangers of this situation. As soon as polyuria is observed (it is usually present on admission) potassium chloride should be added at a rate of 2 g (26 mmol)/litre of i.v. fluid given hourly. In severe cases (serum bicarbonate <5 mmol/litre) some would give 250 mmol of bicarbonate and 3 g (39 mmol)/litre of potassium every hour if the serum potassium is <3 mmol/litre. A few patients will nevertheless have hyperkalaemia, and infusion should then be withheld whilst monitoring serum levels hourly. (Acidosis will have caused a shift of intracellular potassium into the blood, and treatment causes it to move back in again.) The potassium may be monitored by the ECG, though this is not fully reliable—if signs of hyperkalaemia are present on the ECG (page 83), potassium is withheld until plasma results are known. Aim to keep plasma potassium between 4 and 5 mmol per litre.

4 *Insulin.* Soluble insulin must be given immediately, preferably using the low-dose technique.

After a loading dose of about 8 units, soluble insulin is given at a rate of between 4 and 12 units per hour by intravenous infusion in dilution. The blood sugar falls at a rate of about 4.0 mmol/litre each hour. Insulin is rarely required at blood sugar levels below 14 mmol/litre unless ketosis persists when the insulin should be continued giving adequate carbohydrate.

At this stage it is usually feasible to return the patient to his normal insulin dosage divided into 2–4 doses per day. If the patient is awake, fluid and food are given by mouth.

5 *Catheterisation.* Urinary catheterisation is unnecessary in mild cases where confusion is minimal, but is required in those who are in coma as it is otherwise not possible to assess urine output. A diabetic urine chart and fluid balance chart are started and urine sent to the laboratory for bacteriology.

6 *Acidosis.* The use of bicarbonate to correct acidosis is disputed. Some consider that correction results in quicker control of symptoms, whilst others underline the danger of inducing further hypokalaemia. It would seem reasonable to correct partially, at a rate not exceeding 50 mmol/15 min to achieve a pH of 7.1 in adults (7.2 in children). A rough guide in adults is 50 mmol of bicarbonate for every 0.1 units of pH below 7.1 given at a rate of 50 mmol/30 min + 10 mmol KCl extra.

7 *Infection.* Intercurrent infection must always be considered and treated. In the absence of obvious infection, it is advisable to perform urine microscopy and culture, chest X-ray and blood culture.

Hyperosmolar non-ketotic coma

This occurs in the elderly obese diabetic, often previously undiagnosed and may be precipitated by myocardial infarction or stroke. The onset is slow with polyuria over 2–3 weeks and progressive dehydration. Blood glucose levels are very high (often above 45.0 mmol/litre), plasma osmolality is increased (often above 400 mosmol/litre). Plasma bicarbonate is usually normal and there is little or no ketonuria. These patients require insulin—often in small doses over the acute episode (10–20 units may suffice)—and hypotonic (e.g. 0.5 normal saline) fluid replacement given slowly but usually in large quantities. The mortality is high (50%) and cerebral oedema from overhydration a real risk. Prophylactic heparin may help to reduce the increased risk of thrombosis, arterial and venous.

Lactic acidosis

This occurs in the elderly diabetic and is precipitated by biguanides and alcohol. It may occur in shocked patients and with uraemia. The patients are very acidotic and hyperventilating. Blood glucose may be normal and there is little or no ketonuria. Blood lactic acid levels are raised and serum bicarbonate levels reduced.

There is an increased 'anion gap' in which the cation total (Na^+ plus K^+) exceeds the anion total (Cl^- plus HCO_3^-) by up to 25 mmol/litre, the difference being lactate. These patients require insulin (if hyperglycaemic), glucose, bicarbonate (up to 2500 mmol in 24 h), and fluid replacement. Dialysis may be required to remove excess sodium (from the bicarbonate). The mortality is very high (80%).

NB Cerebrovascular accidents and aspirin overdosage may both produce a combination of coma plus glycosuria.

Diabetics also have strokes, take overdoses and become concussed.

Diabetes in surgery and in pregnancy

See pages 106, 107

CARCINOID SYNDROME

Aetiology

This is a rare disorder and results from a malignant carcinoid tumour usually of the ileum which has metastasised to the liver. Carcinoid of the appendix rarely metastasises. The majority of bronchial adenomas are carcinoid but only a few metastasise and produce the syndrome.

Clinical presentation

The symptoms of the primary tumour may be present, e.g. episodic diarrhoea or recurrent haemoptysis. The carcinoid syndrome is due to the secretion of 5-hydroxytryptamine and kinin peptides. Attacks are episodic and symptoms include facial flushing, fever, acute dyspnoea from bronchospasm, nausea, vomiting, colic and diarrhoea. Later valvular stenosis of the pulmonary and tricuspid valves may develop, There may be evidence of malignancy with cachexia and irregular hepatomegaly from metastases.

Investigation

The 24-hour urinary excretion of 5-hydroxyindole acetic acid (5-HIAA) is estimated on a low serotonin diet (excluding bananas, tomatoes, walnuts, etc.). Normal range: 2–10 mg in 24 h.

Management

Cyproheptadine 4 mg tds, α-blockade, octreotide (somatostatin analogue) or methysergide 1–2 mg qds (serotonin antagonists) and tumour chemotherapy, e.g. streptozotocin, are usually given but give disappointing results. Hepatic arterial embolisation is helpful in some. Treat diarrhoea symptomatically.

PORPHYRIA

This describes six syndromes in which there is increased intermittent excretion of porphyrins in the urine and/or faeces. The first four below are hepatic porphyrias with excess hepatic production of porphobilinogen. They are all rare. In the erythropoietic porphyrias (five and six below) there is increased production of porphyrins in the red cells due to enzyme deficiency. (RBC porphyrin levels are normal in hepatic porphyrias).

There are acute episodes in three important inherited (autosomal dominant) varieties (acute intermittent and variegate porphyria, and hereditary copropophyria) with gastrointestinal, neuropsychiatric and cardiovascular features often precipitated by administration of drugs—usually barbiturates (especially intravenous general anaesthetics), phenytoin, sulphonamides, griseofulvin, rifampicin, alcohol or the contraceptive pill. All are metabolised by hepatic microsomes (P450) and lead to increased δ-amino-laevulinic (ALA)-synthetase activity and the urinary excretion of large amounts of ALA and phorphobilinogen (PBG) in patients with acute intermittent porphyria. Fasting may also precipitate an acute attack. The clinical features (which bear a superficial resemblance to lead poisoning) are:

- abdominal pain, vomiting or constipation
- peripheral neuropathy with weakness or paralysis
- confusion and psychosis
- tachycardia and hypertension

During attacks there is increased urinary PBG and ALA, and increased faecal porphyrins. PBG is detected by Ehrlich's aldehyde reagent and porphyrins recognised by fluorescence in ultraviolet light. PBG in urine darkens on standing (oxidation).

1. *Acute intermittent porphyria* (AIP)

    This is the 'Swedish' type, the most severe and the commonest in the UK. Onset is usually between 15 and 35 years. The skin is 'never' affected. In remission the urine still has excess PBG and ALA but the faeces are relatively normal. The best screening test is the urinary PBG.

2. *Variegate porphyria* (VP)

    This is the 'South African' type. Onset is usually between 10 and 30 years. The skin, photosensitised by porphyrins, is fragile, particularly on the backs of the hands. In remission the faeces contain excess porphyrins but the urine may be normal. The best screening test is thus for faecal porphyrins and protoporphyrin. Latent forms are common.

3. *Cutaneous hepatic porphyria* (porphyria cutanea tarda)

    This is an important variety which may be acquired or, less commonly, inherited and present at any age. This is usually secondary to liver disease from alcohol (hence 'symptomatic' porphyria) but perhaps only occurs in genetically predisposed subjects. There are no acute attacks (except in the hereditary type) and the patient is usually not sensitive to drugs (except occasionally barbiturates). The patient may present after an alcoholic binge. The signs are predominantly cutaneous with porphyrin-induced photosensitivity leading to bullae on exposed areas and hyperpigmentation. There is no family history of porphyria and the liver function tests are usually abnormal. There is no excess porphyrin in the stool and no excess PBG or ALA in the urine. There is excess uroporphyrin in the urine. There is clinical, biochemical and histological evidence of liver disease.

4. *Hereditary coproporphyria* (HC)

    Very rare. Clinically like AIP but urinary coproporphyrin always raised.

Management of hepatic porphyrias (1–4)

    Avoid the usual precipitant drugs (the patient should carry a complete list) and alcohol. Shield the skin in photosensitive patients. Pregnancy can be dangerous in acute intermittent porphyria.

    During attacks, use morphine, diazepam, promazine and propranolol as necessary. Circulatory and respiratory failure may occur and artificial ventilation may be necessary. Intravenous fluids are given if vomiting is severe, and intravenous glucose loading (400 g/day) may help terminate an attack. Repeated venesection is useful in the management of porphyria cutanea tarda and possibly small doses of chloroquine.

5. *Congenital erythropoietic porphyria*

    It is extremely rare, inherited as an autosomal recessive and characterised by extreme skin manifestations plus red-staining of the teeth and bones which presents before the age of 5 years. There are no acute attacks. There is increased uroporphyrin and coproporphyrin.

6. Erythropoietic protoporphyria

It is relatively common and inherited as an autosomal dominant. It presents at any age with cutaneous photosensitivity of varying severity. It is distinguished by the presence of free protoporphyrin in the red cells.

HYPERLIPIDAEMIA

Definition

Hyperlipidaemia is present when serum levels of cholesterol or triglyceride, or both, are raised above those accepted as treatment goals for patients. 'Normal Levels' in the UK are associated with a high morbidity which can be reduced by bringing the levels down. Thus, 25% of the UK population has a serum total cholesterol above the accepted upper limit of 6.5 mmol/litre (and the mean, in UK, is 5.7). Serum triglyceride should be below 2 mmol/litre. The 'HDL ratio' is the ratio of serum HDL cholesterol (see below) to the rest of the cholesterol (total-HDL), and should be <0.2.

Background

Lipids are insoluble in water, so cholesterol and triglyceride circulate bound to proteins as water-soluble lipoproteins. The conventional measurement of these serum lipids is thus an indirect measurement of the circulating pathological agents, the lipid-carrying particles, (chiefly LDL and IDL), which are deposited in vessel walls and cause atheroma. It is best to think of the lipoprotein particles as the pathogens, and the measurement of cholesterol and triglyceride as a guide to them.

Classification of particles

The particles were originally separated and classifed by centrifugation. The smaller the complex, the denser it is and the higher the proportion of cholesterol to triglyceride. In order of size (big to small), and density (low to high) the particles are as follows:

• Chylomicrons are very large particles which transport absorbed dietary fat, mainly triglyceride, from the gut to adipose tissue and muscle cells where triglyceride is removed by lipoprotein lipase, Chylomicrons are normally absent after a 10-h fast. Non-fasted blood samples give an accurate cholesterol but an unrepresentatively high triglyceride level

• Very low density lipoprotein (VLDL) transports endogenous triglyceride from liver to cells for storage for metabolism. It is converted to LDL (via IDL—intermediate density lipoprotein) by the removal of triglyceride

• Low density lipoprotein (LDL) is the result of removal of triglyceride from VLDL and hence is chiefly cholesterol which is transported in this way to peripheral cells for use as energy or for storage

• High density lipoprotein (HDL) carries cholesterol from peripheral cells to the liver for excretion as bile. HDL is thus anti-atherogenic. It is normally 20–25% of the total cholesterol

Hence, LDL is the chief form of cholesterol in the blood, and VLDL the chief form of fasting serum triglyceride.

Classification of diseases (figure 47 and table 21)

The hyperlipidaemias are now usually classified clinically rather than by the WHO/Fredrickson classification which referred to primary hyperlipidaemias and was based on phenotypes. It ignored HDL cholesterol and is of less practical use than the clinical classification.

• *Familial hypercholesterolaemia.* LDL receptor deficiency results in an increase in LDL particles in the circulation. The triglycerides are relatively normal. Homozygotes have a grossly elevated serum cholesterol, develop coronary artery disease in their teens, and usually die in their twenties

• *Polygenic hypercholesterolaemia.* The LDL receptor is usually normal but too much LDL-cholesterol is produced. It may be secondary to hypothyroidism, nephrotic syndrome or prolonged obstructive jaundice

• *Familial hypertriglyceridaemia.* It may also be secondary to diabetes mellitus and obesity, when the cholesterol may be normal and the triglyceride not more than 10 mmol/litre. It is associated with gout, alcoholism and pancreatitis

• *Familial combined hyperlipidaemia* (so-called because cholesterol and triglycerides are both roughly equally increased). It is associated with coronary heart disease, hypertension and diabetes mellitus. It may produce xanthelasmata but not tendon xanthomata. Corneal arcus are frequently present

• *Remnant particle (or 'dysbeta') lipoproteinaemia.* This is characterised by abnormal (IDL) particles, and raised cholesterol and triglyceride. There is widespread atheroma. Patients may have fat deposition in the palm creases, or tuberous xanthomata on the elbows

• *The chylomicronaemia syndrome* is due to deficiency of extrahepatic lipoprotein lipase (or of its co-factor apoprotein C-II). There is a failure to clear fat from the circulation, and the serum is milky in appearance even in the fasting state. It is autosomal recessive and presents in childhood

Particles	Diameter (nm)		Proportion	Atheroma?
Chylomicrons (exogenous triglyceride)	80–500	LARGE	Triglyceride	0
VLDL	30–80			+
IDL	25–35			+ + +
LDL	20			+ + +
HDL	10	SMALL	Cholesterol	Protects

Figure 47. Blood lipids.

Table 21. Classification of hyperlipidaemias. Modified from *Mims* (Supplement) 1989, by permission of Haymarket Medical Publications, London.

Type of hyperlipidaemia	Prevalence	Frederickson/WHO lipoprotein phenotype	Typical lipid levels (mmol/litre)	Lipoproteins	Chronic heart disease risk	Pancreatitis risk	Clinical signs
Polygenic hypercholesterolaemia	—	IIa	Cholesterol: 6.5–9.0 Triglyceride: normal	LDL↑ HDL→↓	+	—	Xanthelasma, corneal arcus
Familial combined hyperlipidaemia	1 : 200	IIb (IIa or IV)	Cholesterol: 6.5–10.0 Triglyceride: 2.5–12.0	VLDL↑→ LDL↑→ HDL→↓	+ +	—	Corneal arcus, xanthelasma
Familial hypercholesterolaemia (heterozygous)	1 : 500	IIa (or IIb)	Cholesterol: 7.5–16.0 Triglyceride: <5.0	LDL↑ VLDL→↑ HDL→↓	+ + +	—	Tendon xanthomata, corneal arcus, xanthelasma
Remnant particle disease	1 : 10 000	III	Cholesterol: 9.0–14.0 Triglyceride: 9.0–14.0	IDL↑ HDL→↓	+ + +	+	Palmar tuberous and occasional tendon xanthomata
Chylomicronaemia syndrome	—	I	Cholesterol: <6.5 Triglyceride: 10.0–30.0	Chylomicrons ↑	—	+ + +	Eruptive xanthomata, lipaemia retinalis, hepatosplenomegaly
Familial hypertrigyceridaemia	—	IV (or V)	Cholesterol: 6.5–12.0 Triglyceride: 10.0–30.0	VLDL↑ Chylomicrons →↑	?	+ +	Eruptive xanthomata, lipaemia retinalis, hepatosplenomegaly

Screening

The greatest benefit is to those at greatest risk. It is important to identify high-risk patients. Modifiable risks, which characterise secondary hyperlipidaemias, include smoking, hypertension, inappropriate diet, diabetes mellitus, obesity, hypothyroidism, alcoholism, some therapy (e.g. thiazides, corticosteroids, oestrogens and some β-blockers), and possibly a sedentary life style and emotional stress. Non-modifiable factors include age, and a family history of hypercholesterolaemia or of premature coronary heart disease, cerebrovascular disease or peripheral vascular disease. In any individual high-risk approach to screening, people should be selected by:

First-degree relatives with disease.

Any relative <55 years old with atheromatous disease.

Presence of the risk factors given above.

Physical signs of lipid deposits.

Treatment

The cornerstone is diet. Calories should be reduced to achieve a satisfactory body weight. Fat should constitute <30% of energy intake and be predominantly polyunsaturated or mono-unsaturated. Daily intake of cholesterol should be <300 mg. Vigorous exercise at least twice a week may help. The other modifiable risk factors given above should be assessed and treated.

If serum lipid levels are still abnormally raised after at least 3 months adherence to a satisfactory regime, drug therapy may become necessary.

Drug treatment

- *Resins.* Cholestyramine and colestipol bind bile acids in the gut and prevent their reabsorption. The liver uses more cholesterol to make bile acids and LDL receptor activity is increased. HDL levels tend to increase. Gastrointestinal side-effects are common and compliance is low. Very low density lipoproteins increase so the resins should not be used in combined hyperlipidaemias. They may be combined with the following drugs to obtain increased effect:
- *Fibrates.* Bezafibrate and gemfibrozil reduce VLDL and therefore tend to be used primarily in hypertriglyceridaemia and the combined hyperlipidaemias
- *Nicotinic acid and derivatives* (acipimox, nicofuranose) reduce VLDL synthesis and tend to increase HDL cholesterol. They are used for the combined hyperlipidaemias and, in combination with resins, for hypercholesterolaemia. Compliance is low because of flushing, which may be reduced with aspirin. Uric acid and glucose should be monitored
- *Probucol.* This tends to decrease both LDL and HDL cholesterols, but is nevertheless associated with resolution of xanthomata. Its place requires further evaluation
- *Vastatins.* These, by competitively inhibiting hydroxy-methyl-glutaryl coenzyme A (HMG CoA) reductase in the liver, decrease cholesterol synthesis. As a consequence, the number of LDL receptors increases with time. They are more effective than the resins in reducing LDL cholesterol, but less effective than the fibrates in raising HDL cholesterol and reducing triglycerides. They may be

combined with resins but not, at present, with the other hypolipidaemic drugs. Simvastatin, 20–40 mg once daily, is often given to those with serum total cholesterol levels above 8 mmol/litre

- *Omega-3-triglycerides* may be used in patients with combined hyperlipidaemias particularly when the patient is prone to recurrent pancreatitis, which tends to occur with triglyceride levels >11 mmol/litre. Triglyceride may be an independent risk factor for coronary heart disease

NB Blood samples for a full lipid screen should be taken after an overnight fast, e.g. 14 h. Results tend to be misleading within 3 months of a myocardial infarction, but useful if taken within 24 h.

METABOLIC BONE DISEASE

Bone normally consists of 60% mineral and 40% organic matter (matrix). The former is mostly calcium and the latter mostly collagen.

Osteoporosis

This refers to a loss of bone mass rather than an alteration in its constituents. It may be determined chemically or histologically on bone biopsy, but this is subject to considerable sampling errors. Osteoporosis as judged by these criteria increases steadily with age in the normal person. 'Osteoporosis' also describes the clinical syndrome of a spinal disorder characterised by intermittent severe backache with non-traumatic crush fracture of vertebral bodies and kyphosis with loss of height or femoral fractures with trauma. The lumbar spine is the area most involved, and the discs may rupture into the vertebral bodies (Schmorl's nodes). X-rays of the lumbar spine in this syndrome show loss of bone density, the bodies being nearly as transradiant as the discs, with increased trabeculation and biconcavity of the bodies with anterior wedging and kyphosis. Bone densitometry, e.g. of the lower forearm, is relatively reliable. The diagnosis in the age chiefly at risk (i.e. the elderly) is from myelomatosis and secondary carcinoma.

Aetiology

Clinically important osteoporosis, i.e. fractures, develops as a result of inexorable normal bone loss with ageing. It is also affected by sex (female—especially postmenopausal), race (white and Asian), drug (steroids), nutrition (leanness), and physical inactivity. It seems important to start this ageing process with as high a peak bone mass as possible. Nearly all cases are of unknown cause and generalised. Decreased bone density is more marked in women than men, particularly following the menopause. The roles of calcium intake, calcium absorption, vitamin D, oestrogens, and gonadotrophins remain controversial. A negative calcium balance due to reduced intake or absorption, or excessive excretion has been suggested, and the roles of calciferol and oestrogens emphasised. Immobilisation (and weightlessness!) often due to arthritis appears to contribute. Some drugs may encourage osteoporosis, such as diuretics, some antacids, thyroid hormones and steroids.

Classification

Generalised

Normal ageing especially in women:
1 *Postmenopausal (Type 1)* with trabecular bone loss giving vertebral lesions of end-plate collapse, wedging and crush fracture, up to about 70 years.
2 *Senile (Type 2)* with additional cortical bone loss giving fractures characteristically of the neck of femur, usually in women over 75 years old. This fracture is partly due to the normal increase in body sway with age and resultant instability with falls.
Idiopathic—any age, but excessive in degree when compared within the age group. It is usually more dramatic, therefore, in the young.

Secondary

Endocrine
- Cushing's syndrome (including steroid therapy)
- Thyrotoxicosis (including thyroid therapy)
- Pregnancy
- Hypogonadism
- Chronic liver disease and alcoholism

Localised

- Immobilisation and paralysis
- Rheumatoid arthritis

Diagnosis and treatment

If the point of diagnosis is to allow prognosis and treatment, then there is quite correctly little attention paid to the diagnosis of idiopathic osteoporosis in the elderly. The condition usually presents with fracture—vertebra or femoral neck (in both sexes) and Colles' fracture (especially in the female). The treatment of these fractures is little altered by the diagnosis of coexistent osteoporosis. There is no convincing evidence yet of successful results from treatment with oestrogens, anabolic steroids, calcium supplements, microcrystalline hydroxyapatite, exercise, calcitonin, fluoride, diphosphonates or vitamin D metabolites, though further loss of bone mass may be prevented by some of these. Hormone replacement therapy (HRT) appears to maintain cortical bone mass if started within a few years of the menopause, though it will replace little if any of that which is already lost. Treatment should be directed at those with identifiable risk factors including late menarche, early menopause, oophorectomy before 50 years, slimness, cigarette smoking and physical sluggishness. Accelerated bone loss occurs on stopping HRT though net benefit is maintained. Therefore aim to continue treatment for 5–10 years. Breast and uterine malignancy must be excluded first and the patient warned of possible mastalgia and the return of periods. There should be a good calcium intake of 1–1.5 g/day (1 pint of milk, skimmed or whole, contains about ¾ g).

For the postmenopausal woman, the treatment of choice outside specialist centres is cyclical oestrogen therapy with good calcium and vitamin D intake or cyclic diphosphonate therapy alternating with supplementary calcium. It is important to avoid immobilisation (including the use of corsets) and treat pain symptomatically. Even correction of Cushing's syndrome is not followed by clear evidence of healing of osteoporosis, though its progress may be arrested.

Investigation

Biochemistry. Serum calcium, phosphorus and alkaline phosphatase and urinary calcium are normal.

Radiology. Lateral lumbar spine and indices of cortical narrowing (e.g. metacarpal index).

Histology. This is not indicated routinely but shows a diminished number of normally calcified trabeculae, the changes being most marked in the vertebrae. Bone mass can be estimated using photon absorptiometry (single or dual) quantitative CT or DEXA (dual energy X-ray absorptiometry).

Osteomalacia and rickets

This refers to the situation in which there is inadequate mineralisation of bone. There is usually a reduced serum phosphate level and (less commonly) a reduced serum calcium level. The alkaline phosphatase tends to be raised (biochemical osteomalacia or rickets).

Adult osteomalacia may present with:
Bone pain ('rheumatism' in the elderly) and tenderness.
Pathological fracture.
Weakness, said to be most marked in the quadriceps and glutei which results in a waddling gait and difficulty in rising from a chair.
The signs of underlying disease e.g. malabsorption—the osteomalacia being diagnosed in the course of investigation.

Rickets (juvenile osteomalacia) present differently because the reduced mineralisation can affect the epiphyses, as yet unfused, and the modelling of bones, with:
- Deformities in the legs (bow-legs, knock-knees)
- Deformities in the chest (early sign—ricketic rosary)
- Deformities in the skull (craniotabes, open fontanelles and delayed eruption of the teeth)
- Hypotonia, weakness, tetany

NB Rickets in Britain occur chiefly in Asian immigrants due to a combination of poor sunlight and a diet poor in vitamin D.

Aetiology

- Reduced intake of vitamin D—either dietary calciferol or cutaneous cholecalciferol (from 7-dehydrocholesterol), but usually both (dark skin, northern climate, poor diet)
- Malabsorption (page 270), especially gluten-sensitive enteropathy and postgastrectomy states

- Vitamin D resistance, i.e. osteomalacia or rickets despite a normal intake and blood level of vitamin D. In chronic renal failure, the osteomalacia due to deficient calciferol hydroxylation in the kidney is added to the bone disease from hyperparathyroidism secondary to renal phosphate retention
- Increased vitamin D inactivation with chronic anticonvulsant therapy

Diagnosis and investigation

Biochemistry. Reduced serum phosphorus and calcium with increased alkaline phosphatase. Urinary calcium is reduced and there is a tendency to mild renal tubular acidosis.

X-ray. Deformities, especially rickets with slight biconcavity of the vertebral bodies in the lumbar spine with normal or even increased density.

Pseudofractures (Looser's zones). These are translucent 2 mm bands perpendicular to the surface of the bone extending from the cortex inwards, best seen in the pubic rami, the necks of the humeri and femurs and in the outer borders of the scapulae which are 'points of stress'.

Secondary hyperparathyroidism which occurs as a consequence of the lower serum calcium level.

Rickets. In addition to the deformity there are cupped and irregular epiphyses ('cupping, splaying and fraying') which are delayed in appearance.

Bone scan. There is a generalized diffuse increase in uptake. Occasionally Looser's zones may show multiple areas of increased uptake of tracer simulating metastases. The scan is normal in osteoporosis and shows strongly focal uptake in Paget's disease.

Histology. The number of bone seams is normal. There is excess volume of osteoid tissue.

There are an absent calcification fronts.

There is usually some evidence of hyperparathyroidism.

Investigate the underlying disease, e.g. malabsorption, uraemia.

Differential diagnosis

In the elderly, rheumatism and polymyalgia rheumatica.

Paget's disease (because of the raised alkaline phosphatase).

Osteoporosis which often coexists.

Treatment

Vitamin D (calciferol). The dose depends upon the aetiology. The serum calcium must always be monitored.

NB   Calciferol 10 µg equals 400 units.

- In deficiency states: 1000 units per day. Maintenance requirements for health in the normal individual are probably about 500 units per day, including children
- In vitamin D resistance—see uraemia
- In malabsorption states: alfacalcidol 1–6 µg daily
- In post-parathyroidectomy maintenance: alfacalcidol (1 µg daily) is not always required

Calcium. 1–3 g per day.

NB   About 1 g of clacium is contained in 1½ pints of milk, 1 tablet Sandocal 1000, 20 tablets calcium gluconate, and 25 tablets calcium lactate.

Treat the underlying disease, e.g. malabsorption or uraemia.

Uraemic bone disease (renal osteodystrophy) (*see* mechanisms **1–4** below)

Vitamin D and parathyroid hormone (PTH). Calcium homoeostasis depends on two hormones, PTH and the active form of vitamin D_3: 1-25-$(OH) 2D_3$, referred to here as dihydroxy-cholecalciferol (DHCC). Both mobilize calcium from bone. PTH increases reabsorption of calcium from the renal tubule. DHCC increases absorption of calcium by the intestine. DHCC enhances the effect of PTH on bone. By stimulating 1-α-hydroxylase activity in the kidney, PTH enhances production of DHCC. In turn, DHCC may reduce production or release of PTH.

In renal failure, there is reduced DHCC (because of reduced 1-α-hydroxylase activity in the kidney) with increased PTH. This increased PTH may be because the slight phosphate retention leads to a small decrease in ionised calcium level which is the standard stimulus to release of PTH. Bone is resistant to the effects of PTH because of the lower level of DHCC. Reduction in dietary phosphate and therefore renal tissue phosphate might reduce PTH levels in renal failure by increasing ionised calcium and DHCC.

Phosphate retention

This has two secondary effects:

1   Reciprocal depression of serum calcium level (mediated at the bone surface)
2   Rise in the calcium × phosphorus product (despite the serum calcium depression) which may lead to ectopic calcification and pseudogout

Vitamin D resistance

The diseased kidneys fail to hydroxylate 25-hydroxycholecalciferol (25-HCC) to 1-25-DHCC which is the most active form of the vitamin.

This failure is expressed at two important sites:

3   The gut where there is reduced calcium absorption
4   The bone to produce osteomalacia and hypocalcaemia

The ionic hypocalcaemia produced by the first and fourth mechanisms is a physiological stimulus to the parathyroid glands (phosphate has no direct effect on parathyroid activity) which are thus in a state of chronic hypersecretion, tending to return the serum calcium level (and phosphate level) towards normal but doing so only incompletely. This (secondary) hyperparathyroidism (page 220) may be demonstrated on bone X-rays and the serum level of parathyroid hormone is raised. The hypocalcaemia only rarely leads to tetany because of two other biochemical changes which may occur in chronic renal failure:

• acidosis reduces the protein binding of calcium and thus increases the levels of ionised calcium
• hypoproteinaemia has a similar effect

The clinical consequences of renal failure on calcium metabolism are thus:

- osteoporosis produced by hyperparathyroidism
- osteomalacia due to vitamin D resistance
- ectopic calcification
- hypocalcaemic tetany (with correction of acidosis)

Management

There are five chief therapeutic manoeuvres:

- *Vitamin D* may be given to treat muscular weakness, bone pain and biochemical or radiological osteomalacia. The rise in serum calcium level should reduce hyperparathyroidism. The unwanted effects which must be monitored during therapy are increased absorption of phosphate from the gut (see above) which may lead to metastatic calcification, and hypercalcaemia. It should not normally be used if the phosphate is much raised. Alfacalcidol (1-α-hydroxycholecalcifrol) 1–2 μg/day is more reliable in effect than calciferol

- *Restriction of dietary phosphate* with oral aluminium hydroxide gel (dose 10 ml qds) reduces the absorption of phosphate from the gut and thus lowers the serum phosphate level (and the calcium × phosphorus product). Though this reduces the risk of metastatic calcification there is a risk of hypercalcaemia developing since the calcium cannot be incorporated into bone (insufficient phosphate to make the mineral).

- *Parathyroidectomy* should reduce calcium and phosphate levels and permit vitamin D therapy without the risk of metastatic calcification but is very seldom necessary.

- *Chronic dialysis* against a suitable calcium concentration (about 1.5 mmol/litre in the dialysis fluid should return the calcium (and phosphate) levels towards normal.

- *Renal transplantation*, if successful, will return renal function and calcium metabolism to normal. However, the side-effects of immunosuppressive drug therapy may influence the skeleton adversely.

NB   No attempt should be made to treat the metabolic acidosis directly since the ionised calcium level will fall and may easily result in tetany. Fracture of the weakened bones may occur in the convulsion.

Vitamin D

The term *vitamin D* refers to two related sterols. Calciferol (D_2) is a compound used therapeutically but is not important physiologically. Cholecalciferol (D_3) is the substance normally absorbed either as such in diet (eggs and fatty fish) or converted from 7-dehydrocholesterol by ultraviolet light in the skin. This has antirachitic activity itself but is normally hyroxylated by the liver to 25-hydroxycholecalciferol (25-HCC) with some increase of potency. The kidney is responsible for a further hydroxylation to 1-25-dihydroxycholecalciferol (1-25-DHCC) which increases calcium absorption from the gut (24-25-DHCC may affect bone mineralisation acting via the parathyroids). The production of 1-25-DHCC is increased by a low serum calcium level which thus forms a feedback mechanism for serum calcium regulation.

Vitamin D resistance thus appears to be due partly to a failure of the kidney to perform the second hydroxylation of 25-HCC. Dialysis would thus not be expected to improve calcium absorption and indeed does not (though it does improve bone mineralisation).

The synthetic calciferol analogue, alfacalcidol, (1-α-HCC) has been used chiefly in the treatment of renal bone disease, the usual daily dose being 1 μg.

Paget's disease

James Paget, 1814–1899, Great Yarmouth. This is characterised histologically by increased bone resorption associated with abnormal new bone formation. The osteoclast dysfunction may be due to a slow virus—an RNA virus similar to measles, or a paramyxovirus have been suggested.

Histology shows abnormally active osteoclasts (with the production of increased urinary hydroxyproline), followed by increased bone formation (wtih increased serum alkaline phosphatase). The bones most commonly affected are those of the axial skeleton and the femora. The early changes show large resorption cavities with increased vascularity and softened bone. The subsequent sclerotic areas are dense and disorganised (mosaic pattern). In Britain this occurs in 1% of the population at 50 years old, rising to 10% by 100 years (males more than females). In only about 5–10% is the disease clinically important. It appears to have a familial incidence.

Clinical features

Bone pain and tenderness in 40% of patients sometimes with a rise in temperature over the lesion. This may mimic osteoarthritis of the hip in up to 10% of patients.

Bone deformity with enlargement of the skull and bowing of the legs.

Complications:

* fracture of a long bone (immobilisation is said to produce hypercalcaemia)
* progressive occlusion of the foramina of the skull, e.g. deafness and basilar invagination and cervical cord stenosis with paraparesis
* about 2% develop bone sarcoma
* high output cardiac failure is rare
* osteoarthritis of related joints

Investigation

Radiology. Coarsening and disorganisation are characteristic and produce bones with thick trabeculae unrelated to the usual stress lines and thick cortices with an enlarged irregular outline. The sacrum and lumbar spine are most frequently affected followed by skull, pelvis, lower limbs and upper limbs. The clavicles may also be affected.

Biochemistry. The alkaline phosphatase (AP) is often over 1000 iu/litre and the 24-h urinary hydroxyproline (OHP) output raised from about 50 mg in the normal up to 1 g or more. These two measurements tend to reflect the severity and extent of the disease and can be used to follow treatment. Immobilisation may produce hypercalcaemia.

Treatment

Both during, and indefinitely after treatment, both AP and OHP are monitored. Bed rest must be avoided.

Analgesics are given for pain. Specific treatment for the Paget's disease with either calcitonin or diphosphonate is indicated:
• For bone pain even when there is associated osteoarthritis for instance of a hip
• For neurological involvement such as basilar invagination syndrome, and spinal cord or nerve root compression. Deafness might not improve
• For deformity, fissure fractures, or osteolytic lesions in weight-bearing bones
• To treat immobilisation hypercalcaemia or to avoid it before orthopaedic surgery. Bone quality is also improved
• For high output cardiac failure

Diphosphonates. Disodium etidronate 5 mg/kg/day as a single dose orally at least 2 h before food for 6 months: usually 400 mg/day. This should not be repeated for 9 months because of the risk of focal osteomalacia. Remission occurs in 90%. Biochemical and clinical improvement can continue for many months after treatment has ceased. Less suitable for osteolytic lesions.

Calcitonins. Salcatonin subcutaneously from 100 iu daily to three times a week especially for osteoclastic disease and hypercalcaemia, and for up to a year depending on response.

Plicamycin (Mithramycin). 15 µg/kg/day in a 6-h diluted infusion, for 5 days, repeated after a week, with haematological, liver, and renal monitoring. Combination therapy can help in resistant disease.

ENDOCRINE BONE DISEASE

Osteogenesis imperfecta

A hereditary connective tissue abnormality with involvement of collagen-containing tissues such as the skeleton (fragile), sclerae (blue), skin (thin), teeth (thin dentine), tendons (hypermobile joints), heart (valve disorders) and ear (deafness).
Osteogenesis imperfecta tarda is a commoner, mild, autosomal dominant disease and fractures are rare.
Osteogenesis imperfecta congenita is a rare, severe, autosomal recessive disease with the above features plus scoliosis and bowed legs and multiple fractures.

Hyperparathyroidism

Parathyroid hormone (PTH) increases serum calcium by:
• increasing calcium absorption from the gut
• increasing mobilisation of calcium from bone

• reducing renal calcium clearance

It also increases renal phosphate clearance and this may also indirectly increase mobilisation of calcium from bone.

Primary hyperparathyroidism results from an adenoma (85%) or hyperplasia of the parathyroid glands. Very rarely a functioning carcinoma may occur. Ectopic PTH may be produced by carcinoma elsewhere, particularly of the lung and kidney. A parathyroid adenoma may be part of a MEA syndrome (page 197).

Secondary hyperparathyroidism is a physiological response to hypocalcaemia produced by another disease, e.g. chronic renal failure and hypovitaminosis D (dietary deficiency or malabsorption). Hypocalcaemia persists.

'Tertiary hyperparathyroidism' refers to the situation where chronic secondary hyperparathyroidism has resulted in an autonomous adenoma. This, as in primary hyperparathyroidism, is characterised by hypercalcaemia, though the hyperphosphataemia of renal failure may persist.

Clinical presentation

'Bones, stones, groans (peptic ulcer) and moans (psychiatric disease).' Hypercalcaemia may be found on routine screening (0.1% of the general population; higher in hospital admissions: up to 8%).

Hypercalciuria produces renal calculi, nephrocalcinosis and later renal failure. X-ray changes (see below).

Severe hypercalcaemia may produce anorexia, nausea, vomiting, thirst, polyuria, constipation, muscle fatigue and hypotonicity and calcium deposition in the conjunctiva, usually at the medial limbus of the eye (3%). Dyspepsia and peptic ulceration may occur (5%).

Psychiatric disorders (3%) include depression and confusion.

Differential diagnosis

This is from other causes of hypercalcaemia (page 223) and hypercalciuria.

Investigation

Biochemistry. In primary hyperparathyroidism the serum calcium is raised and the phosphate reduced. A raised serum alkaline phosphatase indicates increased bone activity. There is a high renal clearance of phosphate and a mild renal tubular acidosis (with a high serum chloride level). The serum calcium level is not reduced by corticosteroids. The serum PTH is raised. In the secondary hyperparathyroidism of renal failure, the serum phosphate is high and the serum calcium tends to be low.

Radiology. More specific changes include loss of the lamina dura of the teeth (25%) and small subperiosteal bone resorption cysts most marked in the middle phalanges of the hands (and feet). Osteitis fibrosa cystica with bone cysts is relatively rare. CT scan and isotopic subtraction scan of the neck and mediastinum (up to 20% are ectopic) seldom helps to localise the abnormal gland.

Treatment

Surgical resection of the diseased parathyroid glands is indicated for a serum calcium persistently over 2.75 mmol/litre (after correction for serum albumin level) or for patients with lower levels plus any of the clinical presenting features given above if more than minor. It is important to visualise and probably biopsy all four parathyroid glands to determine whether they are normal or hyperplastic. A single enlarged gland is removed or, if all are enlarged, three and a half, the remaining half either being left in situ or implanted in the forearm. Some advocate the removal of all hyperplastic glands and subsequent treatment with alfacalcidol. A post-operative 'hungry bones syndrome' can develop with tetany and hypomagnesaemia.

Hypoparathyroidism

Aetiology

Secondary to thyroid surgery
Primary 'idiopathic'. This appears to be an organ-specific autoimmune disease (page 168) and is associated with an increased incidence of Addison's (hypoadrenal) disease, pernicious anaemia and malabsorption. Parathyroid agenesis occurs in DiGeorge's syndrome with thymic hypoplasia as a result of maldevelopment of the third and fourth pharyngeal pouches. There is T-cell deficiency and children die from infection in infancy.

Pseudohypoparathyroidism (very rare) is due to a failure of end-organ response in bone and kidney to endogenous parathyroid hormone which is thus present in excess amounts. Unlike patients with true idiopathic hypoparathyroidism, there is no increase in urinary cyclic AMP when parathyroid hormone is injected.

Clinical presentation

This depends upon its speed of onset and its degree. Acute hypocalcaemia gives paraesthesia around the mouth and in the extremities followed by cramps, tetany, stridor, convulsions, and death if untreated.
Trousseau's and Chvostek's signs may be present.
Ectodermal changes: teeth, nails, skin and hair. There is an excessive incidence of cutaneous moniliasis in primary hypoparathyroidism.
Ocular changes: cataract and occasionally papilloedema.
Calcification in the basal ganglia and less commonly other soft tissues.
NB   The hereditary syndrome of pseudohypoparathyroidism is caused by tissue resistance to PTH and usually presents in childhood. The patients have a moon face, are short, mentally retarded, have calcification of the basal ganglia and

often have short fourth or fifth metacarpals. The biochemistry is similar to idiopathic hypoparathyroidism. Pseudo-pseudohypoparathyroidism refers to patients who have the somatic manifestations of pseudohypoparathyroidism but normal biochemistry.

Tetany may also occur rarely in rickets, the malabsorption syndrome, alkalosis especially hyperventilation (page 305) and very rarely in osteomalacia and uraemia.

Investigation

There is a low serum calcium and a high serum phosphate level with normal alkaline phosphatase. There is no common diagnostic radiological skeletal abnormality. X-ray of the skull may show calcification of the basal ganglia. If the patient is thought to have idiopathic hypoparathyroidism investigate for the associated pathologies.

The differential diagnosis of hypocalcaemia is that of the causes of parathyroid hormone deficiency (page 217) and of hypovitaminosis D—reduced intake or absorption, and resistance (page 217).

Treatment

Emergency. Treat tetany with 10–20 ml of 10% calcium gluconate intravenously.

NB   Re-breathing from a bag if there is hyperventilation.

Intravenous magnesium chloride may also be required if there is also hypomagnesaemia.

Long-term therapy involves the use of vitamin D analogues, alfacalcidol or calcitriol supplements to raise the serum calcium towards normal (page 216).

HYPERCALCAEMIA (see hyperparathyroidism, page 220)

The physiologically relevant measurement is of ionised calcium but this is seldom performed. Some measure of this is obtained by determining what proportion of the serum calcium is protein-bound. There are a number of techniques for 'correcting' serum calcium levels (normal range: 2.2–2.6 mmol/litre) for serum protein or albumin concentration, e.g. for every 10 g/litre serum albumin over 40 g/litre subtract 0.2 mmol/litre from the measured total calcium level (or add on, if albumin low). These are inaccurate compared with laboratory values of ionised calcium.

Aetiology

Malignant involvement of bone. Carcinoma, myeloma, reticulosis.

Excess PTH. Primary and tertiary hyperparathyroidism and ectopic PTH syndromes (carcinoma).

Excess vitamin D effect

- medication (self-administered or iatrogenic)
- increased sensitivity (sarcoidosis, granulomatous disease)

Bone diseases (all rare)
- thyrotoxicosis
- immobilised Paget's disease
- Addison's disease
- milk–alkali syndrome

Investigation

A detailed history and examination should eliminate most of the differential diagnoses listed above. Bone X-rays may be diagnostic. Phosphate clearance studies and the hydrocortisone test (40 mg orally 8-hourly for 10 days) are not often required or diagnostically conclusive. Routine measurements of urine calcium are not usually helpful. Sarcoid, myeloma and occult carcinoma should not be overlooked. Serum PTH levels are useful when available and reliable.

Treatment

Emergency. Rehydrate with intravenous infusion of saline and give frusemide. Parenteral calcitonin (4 MRC units per kg per day or more).
Corticosteroids (ineffective in parathyroid disease).
Oral sodium phosphate
Intravenous or oral diphosphonates (disodium etidronate, clodronate) inhibit osteoclast-mediated bone resorption and can be used with rehydration to treat the hypercalcaemia of malignancy. Peritoneal dialysis using a calcium-free dialysate, and haemodialysis are also effective.
Long-term. Remove the cause by specific therapy.

GOUT AND HYPERURICAEMIA

A disease characterised by episodes of acute arthritis, at first affecting only one joint and associated with hyperuricaemia. Hyperuricaemia is 10 times commoner without clinical gout than with it.

Primary gout
An error of purine metabolism which occurs in men and postmenopausal women (10 : 1) with a prevalence in the UK of 3/1000. The hyperuricaemia is familial and there is a family history of gout in 30%. Hyperuricaemia can also result from increased consumption of purine-containing foods and excess alcohol, especially in predisposed individuals who are often also obese.

Secondary gout
This occurs at all ages in both sexes.
Ten per cent of all gout is associated with myeloproliferative disease which causes increased purine turnover and release and hence a rise in serum uric acid (e.g. myeloid leukaemia, myelofibrosis, polycythaemia rubra vera, multiple myeloma and in Hodgkin's disease). This occurs particularly after treatment with

anti-metabolite drugs when the serum uric acid and urea rise as a result of tissue destruction.

Drug-induced hyperuricaemia may follow treatment with diuretics, particularly thiazides, and salicylates in small doses.

Chronic renal failure may be associated with hyperuricaemia and rarely clinical gout, secondary to reduced renal uric acid excretion.

Clinical features

In the first attack, the big toe is affected in 75% of cases, the ankle or tarsus in 35%, and knee in 20%. In 40% it involves more than one joint. The onset is usually sudden and the joint is red, hot, shiny and exquisitely tender. The patient is febrile, irritable and anorexic. Attacks, at first monarticular in most patients, tend to be recurrent and to become polyarticular. They may be precipitated by trauma (including surgery), exercise, dietary excess, alcohol and starvation. Chronic gouty arthritis remains asymmetrical and tophi appear, especially on the cartilages of the ears and close to joints in 20% of untreated patients.

Complications

Renal disease. Uric acid stones occur in 10% of patients in the UK and may produce renal colic. Chronic renal failure may follow longstanding hyperuric-aemia (chronic urate nephropathy).

Hypertension, obesity, coronary artery disease are more common in patients with hyperuricaemia. Secondary pyogenic infection of gouty joints is uncommon.

Investigation

The serum uric acid is raised.

NB Five per cent of men have levels of 0.42 mmol/litre or more but only 0.6% have clinical gout.

Leucocytosis is common and the erythrocyte sedimentation rate (ESR) is raised.

Radiology: asymmetrical soft tissue swelling may be the only abnormality in acute gout. Chronic disease produces irregular punched-out bony erosions near but not usually involving the articular margins. Tophi may be seen if calcified. Osteoarthritic changes are common in gouty joints. Uric acid renal stones are radiolucent.

Aspirates of joint fluid contain negatively birefringent needle crystals of monosodium urate when viewed by polarised light.

Differential diagnosis

Acute gout must be distinguished from other causes of acute arthritis, particularly septic staphylococcal arthritis and rheumatic fever. Pseudogout may occur in chronic renal failure.

Chronic gout, particularly if widespread, may resemble rheumatoid or osteoarthritis.

Hyperuricaemia may be secondary to diuretic therapy.

Management

Acute episodes

Indomethacin 100 mg followed by 25 mg tds or naproxen 750 mg followed by 250 mg tds. Hydrocortisone, 100 mg i.m. repeated as required, may be given in resistant cases and may relieve pain almost instantaneously.

Colchicine (0.5–1 mg 2-hourly until pain is relieved, vomiting and diarrhoea begin or a total of 8 mg) may be given if non-steroidal anti-inflammatory drugs are contraindicated. Allopurinol may be started a fortnight after the acute attack has subsided but must be covered by continuation of non-steroidal anti-inflammatory drug (NSAID) therapy or colchicine 0.5 mg bd for the first 3 months because acute gout may otherwise be precipitated.

Chronic recurrent gout and hyperuricaemia

Probenecid, 0.5 g two or three times a day and sulphinpyrazone 100 mg tds act by increasing renal clearance of uric acid and urates.

Allopurinol, 300 mg daily, is of particular value in treatment of chronic tophaceous gout or chronic hyperuricaemia and when renal disease is present. It blocks the metabolic pathway at xanthine and hypoxanthine (by inhibiting xanthine oxidase), both of which are more soluble than uric acid and less liable to form stones. The dose is adjusted between 200 and 900 mg daily to keep the serum uric acid normal. It should be given well before starting cytotoxic chemotherapy otherwise the release of uric acid in the tumour lysis syndrome can precipitate acute renal failure.

These drugs may precipitate an acute attack and 3 months cover with colchicine or anti-inflammatory agent (steroidal or non-steroidal) is advised.

Indications for long-term therapy are the presence of clinical gout, urate nephropathy, tophaceous gout, myeloproliferative disorders under therapy, or non-symptomatic but persistent plasma uric acid levels over 0.8 mmol/litre.

Overeating and overdrinking (of alcohol) should be corrected (not only for gout), the obese should lose weight, and drug therapy, particularly thiazides and aspirin-containing drugs, assessed and modified where necessary.

Pseudogout (articular chondrocalcinosis or calcium pyrophosphate gout)

This is rare and sometimes familial. It is less uncommon in females (M/F 2 : 1) than gout. The patients are usually elderly. It is associated with diabetes mellitus (40%), hyperparathyroidism (page 220) and haemochromatosis (page 257). It may occur in chronic renal failure. Chondrocalcinosis is frequently found by chance on X-ray of the knees and may be symptom-free. It may present as osteoarthritis. However, there may be episodic pain and effusions into large joints and it may thus mimic gout, though the big toe is seldom affected and the symptoms are usually less acute, less severe and more prolonged. The effusions contain calcium pyrophosphate crystals which are rod- or brick-shaped and positively birefringent (whereas crystals in gout are negatively birefringent). The disease is associated with radiological calcification of the joint capsule and cartilage. The cartilages of the knee are characteristically outlined by calcium but calcification may occur in any cartilaginous joint. The patient may develop osteoarthritis secondary to the destruction of joint cartilage. Intra-articular steroids have been used. Indomethacin may be needed in acute episodes.

Diagnosis is established by calcification on X-ray of the joint, a normal serum uric acid and the characteristic crystals in the aspiration of joint fluid.

NUTRITION

Obesity

Excess body fat can be measured only indirectly and weight in relation to height and age is used as the measure. Experimentally skin fold thickness of over 20 mm in men and 28 mm in women denotes obesity. The BMI (body mass index) = weight (kg)/height^2(m) is increasingly used. Normal range is up to 25.

Prognosis

Mortality is markedly increased in obesity, death being associated mainly with diabetes mellitus (15–25%) overweight (mortality ratio—MR of 200–500% of the approximate normal of 100%), hypertension (15–25% overweight = MR 250%), myocardial infarction (15–25% overweight = MR 130%). Acturail figures suggest that weight-reduction alone to normal reduces the increased mortality to normal.

Other common complications include risk from surgery, osteoarthritis, herniae, gall-stones, hiatus hernia, and varicose veins. In women there is also an increased incidence of hirsutism and breast and endometrial cancer. Perhaps the saddest complications are psychological. Many fat people particularly women are depressed and so displeased with their appearance that they may shun society.

Aetiology

It is impossible clearly to differentiate between genetic, environmental and socio-economic factors. Most fat people have at least one fat parent, usually the mother. There are likely to be controlling endocrine factors yet to be determined—fat people have high plasma insulin and cortisol with low levels of growth hormone. The presence of less brown fat in the obese remains of uncertain significance.

Ultimately obesity is perpetuated by ingestion of calories in excess of needs and reduced by lowering the calorie intake and maintaining this reduced level.

Differential diagnoses. Weight gain is a feature of myxoedema, and Cushing's syndrome and a rapid weight gain occurs with fluid retention in heart failure and renal failure and hypoalbuminuria of chronic liver disease.

Therapy is aimed at encouraging and supporting the patient during the period when they readjust to a reduced calorie intake. Many patients lose 5–10% weight after starting a diet and this is mainly water. Losing more weight is often very difficult but the initial weight loss is always encouraging.

The embarrassment and sometimes depression felt by the patient, and the irritation of most clinicians based on poor results and poor patient compliance makes successful treatment very difficult. Self-care groups, e.g. Weight Watchers, are usually more successful in the short term. If depression is a feature this will invariably prevent successful attempts at weight reduction unless the cause disappears or it responds to therapy. There is probably no role for anorectic drugs and thyroxine.

Malnutrition

This is a major problem of the developing world. In the developed countries, malnutrition occurs during any acute illness but particularly of the gastrointestinal tract, e.g. carcinoma of the stomach, ulcerative colitis, Crohn's disease, malabsorption. Protein loss is marked following burns from cutaneous loss, and also postoperatively from reduced intake and increased catabolism. Enteral feeding either via a nasogastric tube, or intravenous feeding through a tunnelled line may speed recovery in selected patients.

The elderly, when living alone, often become lonely and depressed and though their calorie intake may be sufficient it is often nutritionally poor: bread, margarine, jam and tea. Iron, folate and vitamin C deficiency may cause anaemia and, occasionally, scurvy.

Vitamin D deficiency leading to rickets has occurred in children of Asian immigrants to the UK who do not take vitamin D in their diet and have inadequate skin exposure to sunlight.

Anorexia nervosa

This is a relatively common disease of young women (incidence 1/250 schoolgirls aged 16 or under in UK) who fast, vomit and/or purge to maintain a markedly low weight and is associated with extreme thinness, anovular amenorrhoea and fine hairs on the arms and legs (lanugo). They have a markedly altered body image and a craving to be very thin after considering themselves overweight. The cause is not known and the disorder may be considered as a hysterical-compulsive disorder.

There is evidence of hypothalamo-pituitary dysfunction with low levels of luteinising hormone (LH), follicle-stimulating hormone (FSH) and oestradiol. LH and FSH levels respond to gonadotrophin releasing hormone (GnRH) injections indicating an intact anterior pituitary. The levels of circulatory hormones return to normal with recovery.

Treatment is extremely difficult and requires expert psychiatric advice and often periods of hospitalisation with the aim of readjusting abnormal psychopathology, and increasing weight. Improvement of varying degrees and often complete occurs in most patients, though treatment is often necessary for many years. The mortality is about 5%, often from suicide.

Renal disease

The commonest disease, especially in females, is urinary tract infection; and in males, prostatic hypertrophy and its consequences.

Clinically, disease of the kidneys presents in only a few ways:
- Proteinuria and its consequences. It may be mild to severe (nephrotic syndrome).
- Haematuria.
- Disorders of excretory function (uraemia): (a) acute renal failure; and (b) chronic renal failure and its consequences, e.g. hypertension. It may be mild to severe.

The underlying aetiology may produce one, more, or all of these clinical manifestations. The prognosis and the management of the patient depend upon both the clinical presentation and the underlying cause.

PROTEINURIA

Proteinuria results from severe urinary tract infection or leakage of protein from the glomeruli or tubules. In glomerular proteinuria, the smaller molecules, e.g. albumin, usually pass through in greater quantities than the larger molecules, e.g. globulins. Bence-Jones proteins are very small in comparison (they are light-chain dimers) and pass through a normal glomerulus. They are not detected by dipsticks. Proteinuria of <150 mg/24 h (1000 mg/litre) may occur from normal kidneys.

Tubular proteinuria is very rare (Fanconi syndrome, heavy metal poisoning, recovery phase of acute tubular necrosis) and is usually of globulins.

Aetiology

Acute and chronic pyelonephritis, acute and chronic glomerulonephritis, obstructive nephropathy, congestive cardiac failure, postural proteinuria, diabetes mellitus, myelomatosis, the causes of nephrotic syndrome (page 230) and analgesic abuse.

Clinical presentation

Patients may have obvious urinary tract infection, symptomless proteinuria, glomerulonephritis or the nephrotic syndrome.

Assessment

The history should include enquiry about previous urinary tract infection, sore throats, skin infections, renal disease, toxaemia in pregnancy, drugs (particularly analgesics), occupational and family history.

Examination may be normal but there may be evidence of uraemia, nephrotic syndrome, heart failure, or hypertension.

The kidneys are large and palpable in polycystic disease. Postural protein-uria, absent after lying down, may be present in young patients (up to 30 years) on standing. Early morning specimens should be normal. About 30% of these patients have persistent proteinuria 10 years later and full investigation or long-term follow-up may be indicated.

Investigation

Mid-stream urine (MSU) for microscopic haematuria (page 231), urinary tract infection, urinary sugar, and Bence-Jones protein.

Twenty-four-hour urine collection for protein content, creatinine clearance and differential protein clearance if nephrotic.

Blood urea and electrolytes. Serum proteins for nephrotic syndrome and protein strip and urine Bence–Jones protein for myeloma.

Blood glucose (and glucose tolerance test for diabetes), if indicated.

Straight X-ray of abdomen or ultrasound for renal size (13 ± 2.5 cm: kidneys are normally the same length as the adjacent 2½–3 vertebrae) and stones, and if necessary intravenous urogram (IVU) or infusion pyelogram (if the blood urea is much raised) to assess structural abnormalities.

IVU is dangerous in myeloma and renal failure unless the patient is kept well hydrated.

If the diagnosis remains obscure and the proteinuria persists, proceed to renal biopsy. This allows classification of glomerulonephritis with appropriate early treatment and the detection of polyarteritis nodosa and interstitial nephritis.

Other investigations which may be required include:
- serum uric acid, calcium, phosphate and alkaline phosphatase
- ASO titre, serum complement (if low, suggests glomerulonephritis)
- bone X-rays for 1° and 2° hyperparathyroidism and myeloma

NEPHROTIC SYNDROME

This may be regarded as a severe proteinuria sufficient to lower the serum albumin so far that sodium and water excretion are affected. It is usually considered separately because it is the presenting syndrome of a different range of renal disease. Renal function, as determined by serum urea and creatinine, is usually normal though renal failure can develop, depending on the cause. It is rare.

The nephrotic syndrome is defined as:
- severe proteinuria (usually >5 g/24 h), with
- hypoalbuminaemia (usually <20 g/litre), and
- peripheral oedema

Hypercholesterolaemia is commonly present.

Aetiology

Up to 80% of cases in children (and 25% of adults) are associated with minimal change glomerulonephritis (page 239). About half of adult cases have other primary glomerular disease. Other causes include diabetes mellitus, amyloidosis, systemic lupus erythematosus, myelomatosis, drug therapy (gold, penicillamine) and renal vein thrombosis.

Management

Treat the underlying cause.

In glomerulonephritis, renal histology and the selectivity of the proteinuria give a guide to the use of steroids and immunosuppression. When the protein loss is >3 g/24 h, a differential protein excretion index may be performed. It is usual to measure the renal clearance of endogenous transferrin (small molecule) and IgG (large molecule). The ratio of these, if <0.2, shows a selective protein loss, and this finding correlates with 'minimal change' on light microscopy and with a good response to steroid therapy and a good prognosis. Ninety per cent of children with 'minimal change lesions' respond initially to a short steroid course with complete remission, but half relapse. Cyclophosphamide therapy has been used in children. It is more dangerous but has a lower relapse rate. Spontaneous remission is common in adult nephrotics with 'minimal change' lesions on histology. 'Proliferative' and 'membranous' glomerulonephritic changes are usually unresponsive to steroids, cyclophosphamide or azathioprine, but exceptions have been described.

General management is aimed at:

• increasing oral protein intake to compensate for the renal loss—but urea levels must be carefully monitored
• reducing oedema with a low salt diet and diuretics and possibly salt-free albumin and intravenous diuretics in resistant cases
• treatment of intercurrent infection

HAEMATURIA

Haematuria must always be considered abnormal and fully investigated.

Aetiology

Common

Renal tract stones (in the UK, calcium oxalate 85%, triple phosphate 10%, urate 5%, cystine <1%).
Tumours of the bladder, kidneys and prostate.
Renal tract infection especially cystitis. Tuberculosis may produce 'sterile' pyuria. Schistosomiasis is common world-wide.

Uncommon

Acute papillary necrosis.
Renal trauma and infarction.
Acute glomerulonephritis.
Malignant hypertension.
Benign recurrent haematuria—sometimes related to benign prostatic hypertrophy.

Polyarteritis nodosa, lupus erythematosus, Henoch–Schönlein purpura, and infective endocarditis.

Haemorrhagic disease, usually caused by anticoagulant drugs.

Polycystic disease.

Investigation

Mid-stream urine for infection (including early morning specimen for tuberculosis if sterile pyuria present). Examine the deposit for casts, cells and microliths. The presence of red cells distinguishes haematuria from haemoglobinuria and also from other causes of red-coloured urine and drugs (phenolphthalein in alkaline urine, rifampicin and senna derivatives), food (beetroot and red sweets) and porphyria. Urine should also be sent for cytology.

Plasma urea and electrolytes.

Straight X-ray of abdomen to assess renal size proceeding to ultrasound and possibly IVU as in proteinuria.

Ultrasound will help in differentiating solid from cystic lesions and CT scan may be even more precise.

Cystoscopy (early) and retrograde pyelography for tumours and structural abnormalities.

Renal biopsy may be required to provide histological diagnosis.

Renal arteriography may occasionally be required to differentiate renal carcinoma (95% have an abnormal vascular supply) from benign avascular cysts but ultrasound usually gives the answer.

Mid-stream urine (MSU)

NB Normal urine (centrifuged deposit) contains:

Red blood corpuscles (RBC) 1×10^6 cells/24 h (2 per high power field).
White blood corpuscles (WBC) 2×10^6 cells/24 h (4 per high power field).
Hyaline casts arise from the tubules and may not be significant.
Granular casts are composed of protein leaked from tubules in which RBCs and WBCs from glomerular leakage adhere. They are virtually always significant.

ACUTE RENAL FAILURE (acute uraemia) (page 50)

Definition

Urine output <400 ml/24 h (the normal urine production is approximately 1 ml/min, i.e. 1.5 litre/24 h).

NB Non-oliguric renal failure can occur.

Anuria usually indicates obstruction (examine the pelvis and for enlarged bladder and prostate). Remember anticholinergic drugs (e.g. tricyclics). Check for blocked catheter!

Aetiology (pre-renal, post-renal, renal).

Pre-renal uraemia

Following severe hypotension from:

- hypovolaemia (road traffic accidents, burns, postpartum haemorrhage, blood loss at operation, severe diarrhoea, vomiting or polyuria with salt-losing kidneys)
- myocardial infarction and shock
- septicaemic shock
- drug overdosage

If hypotension is severe and prolonged, acute tubular necrosis may follow.

Post-renal uraemia

Acute urinary tract obstruction from:
- prostatic hypertrophy
- renal and ureteric stones
- pelvic carcinoma
- surgical mishap (e.g. ureteric involvement in hysterectomy)
- retroperitoneal tumours and fibrosis

NB In ureteric conditions, both must be blocked.

Intrinsic renal parenchymal disease (renal uraemia)

This includes acute glomerulonephritis, eclampsia, acute tubular necrosis, poisoning with heavy metals or barbiturates, papillary necrosis, malignant hypertension, polyarteritis nodosa, leptospirosis, septicaemia and disseminated intravascular coagulation (DIC), including the haemolytic–uraemic syndrome, prolonged hypotension and severe acute hypercalcaemia.

NB Acute renal failure may complicate chronic renal parenchymal disease.

Assessment

Rapid correction of hypovolaemia with blood or plasma after haemorrhage or saline may prevent renal failure. Measurement of central venous pressure will confirm the diagnosis and monitor replacement of fluids.

Where there is no obvious cause for oliguria and uraemia it becomes necessary to:
- ensure that hypovolaemia, if present, is corrected
- check that there is no obstruction to the urinary tract
- assess the presence of previous intrinsic renal disease (suggested by hypertension, skin pigmentation, calcium, phosphate, metabolic acidosis, a normochromic normocytic anaemia, bone X-ray changes and small renal shadows)

Clinical history and examination

A full history is taken with particular attention to previous renal disease, acute infection (malaria in the tropics), stones, prostatism and abdominal operations. There may have been previous hypertension or a history of analgesic abuse.

Examination includes an assessment of the state of hydration. Hypovolaemia causes postural hypotension, rapid small-volume pulse, cold extremities, reduced tissue turgor and thirst. The bladder is enlarged in urethral obstruction. Rectal examination is obligatory to exclude prostatic disease in men and pelvic carcinoma in women—vaginal examination may be necessary.

Investigation (table 22)

Urine

Culture for infection.

Oliguria following hypovolaemia and before the onset of tubular necrosis is indicated by the absence of casts, urine osmolality >450 mOsm/kg (specific gravity >1015), sodium <10mmol/litre, and urea concentration above 330 mmol/litre.

In intrinsic renal disease (including acute tubular necrosis) casts are present, the tubules are unable to concentrate the glomerular filtrate producing an osmolality of filtered plasma (250–300 mOsm/kg) and a specific gravity of 1010 and urea concentration of usually <100 mmol/litre.

Blood

Serum urea, creatinine and electrolytes are estimated as a baseline to measure the degree of uraemia, hyperkalaemia and acidosis. In hypovolaemia (in the absence of tubular necrosis) the ratio of urine to blood urea concentration is over 10:1 and the urine–blood osmolality ratio is over 1.5:1. A sodium excretion >20 mmol/litre suggests good tubular function.

Urine flow

It is almost invariably necessary to catheterise the bladder if anuria is present in the absence of known previous intrinsic renal disease, despite the risk of introducing infection. This may be the only way to ensure that the bladder is not full (i.e. there is no obstruction distal to the bladder), of obtaining a urine sample

Table 22. Differentiation between pre-renal uraemia in a person with healthy kidneys and acute tubular necrosis.

Pre-renal (volume depletion)	Acute tubular necrosis
Reduced skin turgor, low occular tension, empty neck veins, postural hypotension, weight loss, dry tongue, raised plasma haematocrit	Well hydrated or fluid overloaded with visible or raised neck veins
Urine osmolality >450	Urine osmolality <310
Concentrated urine, with urine : plasma osmolality >1.5	Dilute urine, with urine : plasma osmolality <1.1
Urine : plasma creatinine ratio >40	Urine : plasma creatinine ratio <40
Urine urea >330	Urine urea >150
Urine : plasma urea ratio >8	Urine : plasma urea ratio <3
Urine$_{Na}$ <10–20 mmol/litre	Urine$_{Na}$ >20–40 mmol/litre

and of accurately estimating urine flow. A persistent urine flow of 0.3–0.5 ml/min or less after correction of hypovolaemia may indicate the onset of tubular necrosis. Monitoring urine output is the simplest means of assessing changes in renal function.

Radiology

A plain X-ray of the urinary tract may demonstrate small kidneys (normal 13 ± 2.5 cm or 2½–3 adjacent vertebrae) if pre-existent renal disease was present, large kidneys in polycystic disease, and asymmetrical kidneys in unilateral renal disease. It may demonstrate renal and ureteric stones. Ultrasound may show kidney size, stones and dilatation of the pelvicalyceal system in outflow obstruction. If renal outflow obstruction is suspected—usually on the basis of total anuria and/or a history of ureteric colic—isotope renography may confirm the diagnosis, and indicate if both kidneys are functioning. It may be necessary to proceed to cystoscopy with ureteric catheterization. X-ray of the hands may suggest hyperparathyroidism and therefore chronic renal failure.

Infusion urography with tomograms for renal size (small scarred kidneys suggest previous renal disease) and for the 'negative pyelogram' of acute outflow obstruction. An early nephrogram within 5–10 min shows that the renal blood supply is adequate but if it persists for hours—or even days—this suggests acute tubular necrosis.

Management

Hypovolaemia

Replacement of circulating volume with blood or saline may be sufficient to prevent tubular necrosis. Fluid replacement is most easily monitored by daily weighing and with a central venous pressure catheter (central venous pressure at 10 cm H_2O). Mannitol (50 ml of 25% mannitol (i.v.) or frusemide (200 mg increasing to 1–2 g i.v.)) may reverse the onset phase of acute tubular necrosis.

Outflow obstruction

Remove mechanical obstruction, e.g. prostatic stones and tumours. It is occasionally necessary to cannulate the dilated renal pelvis percutaneously to drain it. If surgery is contraindicated in benign prostatic hypertrophy, use a catheter.

Infection and systemic disease

Treat septicaemia (after taking blood culture) and any other systemic disease, e.g. systemic lupus erythematosus (SLE).

Nutrition

Maintain with fine bore nasogastric tube, or otherwise a subclavian line to include glucose, essential amino acids with or without vitamins and with or without trace elements.

Non-protein high carbohydrate diet

Non-protein high carbohydrate diet (e.g. Hycal 2000–2500 cal/24 h) for 1–2 days.

Fluid replacement. Give as water or glucose solution orally 500 ml (insensible loss) plus volume of urine output from previous 24 h (ml for ml). Ice cubes (from 24 h allowance) or lemon slices relieve a dry mouth.

Assess the following daily:
- weight to assess fluid retention—on the above regime patients should lose 0–0.5 kg per day (easiest with a weigh-bed)
- clinical degree of hydration (thirst, tissue turgor, oedema and blood pressure)
- serum urea and electrolytes, and creatinine and 24-h urinary excretion of sodium and potassium.

Electrolytes. No electrolytes should be given in the first 24 h. After that, if hydration is normal, replace the previous 24-h urinary sodium loss. Potassium is usually raised in acute tubular necrosis and tends to rise. ECG changes of 'tenting' of the T wave may be the first indication of serious hyperkalaemia. This may be reduced by glucose/insulin or oral calcium-resonium resin.

Recovery is indicated by the onset of a variable degree of polyuria, usually after 1–2 weeks. If spontaneous recovery dose not occur, consider renal biopsy for the cause of underlying disease such as glomerulonephritis. There may be marked loss of water and electrolytes and these must be replaced, ml for ml, and mmol for mmol.

Indications for dialysis

Deteriorating clinical state with mental dullness, confusion and hiccough, fits, pulmonary oedema, pericarditis and peripheral neuropathy.

Blood urea above 50 mmol/litre and rising. In anuria the urea rises by about 5 mmol/litre/day. A rise of over 8 mmol/litre/day occurs in hypercatabolic states and indicates the need for early dialysis.

Serum potassium above 6–7 mmol/litre.

Bicarbonate below 10–15 mmol/litre.

Progressive weight gain of fluid retention.

The rates of change are more important than the absolute levels—the above levels are intended as guides and are not absolute.

CHRONIC RENAL FAILURE (chronic uraemia)

This clinical syndrome is common to the later stages of all chronic and insidious renal disease and is characterised by uraemia. The urine osmolality eventually becomes fixed at 250–300 mOsm/kg (the osmolality of filtered plasma) when the number of nephrons becomes too small to alter glomerular filtrate.

In patients presenting with renal failure for the first time, the following features suggest chronic rather than acute renal failure:
- a history of chronic ill-health and urinary symptoms
- anaemia (normochromic, normocytic)
- osteodystrophy (hyperparathyroidism: check alkaline phosphatase)
- small kidneys on X-ray or ultrasound
- brown line on finger nails

Aetiology

Common

Chronic urinary tract obstruction (commonly prostatic hypertrophy).
Chronic glomerulonephritis.
Diabetic nephropathy.
Hypertensive nephropathy.
Interstitial nephritis, including chronic nephritis, analgesic abuse and tuberculosis.

Less common

Polycystic disease.
The collagen diseases.
Hypercalcaemia and hyperuricaemia.
Retroperitoneal fibrosis.
Persisting acute renal failure.

Clinical presentation

The history is usually of lethargy, polyuria and nocturia, and general ill health. In later stages of the disease, symptoms of uraemia with anorexia, nausea, vomiting, hiccough, weight loss, bruising and epistaxis are common. There may be a history of prostatic obstruction, recurrent dysuria sometimes with episodic fever and loin pain, or a known story of acute glomerulonephritis. Analgesic nephropathy may occur when 1–2 kg of analgesic has been taken for arthritis, headache or depression. Polycystic disease is familial (autosomal dominant).

Examination

In the early stages there may be no abnormal clinical signs but anaemia is common and there may be a uraemic line in the finger nail. Urinary tract obstruction secondary to prostatic hypertrophy must be excluded. In the later stages of uraemia the patient shows varying degrees of mental confusion. A pericardial rub is characteristic and a neuropathy not uncommon. There is a characteristic 'dirty' yellow pallor of the skin, bruising is common and hyperventilation of metabolic acidosis occurs. Secondary infection is common. The kidneys are large in polycystic disease. There may be hypertension.

Remember to examine for a large bladder. Rectal examination is obligatory in both sexes.

Investigation

Mid-stream urine may reveal bacterial infection and granular casts.

Blood urea and electrolyte concentrations and creatinine clearance will indicate the degree of renal dysfunction and acidosis. The rise in urea may partly reflect the degree of dehydration. The serum calcium may fall secondary to renal phosphate retention or acquired vitamin D resistance (page 217). Reduced excretion of phosphate, together with reduced calcium absorption from the gut due to lack of the second hydroxylation of vitamin D (from 25-OHD to

1-25-OHD) in the kidney, results in lowering of the serum calcium. Acidosis protects the patient from tetany by increasing the ionised portion of the reduced calcium.

Plasma uric acid is often raised (but clinical gout is rare).

Plain X-ray of the abdomen should define kidney size and ultrasound or IVU outline the renal tract to exclude obstructive lesions. Isotope renography may indicate obstruction to outflow. X-ray of the chest, teeth and hands, may show evidence of secondary hyperparathyroidism. Proceed to cystoscopy and retrograde pyelography if necessary.

Renal biopsy is indicated after pre-renal (hypovalaemic) and postrenal (obstructive) diseases have been excluded to determine the cause of underlying disease, particularly if renal size is normal. Ultrasound or IVU must be performed first. Biopsy is not performed when there is only one functioning kidney, if there is a bleeding disorder or if the kidneys are small—when histology is no longer helpful in determining the aetiology. Investigate for relevant systemic disease.

Management

Exclude or treat prerenal disorders (e.g. sodium or water depletion) and postrenal obstruction.

Treat infection, both renal and intercurrent, which itself induces a hypercatabolic state and hence a rapid rise in blood urea.

Treat hypertension as in patients with essential hypertension. Control may improve or prevent deterioration in renal function. Reduction in dietary sodium may be effective alone. Be aware of altered drug handling in renal failure.

Dietary control. The main purpose of protein restriction is to produce a fall in the blood urea and thus reduce the symptoms of uraemia, in particular anorexia, nausea and vomiting. The protein need not be reduced more than is necessary to relieve symptoms, usually achieved at blood urea levels of about 15–25 mmol/litre. Normal diet contains about 85 g protein per day. In conservative management of chronic renal failure a 40 g protein diet is usually adequate. In severe uraemia the intake may be reduced as far as 20 g protein. At this stage essential amino acids should be added and a high calorie intake is essential to suppress breakdown of body protein, i.e. 2000–3000 Cal per day as carbohydrate (Caloreen or Hycal). Vitamin supplements, particularly B and C, may be required.

Water and electrolyte control. This is aimed at achieving as high a urine output as possible to eliminate urea and other toxic metabolites, without inducing heart failure. This may be achieved with oral fluids alone (up to 2.5–3.0 litres/24 h) or by the addition of frusemide 0.5–1.5 g daily, which may also increase the glomerular filtration rate. The 24-h urinary sodium loss must be measured and replaced if excessive. Hypertension and fluid retention would suggest the need for a reduction in sodium intake. Hyperkalaemia is treated by dietary restriction, followed, if necessary, by ion-exchange resin (calcium resonium 45 g daily in divided doses).

Vitamin D supplements (pages 216, 218) may be required if uraemic bone disease occurs with symptoms of osteomalacia (weakness and bone pain).

Dietary phosphate restriction with or without aluminium hydroxide may reduce serum phosphate levels (page 217) and prevent ectopic calcification.

Anaemia tends to be unresponsive to iron or vitamins (except when on dialysis), but serum iron, B_{12} and folate should be checked. Recombinant human erythropoietin increases the haemoglobin, but may increase the incidence of hypertension and thrombotic events.

Infection. Septicaemic and urinary tract infections are best treated according to the results of bacterial sensitivities in urine and blood culture. The penicillins and 'third generation' cephalosporins are relatively safe. Aminoglycosides (gentamicin, tobramycin, amikacin) are given in reduced doses or less frequently in renal failure and serum levels should be monitored.

Allopurinol may be required for hyperuricaemia and dietary control for Type IV hyperlipidaemia (page 209).

Consider the suitability of intermittent chronic haemodialysis, continuous ambulatory peritoneal dialysis (CAPD) or transplantation.

Haemofiltration can be used as a substitute for dialysis (haemo- and peritoneal) if there is cardiovascular instability and hypotension, or if dialysis is not available. (A reasonable blood pressure is required to 'drive' dialysis machines and dialysis leads to large changes in circulating volume.)

Indications for dialysis

Severe renal failure (creatinine clearance <3–4 ml/min) is most easily managed by dialysis. It seems reasonable to dialyse every new patient with rapidly progressive uraemia of undiagnosed aetiology, to allow time for full assessment including renal biopsy, particularly in the presence of normal-sized kidneys which indicate recent renal disease (acute glomerulonephritis, myeloma, infective endocarditis, polyarteritis nodosa, renal vein thrombosis, malignant hypertension, amyloid).

Indications for long-term dialysis (haemodialysis or peritoneal dialysis) and renal transplantation vary from place to place and time to time. Every reasonable case should be referred, preferably early in their chronic downhill course, for assessment by the dialysis centre.

GLOMERULONEPHRITIS

This describes a number of disorders which affect one or more of the glomerular components in both kidneys (figure 48). Clinically patients present with one or more of the usual features of renal disease, i.e. haematuria, proteinuria, (the nephrotic syndrome if severe) and various degrees of acute or chronic renal failure.

The classification of glomerulonephritis is based on histology and immunofluorescence and is similar to the changes found on renal biopsy in the nephrotic syndrome. Confusion arises because it is impossible to classify glomerulonephritis clinically as any of the histological features may be associated with one or more of haematuria, proteinuria, nephrosis and varying degrees of renal failure. Renal biopsy and histology are sometimes helpful guides to prognosis. The histological changes usually found are:

- Minimal change
- Membranous
- Diffuse proliferative
- Focal nephritis
- Mesangiocapillary
- IgA nephropathy

The diagnosis is invariably confirmed only after the renal biopsy. Contraindications to biopsy include: (a) one functioning kidney, (b) small kidneys, and (c bleeding disorders.

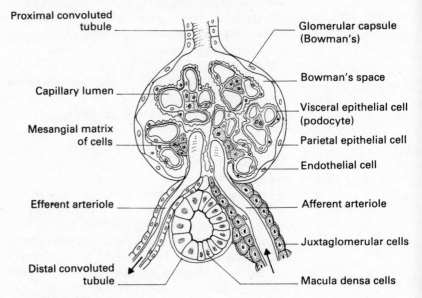

Figure 48. Glomerulus.

- *Minimal change*. This is mainly a disease of children with increased permeability of the basement membrane and often presents with nephrotic syndrome. Light microscopy is normal but electron microscopy (EM) reveal fusion of the epithelial cell foot processes. No immunoglobulin deposition is seer on immunofluorescence. It is associated with selective proteinuria (e.g. ratio o IgG to transferrin). It accounts for 80% of cases of childhood nephrotic syndrome, up to one-third of adult nephrotics and is steroid-responsive.

- *Membranous*. This is mainly a disease of adults and presents with proteinuria or nephrotic syndrome but rarely haematuria. There may be a genetic factor and it may follow infection with hepatitis B virus, treatment with gold, mercury o penicillamine and sometimes occurs with SLE and malignancy (carcinoma of the bronchus). There is diffuse thickening of the glomerular wall, with deposition o antigen–antibody complexes on the epithelium visible on electron microscopy At first the basement membrane contains granular deposits of IgG on immuno fluorescence. Later it appears thickened. About a third of patients improve spontaneously, another third have persistent proteinuria with a variable degree of uraemia and the final third develop progressive uraemia. Response to steroids is usually poor though they are worth trying. Treatment with steroids and chlorombucil may improve the prognosis. Hypertension should be treated.

- *Diffuse proliferative.* Patients present with rapidly progressive renal failure. It is associated with collagen diseases. There is marked proliferation of all the components of Bowman's capsule with crescent formation and fibrinoid necrosis of the glomerular vessels. If crescents are seen in more than 50% of the glomeruli, it may be called crescentic glomerulonephritis. It is associated with SLE, polyarteritis nodosa, Wegener's disease, and Goodpasture's syndrome (antiglomerular basement membrane disease). Treatment is with steroids, cyclophosphamide and plasma exchange to remove antigen—antibody complexes, and is particularly indicated in Wegener's granulomatosis when the antinuclear cytoplasmic antibody is positive, and in Goodpasture's syndrome. The prognosis is poor.
- *Focal nephritis.* Some, but not all, glomeruli are affected with variable degrees of cellular proliferation, hyalinosis, sclerosis and crescent formation. It may be segmental in that only parts of the affected glomeruli are involved.
- It is associated with SLE, polyarteritis nodosa, Wegener's disease, infectious endocarditis and Henoch–Schönlein purpura. The aetiology is usually unknown, and the prognosis is very variable depending on associated diseases.
- *Mesangiocapillary.* There is mesangial cell proliferation and increase in mesangial matrix together with thickening of the capillary walls. It may be associated with the presence of C_3 nephritic factor, an Ig autoantibody which stabilises C_3 convertase in the complement cascade allowing continuous degradation of C_3. Mesangiocapillary glomerulonephritis may also occur with chronic infections such as bacterial endocarditis. Rarely, it is associated with partial lipoatrophy. It may present with haematuria, proteinuria, the nephrotic syndrome or renal impairment. There is no proven therapy. Most patients develop progressive renal failure over a period of years.
- *IgA nephropathy* (Berger's disease). This usually presents with intermittent haematuria in an otherwise fit young man and is sometimes associated with upper respiratory tract infection. Treament is not required and the prognosis excellent though 5–10% may progress. Immunofluorescence shows diffuse deposition of IgA (and usually IgG) with cellular proliferation within the glomerular mesangium.
- **NB** *Goodpasture's syndrome.* Patients present with rapidly progressive renal failure associated with pulmonary haemorrhage. (Chest X-ray changes usually with frank haemoptysis.) There is linear immunofluorescence of IgG along the basement membrane and IgG antibodies are present in the serum. Treatment is as in diffuse crescentic glomerulonephritis. It is worth measuring antiglomerular basement membrane antibodies in acute renal failure because early treatment may achieve complete remission, whereas delayed treatment may allow irreversible renal damage.

Acute streptococcal glomerulonephritis (acute nephritic syndrome)

Clinical presentation. A well-defined clinical syndrome with abrupt onset of haematuria and oliguria. This is rapidly followed by oedema (classically ankle and periorbital), hypertension and varying degrees of uraemia. This is now relatively rare.

Aetiology. The majority occur in childhood and follow 10–15 days after a haemolytic streptococcal (group A, type 12) infection of the throat—antigen–antibody complexes have been demonstrated in the glomerular tufts. (The clinical picture of acute nephritis may also occur in other types of glomerulo-nephritis, Henoch–Schönlein purpura (page 96), polyarteritis nodosa, SLE and Goodpasture's syndrome.)

Investigation. Streptococci may be isolated from the throat if penicillin has not already been given. A rising ASO titre may be demonstrable and serum complement reduced.

Management. As for acute renal failure. Daily weighing and estimation of serum electrolytes are essential. In the large majority severe renal failure does not occur and uraemia is transitory. Penicillin should be given to eliminate the streptococci. Hypertension may be severe and require treatment in the usual way (page 317).

Prognosis. Over 90% of children and 60–70% of adults recover fully. With advances in dialysis technique and management of hypertensive encephalopathy, death in the acute phase is uncommon. Insidious renal failure develops in a very small number of cases.

URINARY TRACT INFECTION

There are two main clinical syndromes:
- Cystitis which is characterised by suprapubic tenderness, dysuria and frequency. These symptoms can also occur without evidence of infection—'the urethral syndrome'
- Acute pyleonephritis is characterised by dysuria, frequency, loin tenderness and fever, often with rigors and vomiting. Fever may be the only feature in children in whom recurrent infection may be associated with vesico-ureteric reflux which tends to diminish with age

Bacteriuria is confirmed by a urinary excretion of more than 100 000 organisms/ml (counts <10 000/ml are usually due to contamination). Infection may be symptom-free.

E. coli is the most frequent organism (70–80% of cases). Other organisms (*Proteus, Staphylococcus, Streptococcus, Klebsiella* and *Pseudomonas*) are usually associated with structural abnormality and reinfection, or previous catheterisation. Tuberculosis classically causes a 'sterile' pyuria.

Urinary white cell counts remain of uncertain value in diagnosis as the normal values are ill-defined. Non-inflammatory disorders may provoke their excretion, and the absence of white cells may still be associated with bacteriuria and clinically significant urinary tract infection.

Management

There may be an obvious predisposing cause, e.g. pregnancy, urinary obstruction or catheterisation. Diabetes mellitus must be excluded. More than two episodes of cystitis in a woman, or a single episode in a man, suggests a structural abnormality of the renal tract and renal ultrasound is performed and, if indicated, intravenous urogram, a micturating cystogram for reflux, and possibly cystoscopy with retrograde pyelography.

A single attack of pyelonephritis should be investigated fully.

The organism should be set up for culture and antibiotic sensitivities before treatment is started.

Augmentin or trimethoprim are probably the drugs of first choice unless the patient is pregnant. 30% urinary coliforms are amoxycillin resistant. Recurrent infection which is often asymptomatic may occur, usually with the same organism. The best treatment for chronic and recurrent infection remains uncertain. It seems reasonable to treat single recurrent episodes as new infections with short courses of antimicrobial drugs. Frequent attacks (symptomatic or asymptomatic) are sometimes prevented or reduced by continuous low-dose chemotherapy, usually taken at night (e.g. nitrofurantoin 100 mg, trimethoprim 200 mg or nalidixic acid 500 mg nightly).

Chronic infection (where the urinary excretion of organisms remains above 100 000/ml) may require continued cyclical therapy (e.g. cotrimoxazole 2 bd, ampicillin 250 mg qds and nitrofurantoin 100–200 mg daily for 10 days each continuously) but the organism must be carefully monitored throughout therapy and drugs chosen appropriately. Structural abnormalities should always be considered in recurrent and chronic infection or infection with uncommon organisms (e.g. *Pseudomonas*).

CHRONIC INTERSTITIAL NEPHRITIS

Clinical presentation

Patients present usually with insidious renal failure, hypertension or proteinuria.

There may or may not be clinical or bacteriological evidence of urinary tract infection. The diagnosis is made on IVP findings of small, scarred kidneys often with cortical thinning overlying calyceal 'clubbing'. If renal biopsy is performed the kidney shows patchy areas of cellular infiltration with plasma cells and lymphocytes between the tubules, which are atrophic or ballooned. There is periglomerular fibrosis. Some glomeruli are normal and others hyalinised.

Aetiology

The clinical, radiological and histological features of 'chronic pyelonephritis' are not necessarily the result of infection, acute or chronic. They may also be given by glomerulonephritis, diabetes and hypertension. Hence the term 'chronic pyelonephritis' with an implied infective aetiology is confusing. The term 'chronic interstitial nephritis' is used instead, and allows the inclusion of other conditions in which interstitial round cell infiltration is a principal reaction. These include obstructive uropathy, analgesic nephropathy, hypokalaemia, hypercalcaemia and amyloidosis.

The roles of recurrent urinary tract infection and ureteric reflux remain uncertain. New kidney scars rarely develop after the age of 4 years. All urinary tract infections in children below this age should be vigorously treated and closely followed up. The value of ureteric reimplantation for urinary reflux to prevent progressive renal damage remains unproven.

Management

Urinary tract infection, if present, must be treated. Congenital structural abnormalities may be present but other common conditions (e.g. prostatic hypertrophy, tumours and stones) must be considered.

Chronic renal failure is managed as described (page 238).

POLYCYSTIC KIDNEY DISEASE

Patients, usually between the ages of 30 and 50 years, present with chronic renal failure. Hypertension (70%), abdominal pain (40%), or urinary tract infection (30%) or haematuria (30%), may also occur. Its inheritance is autosomal dominant. There is a family history in over 50%. Diagnosis is usually obvious clinically. Ultrasound gives a characteristic picture of many small reflections of multiple cysts and an intravenous urogram shows spider calyces.

Prognosis and management

There is progressive renal failure with hypertension and recurrent urinary tract infection. Haematuria, though recurrent, is usually slight and self-limiting. Haemodialysis, and transplantation eventually may become necessary and early referral to a renal unit is advisable. Genetic counselling is recommended.

HEPATORENAL SYNDROME

Acute renal failure may occur following surgery to the lower end of the bile duct for relief of longstanding obstructive jaundice. The causes remain uncertain but the renal failure might be preventable by maintaining mannitol diuresis from before and during surgery.

NB In all patients who have both jaundice and renal failure, leptospirosis should be considered. The clinical picture may also include fever, haematuria, meningitis and conjunctivitis. The organism can be grown from urine and blood and responds to penicillin.

HAEMOLYTIC URAEMIC SYNDROME (diffuse intravascular coagulation)

A disease usually of infants under 3 years old of unknown aetiology often following infections of the gastrointestinal tract. Renal failure is caused by intravascular blood-clotting in small renal arterioles. Fibrin degradation products are detectable in the blood and haemolysis and thrombocytopenia also occur. Treatment is by dialysis for renal failure, anticoagulation with heparin or prostacyclin, with or without plasma exchange. A similar, often fatal, disease occurs in adults (thrombotic thrombocytopenic purpura, page 100).

FLUIDS AND ELECTROLYTES

Minimum daily replacement values in the normal adult (70 kg man) are as follows:

2.5–3.0 litres water per day
80 mmol sodium (0.5 litres normal saline)
80 mmol potassium (6 g potassium chloride)

These are minimum requirements and most patients with normal kidneys are able to maintain sodium and potassium balance with higher intakes. The above schedule forms the basis of postoperative fluid replacement.

Salt and water depletion

In Britain this usually results from:
- gastrointestinal loss: vomiting and diarrhoea and fistulae
- renal loss: chronic renal failure with sodium loss, excess dialysis, acute diuresis due to drugs, recovery from acute renal failure, relief of urinary obstruction (postprostatectomy) and diabetic ketoacidosis, and very rarely Addison's disease
- skin loss: excess sweating (NB cystic fibrosis), burns, exfoliative dermatitis

Clinical presentation

Mental confusion, thirst and dry tongue are common, and tissue turgor is reduced. Oliguria is not universally present, particularly when deficit follows the polyuria of chronic renal failure. In severe depletion hypotension and shock occur.

Investigation

Weight is usually reduced. Blood pressure tends to fall and there is a marked postural drop. Blood urea, haemoglobin and packed cell volume tend to rise. The serum sodium concentration does not necessarily give an accurate indication of total body sodium since it tends to move with water.

Management

In the elderly and ill monitor saline infusion with a central venous pressure line. With continuous salt loss, daily weighing gives an approximate estimate of salt loss but these are more accurately estimated by collection of urine (and faeces or vomit if necessary). Potassium loss is not necessarily associated with body sodium loss from chronic renal disease, but is invariable in losses from the gastrointestinal tract.

Water excess

Clinical presentation

Drowsiness, depression, confusion, fits and coma, headache, anorexia, nausea and vomiting.

Aetiology

Excess water intake (oral or intravenous) or reduced water output, e.g. inappropriate *antidiuretic hormone (ADH) syndrome*, often secondary to carcinoma, usually of bronchus or pancreas, or to drugs, usually chlorpropamide or carbamazepine therapy. It may also follow head injury, acute alcoholism and pneumonia.

Diagnosis

The plasma sodium is <130 mmol/litre and frequently under 120 mmol/litre before the diagnosis is made. The plasma osmolality is under 280 mOsm/litre. The urine osmolality in inappropriate ADH syndrome is always inappropriately high compared with the plasma osmolality. If plasma osmolality test are not available, a single calculation will give a rough approximation: Plasma osmolality = 1.85 (sodium + potassium) + blood urea + blood glucose.

Management

Restrict water intake to <600 ml/24 h. If the patient is seriously ill, it may be necessary to give saline and rarely hyperosmolar solutions such as 2 N saline (300 ml in 2 h, repeated if required). Where possible, the cause should be treated. If not, try demeclocycline 300 mg tds.

Hypokalaemia

Normal potassium intake = 60–200 mmol/day.

Aetiology

This arises from:
- diuretic therapy
- gastrointestinal loss: vomiting and pyloric stenosis, gastrointestinal fistulae, diarrhoea, paralytic ileus
- recovery from acidosis, especially diabetic ketoacidosis: potassium is raised in serum but total body potassium is down
- Cushing's disease

The clinical symptoms are of weakness and lethargy.
The ECG shows flat T and prominent U waves.

Management

Treat the underlying cause.

Give oral potassium supplements as potassium chloride.

In diabetic ketoacidosis potassium is given intravenously: 2 g (26 mmol) per litre of intravenous fluid are usually sufficient to maintain balance through the osmotic diuresis in young patients with healthy kidneys. In the elderly or in the presence of renal disease careful monitoring by ECG and serial serum levels are necessary.

NB Potassium supplements are rarely required when low dose thiazide diuretics are used to treat hypertension even though there is a slight reduction in serum potassium concentration. The serum potassium concentration does not necessarily give an accurate indication of total body potassium, being mainly an intracellular ion.

Hyperkalaemia

Aetiology

This is the result of:
- renal failure, acute or chronic case treated with stored blood, potassium salts of penicillin, and food with potassium content (mushrooms, nuts, instant coffee, wine, beer, dried fruit and vegetables, sodium chloride substitutes)
- excess potassium intake, e.g. Slow-K with potassium retaining diuretics (spironolactone, amiloride, triamterene)
- Addison's disease—very rare

Management

Stop oral or intravenous intake.

Ion exchange resins, e.g. calcium resonium 15 g 6-hourly orally (or rectally).

In emergency states: i.v. calcium 10 ml 10% calcium gluconate (this may be fatal in digitalised patients) or insulin in dextrose, e.g. 100 ml of 50% dextrose with 20 units soluble insulin (1 unit to 2.5 g dextrose) followed if necessary by 20% dextrose containing 1 unit soluble insulin per 2 g dextrose (i.e. 100 units/litre) given at the rate of 2 ml/kg over 1 h.

Renal dialysis should always be considered (page 236).

Metabolic acidosis

This commonly occurs in:
- cardiac arrest
- diabetic ketoacidosis
- salicylate poisoning
- renal failure

Management

Bicarbonate deficit can be calculated but total 'correction' is usually not necessary. Total deficit is the measured serum bicarbonate below normal standard bicarbonate × 30% body weight in kg. Replace as 8.4% sodium bicarbonate solution (contains 1 mmol/ml). This should be rapid (give 50–100 mmol) following cardiac arrest as cardiac arrhythmias are difficult to revert in the presence of acidosis. There is little value in correcting acidosis in renal failure and the value of correcting acidosis in diabetic ketosis, and salicylate poisoning remains doubtful unless the pH is <7.1 (7.2 in children) when partial 'correction' only is required.

Hyperaldosteronism

Primary hyperaldosteronism in Conn's syndrome (page 193). Secondary hyperaldosteronism is associated with cardiac failure, the nephrotic syndrome, severe hypertension and cirrhosis with ascites. It is exacerbated when hypovolaemia has been produced by diuretics used in their treatment. Treatment is of the underlying cause and with spironolactone, sometimes in large doses (over 1 g daily).

Hypercalcaemia

The causes include acute renal failure (page 232), hyperparathyroidism (page 220), sarcoidosis (page 296), bone secondaries, myeloma (page 364), and vitamin D excess (page 217).

Hypocalcaemia

The causes include acute pancreatitis, hypoparathyroidism, vitamin D deficiency (and vitamin D-dependent rickets), chronic renal failure, and cytotoxic agents.

Hypomagnesaemia

Magnesium is the second most abundant intracellular cation. Normal requirement is 150 mg/day. Normal intake is 300–400 mg/day.

*Clinical presentation:*parasthesiae, cramp, tetany, apathy and occurs in starvation, enteral nutrition with or without magnesium malabsorption, prolonged diarrhoea, with fistulae and drugs (diuretics, aminoglycosides, carbenicillin, amphotericin).
Usually associated with hypocalcaemia.
Reduced calcium and magnesium are often found in the seriously ill in intensive care units where nutrition has been inaccurately estimated.

The values given in table 23 may be found useful:

Table 23. Fluid and electrolyte values.

Sodium (mEq = mmol)	Quantity	Na$^+$ mmol
Sodium chloride	1 g	17.1
Sodium bicarbonate	1 g	11.9
Normal saline (sodium chloride injection) 0.9%	1 litre	150
Dextrose/saline (1/5 N saline)	1 litre	30
Sodium bicarbonate		
injection 1.4%	1 litre	167
8.4%	1 litre	1000
Slow-sodium tablets	1 tablet	10.0

Potassium (mEq = mmol)	Quantity	K$^+$ mmol
Potassium chloride	1 g	13.4
Potassium citrate	1 g	9.2
Potassium chloride slow tablets (Slow-K, Leo K)	1 tablet	8.1
Potassium chloride effervescent tablets (Sando-K)	1 tablet	12 (8 Cl$^-$)
Potassium citrate mixture	10 ml	27.6

NB A millimole is the molecular weight of an ion in milligrams.

Liver disease

The commonest disease is acute viral hepatitis. Drug jaundice, gall stones, biliary tract obstruction and carcinomatous secondary deposits are fairly common.

ACUTE HEPATITIS (see pages 45–9)

This refers to inflammation of the liver with little or no fibrosis and little or no nodular regeneration. There may be minor distortion of lobular architecture. If there is extensive fibrosis with nodular regeneration (and hence distortion of architecture) the condition is called cirrhosis. These diagnoses are made histologically and there may or may not be clinical evidence of previous hepatic disease.

Acute inflammation with necrosis of liver cells results from:
- Infection, most commonly acute infectious hepatitis A and B but also with the viruses of Hepatitis C, infectious mononucleosis and yellow fever, and associated with septicaemia and leptospirosis. Amoebic hepatitis is common on a world basis and usually presents as a hepatic abscess or amoeboma
- Chemical poisons and drugs are less frequent causes of acute hepatitis. Toxic chemicals include carbon tetrachloride, vinyl chloride, and ethylene glycol and similar solvents (glue sniffing). Toxic drugs include alcohol (ethanol and methanol), halothane (after repeated exposures), PAS, isoniazid and rifampicin, paracetamol, methotrexate, chlorpromazine and the monoamine oxidase inhibitors
- Pregnancy (rare)

If the patient recovers this is usually complete, but, rarely, progressive necrosis may affect almost the entire liver (fulminant hepatic failure or acute massive necrosis) causing hepatic coma (page 255) and death.

Acute viral hepatitis

There are three major groups:
- hepatitis A (infectious hepatitis [IH], short incubation hepatitis)
- hepatitis B (serum hepatitis [SH], long incubation hepatitis)
- hepatitis C—parenterally transmitted
- hepatitis E—faecal–oral transmitted

Hepatitis A

The disease is caused by an enterovirus (hepatitis A antigen) which is excreted in the stools towards the end of the incubation period and disappears as the illness develops. Antibody appears at the onset of the illness and a rising titre indicates recent infection. The disease is endemic but small epidemics may occur in schools or institutions. Spread is usually via the faecal–oral route. It may be spread by food products such as shellfish. The young (5–14 years) are chiefly involved.

Clinical presentation. After a variable incubation period of 2–6 weeks there is a gradual onset of an influenza-like illness with fever, malaise, anorexia, nausea, vomiting and upper abdominal discomfort associated with tender enlargement of the liver and, less commonly, the spleen. There may be a distaste of cigarettes. After 3–4 days the urine becomes characteristically dark and the stools pale—evidence of cholestasis. Symptoms usually become less severe as jaundice appears although pruritus may develop. Jaundice and symptoms tend to improve after 1–2 weeks and recovery is usually complete, although mild symptoms may continue for up to 3–4 months in a few patients. Recurrent hepatitis is extremely rare and immunity probably lifelong. A rise in specific anti-hepatitis A antibody titre can be detected in the serum.

Differential diagnosis. Obstructive jaundice, either in the early cholestatic phase or in the rare cases where cholestatic jaundice persists after other clinical and biochemical evidence of liver cell damage has settled. It is dangerous to diagnose infective hepatitis in patients over 40 years old—a safeguard against mis-diagnosing major bile duct obstruction.
Drug jaundice (page 259).
Glandular fever.
Yellow fever.
Acute alcoholic hepatitis may present with enlargement and tenderness of the liver and, sometimes, obstructive jaundice. There are usually other signs of alcoholism.
Wilson's disease must not be overlooked (page 133).

Management. If hospitalised, the patient should be isolated. The true period of infectivity is unknown but is probably about 1–2 weeks after the appearance of jaundice. Symptomatic treatment only is required in the active disease state. Most physicians would restrict activity until jaundice has disappeared and allow moderate exertion whilst the serum transaminase levels remain elevated. No food restriction other than alcohol is necessary, Liver function tests (page 47) usually return completely to normal in 1–3 months.

Recovery is the rule in virtually every case. Occasionally jaundice may be prolonged by intra-hepatic cholestasis, and corticosteroids can be used to reduce the jaundice rapidly, particulary if it is associated with pruritus. In a small number of patients (5–10%) a mild relapse occurs, sometimes after the jaundice has disappeared. Acute massive necrosis is an extremely rare complication but invariably fatal.

Prophylaxis. Immune γ-globulin (500–750 mg in adults) protects contacts of infectious hepatitis. It is given to travellers entering endemic areas but the period of effectiveness remains uncertain—probably about 3–4 months.

Hepatitis B

This is spread by infected blood or serum and also occurs in saliva, semen and vaginal secretions. It is most frequently seen in heroin addicts who use contaminated syringes and needles, homosexuals and less commonly in patients and staff in renal dialysis units and those attending centres for tattooing or acupuncture. Blood transfusion units now screen all donor blood for the presence of hepatitis B virus. Recent work has shown that the disease can also be transmitted by ingestion, although this must be very uncommon.

Clinical presentation. After a long incubation period of 6 weeks to 6 months, there is a gradual onset of lethargy, anorexia, abdominal discomfort, jaundice, and hepatomegaly. Arthralgia and skin rashes are common.

Diagnosis. Hepatitis B has a surface antigen (HB_sAg) and a core antigen (HB_cAg). The δ-agent is a transmissable, defective, hepatotrophic RNA virus which depends upon the presence of a replicating hepatitis B virus to replicate. (δ-agent is a protein with a molecular weight of 68 000.) In the West this virus is present in the multitransfusional: addicts and their consorts, haemophiliacs, and thalassaemia patients. It may occur in hepatitis B-infected persons or be superimposed upon it. It appears in the blood about 6 weeks after infection, just before jaundice appears, and has usually gone by 3 months. In about 5% it persists beyond 6 months (carrier status) and the patient can transmit the disease even though well. The prevalence of carrier status varies from 1–2/1000 in UK and USA to 10–15% in parts of Africa and the Far East.

The 'e' antigen, found only in the presence of HB_sAg, appears in the blood at the same time as the surface antigen and indicates high infectivity. Surface antibody (anti-HB_s) appears in the blood about 3 months after infection and remains conferring immunity in 80–90% of cases.

Management and prognosis. While in hospital patients should be isolated, barrier nursed, and all excreta disinfected. Blood samples should be taken wearing gloves, transported in plastic bags and the laboratory informed of the suspected diagnosis.

In uncomplicated cases treatment is symptomatic as for infectious hepatitis. Complications include chronic hepatitis, acute necrosis and liver failure which are more common following serum hepatitis than following infectious hepatitis. Carriers are common (5–10%) and have a high incidence of hepatoma in the developing world. Immunization with treated inert hepatitis B antigen is recommended for those likely to be in contact with infected blood, and travellers to the developing world. Interferon is used to reverse HBS antigen carriage.

Hepatitis C

This is caused by a small RNA virus. The antibody is present in 80% of patients with chronic hepatitis. It constitutes 60% of hepatitis non-A, non-B, and is found in 3% of blood donors and 30% of i.v. drug users. Clinical features are similar to hepatitis B.

CHRONIC HEPATITIS

Though the classification is based on pathology, there are fairly clear clinical correlations. These are characterised by inflammatory infiltration around the portal tracts and may have features of superimposed acute hepatitis. Hepatitis C antibody is present in 80% of cases.

Chronic persistent hepatitis

The lobular architecture is preserved and there is little or no necrosis or fibrosis. It may follow acute viral hepatitis A, B, or C, or acute alcoholic hepatitis, drug toxicity or inflammatory bowel disease and usually carries an excellent prognosis without treatment. The patients may have only fatigue and hepatomegaly, though fat and alcohol intolerance may occur.

Chronic lobular hepatitis

Chronic lobular hepatitis (unresolved or protracted hepatitis) has been defined histologically with chronic inflammatory cell infiltration throughout the liver lobule from the portal tracts to the central veins. The absence of hepatocyte necrosis suggests that it may be a variant of acute viral hepatitis or chronic persistent hepatitis. The clinical importance of this condition remains uncertain because of the mixed aetiology, the variable results on investigation, and the variable outcome from complete recovery (usual) to rapidly developing cirrhosis (relatively uncommon and perhaps chiefly in those who have had hepatitis B infection).

Chronic active hepatitis

Inflammation of the liver for at least 3–6 months. Similar and overlapping syndromes include lupoid hepatitis (in the presence of LE cells) and juvenile cirrhosis. In addition to the periportal inflammatory infiltrate, there is piecemeal cellular necrosis along the interlobular septa and some fibrosis with the formation of intralobular septa and the formation of rosettes of cells. Progression to cirrhosis is usual if untreated. It may follow viral hepatitis with hepatitis B or C, alcoholic hepatitis and some drugs, e.g. isoniazid, methyldopa.

Clinical presentation. The autoimmune variety occurs chiefly in young women with the insidious onset of anorexia, abdominal pain and increasing jaundice. It may follow acute hepatitis. It tends to run a relapsing course culminating in cirrhosis. In 50% of patients, other systems are involved, e.g. fever, arthralgia, skin rashes, ulcerative colitis, lymphadenopathy, haemolytic anaemia and thrombocytopenia. Hepatitis B virus and LE cells are associated with a proportion of cases (10–25%) and smooth muscle antibodies are present in 60%.

Management. Steroids, prednisolone 30 mg daily gradually reduced, and/or azathioprine, e.g. 50 mg daily, improve the symptoms, signs and liver function tests, and may improve the outcome. Steroids are more effective than azathioprine but have more side-effects, may worsen the prognosis if ascites is present and if with disease is due to hepatitis B.

ALCOHOLIC HEPATITIS

Sensitivity to alcohol varies enormously between individuals. Males who take over 80 g of ethanol daily (40 g for females) are at risk from alcohol-related diseases. 8 g (10 ml) of ethanol is present in half a pint of beer, a glass of wine or sherry, or a single measure (25 ml) of spirits (= one 'unit') (page 249).

Clinical features

These vary from no clinical evidence at all, through early morning nausea, acute episodes of right subcostal pain associated with tender hepatomegaly, fever and polymorphic leucocytosis, to cirrhosis with portal hypertension and hepatic encephalopathy (page 254). Marked jaundice is not always present. There may be associated alcoholic pancreatitis, cardiomyopathy, proximal myopathy or peripheral neuropathy. In early alcoholic hepatitis, the liver shows fatty infiltration, swelling of cells, some containing Mallory's hyaline with focal destruction of cells, polymorph infiltration. Later, collagen is laid down around central veins and may spread to the portal tracts. Cirrhosis may result. The MCV and γ-GT may be the best indices of persistent ethanol ingestion. The only effective treatment usually is total abstinence from alcohol if necessary with the help of Alcoholics Anonymous. Vitamin B_1 is given, particularly if confusion is present.

CIRRHOSIS

Cirrhosis is a pathological diagnosis and therefore implies liver biopsy in all suspected cases. It is characterised by widespread fibrosis with nodular regeneration. Its presence implies previous or continuing hepatic cell damage. See liver function tests (page 47); these are normal in inactive disease. Identified causes include viral hepatitis A, B, and C, alcoholic hepatitis, haemochromatosis, hepatolenticular disease, α_1-antitrypsin deficiency, chronic severe heart failure, and a few drugs (isoniazid, methyldopa).

Classification

Micronodular (portal cirrhosis) is characterised by regular thick fibrotic bands joining the portal tracts to hepatic veins, and with small regenerative nodules. The liver is initially large with a smooth edge but subsequently shrinks with progressive fibrosis. It is often alcoholic in origin and is then associated with fatty infiltration.

Macronodular (post-necrotic cirrhosis) is less common and is characterised by coarse, irregular bands of fibrosis and loss of normal architecture and large regenerative nodules. It is believed usually to follow viral hepatitis with widespread necrosis. The liver is enlarged and very irregular due to the large nodules.

Biliary cirrhosis is less common and is characterised by fibrosis around distended intrahepatic bile ducts. It may follow chronic cholangitis and biliary obstruction (secondary), or be idiopathic (primary).

Primary biliary cirrhosis is associated with other connective tissue and immunological disorders such as the rheumatoid syndrome, Sjögren's syndrome,

Hashimoto's thyroiditis, dermatomyositis and CREST syndrome (page 166). It chiefly (90%) affects women between 40 and 60 years of age and presents with pruritus (often first), jaundice, pigmentation, xanthomata and finger clubbing. The liver and spleen are usually palpably enlarged. The intrahepatic cholestasis results in jaundice, pale stools, dark urine and steatorrhoea. Investigation shows a high alkaline phosphatase and usually a high bilirubin. Mitochondrial antibodies are present in 95% of patients and this helps with the differential diagnosis from drug cholestasis, sclerosing cholangitis, carcinoma of the bile duct and biliary cirrhosis from chronic obstruction. Histology shows progression from granulomatous changes around the bile ducts through bile duct proliferation to fibrosis and finally frank cirrhosis. Treatment is with cholestyramine for the pruritus and supplementary fat-soluble vitamins plus calcium. Steroids and azathioprine are contraindicated. Death from hepatocellular failure with or without bleeding varices or intercurrent infection occurs commonly within 5 to 10 years. Liver transplantation may be indicated.

Cardiac cirrhosis may occur in chronic cardiac failure. Centrilobular congestion leads to necrosis and fibrosis, but nodular regeneration is not marked.

Other rare causes of cirrhosis include chronic active hepatitis, haemochromatosis and hepatolenticular degeneration.

NB *Schistosomiasis* causes periportal fibrosis and is not a form of cirrhosis. Liver involvement is more common (50%) in *S. mansoni* (bowel) infections than in *S. haematobium* (bladder) due to the portal rather than systemic drainage of the primary infected area in the former. The schistosomes cause a granulomatous fibrosis in the portal tracts and enlargement of the liver. In severe cases the liver shrinks and extensive fibrosis develops leading to portal hypertension. There is little or no hepatocellular failure since the disease is presinusoidal. Late spread may occur to the lungs (cor pulmonale) and to the spinal cord (paraplegia).

Clinical presentation and management

There may be no abnormal clinical or biochemical features of liver disease. Later, features of hepatocellular failure, portal hypertension, or both may appear. Peptic ulceration is common in alcoholic cirrhosis.

Hepatocellular failure (chronic)

Marked jaundice is uncommon. The oestrogen effects of gynaecomastia, spider naevi, liver palms and testicular atrophy may be present. In alcoholics, other features of alcoholism may be present (wasting, polyneuropathy, Korsakoff's psychosis, dementia, delirium tremens and Wernicke's encephalopathy). Pigmentation, fetor hepaticus, clubbing, white nails, cyanosis and peripheral oedema may occur.

Portasystemic encephalopathy (hepatic coma and pre-coma) may be absent or may completely dominate the clinical picture.

Hepatocellular failure may be precipitated acutely by:
- excess protein in the bowel, e.g. after gastrointestinal haemorrhage

- acute alcoholic intoxication
- intercurrent infection, particularly Gram-negative septicaemia
- morphine and other alkaloids
- minor or major surgical procedures including paracentesis
- electrolyte imbalance (potassium and/or sodium depletion) usually from the diuretics used to treat oedema and ascites

Pre-coma is characterised by irritable confusion, drowsiness, flapping tremor, fetor and other signs of hepatocellular failure. Exaggerated reflexes and upgoing plantar responses may be present. Constructional apraxia may be demonstrated in inability to draw or copy a star. In the EEG, δ waves (3–4 c/s) are characteristic. (They also occur in hypoglycaemia, uraemia, CO_2 retention and cerebral abscess).

Specific management includes:

Identify the site of bleeding by fiberoscopy.
Stop the bleeding from gastric or duodenal ulceration with H_2 receptor blockade, and from varices with fiberoptic injection sclerotherapy or pressure tube, e.g. Sengstaken–Blakemore. Some give vasopressin to lower portal pressure (20 units in 100 ml dextrose in 20 min intravenously—repeated 2-hourly if necessary). It produces colic and diarrhoea and is dangerous in ischaemic heart disease.

Sedation. Oxazepam is suitable. Despite the recognised hepatic complication, chlorpromazine is frequently used.
Stop dietary protein and diuretics.
Remove protein and blood (if present) from the bowel with lactulose 50 ml tds or magnesium sulphate enemas and purgation.
Decrease urea splitting bowel organisms with neomycin (1 g qds) and lactulose.
Replace clotting factors with fresh frozen plasma or clotting factors.

General management includes:

Maintenance of fluid balance. Sodium restriction may be required despite hyponatraemia which may be dilutional. Hypokalaemia should be treated with standard potassium preparations. Diuretics (spironolactone followed if necessary by thiazides or loop diuretics) may be given for ascites. *Calories* are given as dextrose (up to 300 g daily) orally or intravenously (the blood glucose may be very low). Give parenteral vitamins B (particularly thiamine: B_1).

Infection. Take blood cultures and send ascitic fluid for bacteriological examination including tuberculosis. Treat infection as indicated remembering that altered liver function may influence drug choice and dosage.
If transfusion is required use fresh blood for preference to avoid further coagulation failure.

Other techniques include exchange transfusion and perfusion through a charcoal column. Orthotopic liver transplantation is becoming more widely used for all forms of liver failure.

NB A reduced level of consciousness in hepatocellular failure (especially alcoholics) may be due to septicaemia, raise intracranial pressure from cerebral oedema, subdural haematoma, hypoglycaemia or epilepsy. Previously healthy patients without cirrhosis who develop acute hepatocellular failure are managed similarly.

Portal hypertension

In cirrhosis, this is suggested by a patient with anorexia, vomiting, upper abdominal pain, splenomegaly and ascites. The liver may be large or small. Collateral circulation may be evident in the oesophagus (varices), anus (anorectal varices, rather than haemorrhoids) and at the umbilicus (where a venous hum may be heard). Haematemesis is the commonest presenting symptom and may have been induced by non-steroidal anti-inflammatory drugs including aspirin. Some evidence of hepatocellular failure and/or alcoholism may be present. Bleeding is often from peptic ulceration or erosions in the alcoholic, and H_2 blockade is then used. Tests of liver cell function are usually slightly abnormal though not always so, and there may be hypersplenism. The immediate mortality is 50% even in experienced hands.

NB Cirrhosis accounts for 80% of the portal hypertension seen in Britain. The other postsinusoidal causes (which have poor hepatic function) are exceedingly rare and result from cardiac failure, constrictive pericarditis and hepatic vein thrombosis (Budd–Chiari syndrome). Presinusoidal obstruction causes portal hypertension with normal hepatic function in schistosomiasis (granulomatous portal tract fibrosis), and in obstruction to the portal vein by tumours or following venous thrombosis with umbilical sepsis.

If cirrhosis develops in a young person (under 30 years) chronic active hepatitis and hepatolenticular degeneration (Wilson's disease) must be considered.

Management of bleeding varices. The initial aim is to replace blood lost with blood (or dextran). Attempt to stop variceal bleeding with endoscopic sclerotherapy, a pressure tube (e.g. Sengstaken–Blakemore) or argipressin (a synthetic vasopressin analogue). Ligation or transection may then be indicated. Transhepatic obliteration by injection of thrombin into the cannulated portal vein is sometimes attempted. Fresh frozen plasma may be given for coagulation complications. Emergency portacaval anastomosis is now rarely performed: contraindications after the first bleed are serum bilirubin (>35 µmol/litre), serum albumin (<30 g/litre), age (above 45 years) ascites and portasystemic encephalopathy during the bleed (this being accepted as a sufficient protein load).

Avoid factors which may precipitate hepatocellular failure and treat if necessary (see above). Propranolol may help reduce portacaval presure.

Sclerotherapy is used in:

1 Emergency—to arrest haemorrhage.
2 Second prevention after variceal bleed.
3 Prophylactically to avoid future bleeding.

It usually needs to be repeated indefinitely.

Portacaval anastomosis may be performed as an elective procedure after the first bleed if the cause is pre-sinusoidal (schistosomiasis) and after investigation to:

- demonstrate oesophageal varices (endoscopy or barium swallow)
- determine the site of obstruction with splenic venography and pressure studies
- assess liver cell function with a high protein diet (120 g/day). If encephalopathy is demonstrated clinically or by EEG, surgery is contraindicated.

Liver transplantation has superseded portacaval anastomosis except when portal hypertension is present with good hepatocellular function (schistosomiasis)

Management of ascites in cirrhosis

Ascites is due to a combination of factors including portal hypertension, hypoalbuminaemia and secondary hyperaldosteronism. The patient is given a restricted salt (<3 g daily) and water (<1 litre daily) intake while on complete bed rest. If weight loss does not occur (weigh daily), high doses of spironolactone and then a loop diuretic are given. Sodium-poor albumin infusions may be helpful in inducing diuresis. A high protein diet (because of the low serum albumin) may give encephalopathy. Ascites may be due to other causes (page 44), especially bacterial infection including tuberculosis. Fluid should be examined for bacterial and malignant cells.

Budd–Chiari syndrome

This results from thrombosis of the major hepatic veins. In women under 30 years it is usually due to the contraceptive pill. It is also associated with polycythaemia, congenital webs of the suprahepatic segment of the inferior vena cava (IVC), local malignancy and veno-occlusive disease. Patients present acutely with tender hepatomegaly (without hepatojugular reflux), resistant ascites and hepatic failure. Chronic onset is associated with weight loss, upper gut bleeding and spider naevi. All patients have abnormal liver function tests. Only half have the diagnostic liver scintiscan finding of maximum uptake in the caudate lobe (which drains directly into the IVC) with decreased uptake in the rest of the liver. Liver biopsy shows congestion around the hepatic venules. Laparotomy may produce abrupt deterioration. Treatment is surgical by side-to-side portal-caval shunt or orthotopic liver transplantation. If there is a web, surgical correction may be attempted by transatrial membranectomy. Five-year survival is 25%.

RARE CIRRHOSES

Idiopathic haemochromatosis (bronzed diabetes)

An autosomal recessive error of metabolism associated with HLA A3 and HLA B14, resulting in excess iron absorption and deposition chiefly in the liver, pancreas and heart and synovial membranes, but also in endocrine glands. Alcohol seems to predispose to the development of symptoms and signs. First degree male relatives should be screened with serum iron and transferrin saturation. Females may present postmenopausally because continuous menstruation until then reduces the iron load.

Clinical presentation

It occurs almost entirely in men over the age of 30 years who present with:
- diabetes mellitus (80%)
- skin pigmentation (due to melanin rather than iron)
- hepatomegaly (large, regular, firm); portal hypertension and hepatocellular failure are not common
- progressive pyrophosphate polyarthropathy (40%) and chondrocalcinosis
- arrhythmias (30%) and cardiac failure (15%)
- testicular atrophy, loss of body hair and loss of libido
- osteoarthritis of the lst and 2nd metacarpophalangeal joints

Diagnosis

The serum iron, normally 23 μmol/litre, is raised so that the serum iron-binding capacity (which remains normal: 63 μmol/litre) is nearly saturated. The serum ferritin is raised. The patient is not anaemic or polycythaemic. The glucose tolerance test is usually abnormal.

Biopsy of most tissues (skin, marrow, testes) shows excess iron deposits but diagnosis is usually made on liver biopsy which shows iron staining of the liver cells with perilobular fibrosis.

Treatment

Deplete the body of the excess iron (up to 50 g) by weekly venesection of 500 ml (which contains 250 mg iron). This is continued until a normal serum iron is established and/or the patient becomes anaemic (in about 2 years). Maintenance venesection will be required (about 500 ml every 3 months depending upon the serum iron).

Treat appropriately the diabetes, hypogonadism, heart failure and arrhythmias, hepatic cell failure and portal hypertension. High alcohol intake must be stopped. The arthropathy and testicular function tend not to improve but other features do.

NB   Primary hepatic carcinoma occurs in up to 20% of cases whether treated or not. Alphafetoprotein (AFP) is a suitable screen.

Overload of the tissues with iron can follow either repeated blood transfusions (about 100 units), as for instance in thalassaemia, or rarely after excessive iron ingestion. If the iron is in the reticuloendothelial cells only, the patients tend not to develop serious sequelae and the condition is called haemosiderosis. Haemochromatosis refers to iron overload which causes tissue damage and hence cirrhosis and diabetes. There is no absolute difference between them.

Hepatolenticular degeneration (Wilson's disease) (page 133)

An autosomal recessive disorder of copper metabolism. Symptoms appear during adolescence or early adult life. In the UK there are 500 recognised cases (and possibly as many unrecognised).

DRUG JAUNDICE
Drugs are responsible for up to 10% of all patients admitted with jaundice.

Hypersensitivity reactions
These are the commonest causes of drug jaundice. They are dose-independent.

Cholestasis
Clinically and biochemically this is an obstructive jaundice. Histologically there are bile plugs in the canaliculi and there may be an inflammatory infiltrate including eosinophils in the portal tracts.

The classical example is chlorpromazine jaundice which occurs 3–6 weeks after starting the drug. The prognosis is excellent if the drug is discontinued (and never given again).

Other drugs producing cholestasis are: other phenothiazines, carbimazole, erythromycin estolate (but not the stearate), sulphonylureas, sulphonamides, PAS and rifampicin, and nitrofurantoin. Occasionally there may be a more generalised reaction with fever, rash, lymphadenopathy and eosinophilia.

Acute hepatitis syndrome
Occasionally with acute necrosis. This is much less common but much more serious (mortality up to 20%). It occurs 2–3 weeks after starting the drug, and is caused by halothane (after multiple exposure), monoamine oxidase inhibitors, methyldopa (which more commonly gives haemolytic jaundice), and the antituberculosis drugs, ethionamide and pyrazinamide (also page 301).

Direct hepatotoxicity
In some cases this is dose-dependent though individual susceptibility is extremely variable.

The mechanisms are:
- Cholestasis (without inflammatory infiltrate or necrosis). Chiefly due to C-17 substituted testosterone derivatives, i.e. anabolic and androgenic steroids, including methyltestosterone and most contraceptive pills
- Necrosis due to organic solvents, e.g. carbon tetrachloride, paracetamol in suicidal overdose, and antimitotic drugs, e.g. methotrexate, 6-mercaptopurine, azathioprine

Haemolytic jaundice
This is a rare complication of therapy. It may occur with methyldopa (which more commonly gives a positive Coombs' reaction without jaundice), and the 8-aminoquinolines (e.g. primaquine) in patients with glucose 6-phosphate dehydrogenase deficiency.

Gastroenterology

Symptoms arising from the gastrointestinal tract are extremely common, usually due to gastroenteritis or food poisoning. In clinics, most are due to disturbances of motility and/or are psychogenic. Over a third may have the irritable bowel syndrome. Peptic ulcer, hiatus hernia, appendicitis, diverticulitis, haemorrhoids, ulcerative colitis and carcinoma of the colon are common. Carcinoma of the stomach and carcinoma of the oesophagus are less common.

GASTRIC AND DUODENAL ULCERATION

Aetiology
No cause is usually found though duodenal ulcer is associated with gastric hypersecretion and the presence of *Helicobacter pylori*. Anti-inflammatory drugs both steroidal and non-steroidal (NSAID, including aspirin) are the commonest precipitating factors. Rarely ulceration is associated with Zollinger–Ellison syndrome (page 263), MEA syndrome Type 1 (page 197) hyperparathyroidism (page 220) or stress (extensive burns and head injury)—Curling's ulcer.

Clinical presentation
It is usually impossible, on the basis of history and examination alone, to differentiate between duodenal ulceration, benign ulceration of the stomach and carcinoma of the stomach, but carcinoma is much rarer.

Duodenal ulceration is the most common and classically presents with a history of periodic epigastric pain, often waking the patient at 1–3 a.m., relieved by food, milk or alkalis.

Gastric ulcer pain may be epigastric or occur anywhere in the anterior upper abdomen. Anorexia, vomiting and weight loss are more frequent and severe in carcinomatous ulcers of the stomach than in benign peptic ulceration. Food occasionally precipitates pain immediately (as it may in reflux oesophagitis and in nervous dyspepsia).

Examination
The patient characteristically puts his hand over the upper abdomen or may point to the epigastrium with a forefinger when asked where the pain is and this is the point of maximum tenderness. The presence of an epigastric mass suggests a carcinoma. A gastric splash (or succussion) indicates pyloric obstruction due to benign duodenal stricture or to carcinoma of the pyloric antrum.

Complications
Bleeding (page 263)
Perforation (usually duodenal ulcer).

Pyloric stenosis. This presents with recurrent vomiting of food ingested up to 24 h previously with immediate relief. Visible gastric peristalsis may be seen. Conservative management with gastric aspiration and intravenous fluids may sometimes allow time for a benign active ulcer to heal and relieve the obstruction. Surgery is usually required either on the first or subsequent admission. These patients may vomit profusely and become dehydrated and alkalotic. Fluid and electrolyte replacement is obligatory and particularly so prior to surgery.

Investigation

Barium meal. Duodenal ulcers are virtually always benign. Gastric carcinomas are commoner on the greater curve and in the antrum but lesser curve ulcers may nevertheless be malignant. The size of the ulcer is no guide to whether a carcinoma is present. Carcinomas may have a rolled edge and a translucent 'halo' around them.

Endoscopy with biopsy in experienced hands is important in establishing the diagnosis of duodenal or gastric ulceration in patients with abdominal pain and will distinguish benign from malignant ulcers in the large majority of cases. Biopsy and exfoliative cytology can give histological confirmation.

Management

Antacids and diet often ameliorate symptoms but do not hasten healing. The patient should stop smoking and adopt whatever dietary regime suits him best. Antacids, especially in liquid form, relieve symptoms and stay in the stomach longer if given after food.

The H_2-receptor blocking drugs such as ranitidine (300 mg nocte), cimetidine (800 mg nocte) or famotidine (80 mg nocte) are the treatments of choice. Ulcers tend to recur when the drugs are stopped and their place in long-term management is not clear, though maintenance therapy is often advocated for the elderly, those with serious cardiopulmonary disease, and frequent relapsers.

Bismuth chelate (De-Nol) is antibacterial to *Helicobacter pylori* and relapse rates may be lower than with H_2 blockade.

Misoprostil, a prostaglandin analogue used with NSAIDs, has not been shown to be significantly better than these other drugs at healing peptic ulcers. It is better not to use non-steroidal anti-inflammatory drugs in the first place, than to add another drug to counteract its side-effects on gastric mucosa.

Omeprazole, a proton hydrogen ion pump inhibitor, reduces acid secretion from the parietal cells.

Duodenal ulcer

Treatment is only indicated when symptoms are present. Antacids and frequent small meals may relieve symptoms. H_2 blockade relieves symptoms and favours healing.

Gastric ulcer

Investigation is directed towards differentiating benign from malignant ulcers by endoscopy and biopsy. Treatment of benign ulcers includes stopping smoking and H_2 blockade. Where endoscopy is not available a repeat barium meal after 3–4 weeks should show a decrease in the size of the ulcer. If this has not occurred, the presence of a carcinoma becomes more likely and endoscopy with biopsy obligatory.

Indications for surgery

Duodenal ulcer

Acute indications include:
- Perforation
- Pyloric obstruction
- Persistent haemorrhage
- *Failed medical treatment.* Surgery in chronic duodenal ulceration depends upon assessment of the degree of disability produced by the symptoms. Factors to be considered are the severity and frequency of pain, and time off work. There is an increasing tendency to perform highly selective vagotomy, rather than truncal vagotomy with drainage (pyloroplasty or gastroenterostomy) or partial gastrectomy, in an attempt to reduce the incidence of side-effects of diarrhoea, malabsorption and 'dumping.'

Gastric ulcer

Acute indication: persistent haemorrhage (page 263).
Non-acute indications:
- carcinoma
- failed medical treatment either if there is a possibility of carcinoma or for persistent symptoms

Gastric carcinoma

Affects mainly the pylorus and antrum. The symptoms are those of a gastric ulcer in the early stages but pyloric obstruction or dysphagia may occur. Occasionally the patient may complain of no more than weight loss. Suggestive features in a middle-aged person include persistent dyspepsia, anorexia, weight loss and iron deficiency anaemia (especially in a male or postmenopausal female). The prognosis is poor, for the 5-year survival after surgery is only 20%.

ENDOCRINE TUMOURS OF THE GUT

All are very rare.

Apudomas

(Amine precursor: uptake and decarboxylation—APUD) cells. These are the hormone secreting cells found chiefly along the length of the gastrointestinal tract. They have molecular and functional similarities with each other and may form various kinds of functioning tumour. They secrete a number of hormones including gastrin, cholecystokinin, secretin, glucagon and vasoactive intestinal peptide (VIP).

Zollinger–Ellison syndrome

This rare disorder is characterised by multiple recurrent duodenal and jejunal ulceration associated with a very high plasma gastrin level (>300 mg/litre with the patient off H_2 receptor blockade), gross gastric acid hypersecretion and the presence of a gastrin secreting adenoma (which may be malignant), usually in the pancreas but sometimes in the stomach wall.

Diarrhoea sometimes with steatorrhoea may be a feature (lipase is inactivated by the low pH). The volume of gastric secretion is 'enormous (7–10 litres/24 h) and acid secretion persistently raised (and raised little further by pentagastrin). Normal fasting gastrin is <100 pg/ml. In Zollinger–Ellison syndrome there is a rise in serum gastrin level >200 pg/ml after infusion of secretin 2 units/kg.

The presence of an adenoma may be associated with adenomata of other endocrine glands, i.e. adrenals, parathyroids and anterior pituitary (page 197)

Treatment is by removal of the tumour which is usually benign. If it cannot be found, give either omeprazole or H_2 blockade long-term.

Other endocrine tumours of the gut

These are very rare indeed but are sometimes discussed in examinations.

Insulinoma. A tumour of the pancreatic islet β cells which produces episodic hypoglycaemic attacks which may present as epilepsy or abnormal behaviour. Fasting produces prolonged hypoglycaemia with high insulin levels in the serum. 10% are malignant and 5% are multiple.

Glucagonoma. A tumour of the α-cells which produces a syndrome of mild diabetes with diarrhoea, weight loss anaemia, glossitis and a migratory necrolytic rash.

Vipoma (WDHA syndrome). A variant of the Zollinger–Ellison syndrome with severe Watery Diarrhoea, Hypokalaemia with or without Achlorhydria caused by a pancreatic tumour producing a vasoactive intestinal polypeptide. Abdominal pain and flushing are typical features. Vipomectomy may be curative.

- *Benign tumours* account for 40% of cases:
- 30% adenoma, 10% islet cell hypertrophy, and 10% duodenal or resectable
- *Malign tumours* account for 60% of cases. Two-thirds have metastasized at diagnosis

GASTROINTESTINAL HAEMORRHAGE

Upper gut

Aetiology

Acute	
Duodenal ulcer	35%
Gastric ulcer	20%
Gastric erosions	20%
Mallory–Weiss (mucosal tears) and oesophagitis	10%

Oesophageal varices*	5%
Others	10%

*Up to 50% in France and parts of USA.

Half the patients are over 60 years old. Bleeding from gastric ulcers is rare under the age of 50 years, and so is bleeding from duodenal ulcers in females. Melaena as a presenting symptom suggests less severe bleeding than haematemesis.

Clinical presentation

Haematemesis is a reliable indication of bleeding above the duodenojejunal flexure, and bright red rectal bleeding of the lower colon or rectum. The colour of altered blood passed per rectum is related to transit time more than to the site of bleeding.

Faintness, weakness, sweating, palpitation and nausea often precede the evidence of bleeding. The patient is pale and sweating, and has tachycardia and hypotension.

Chronic

Bleeding from hiatus hernia and gastric carcinoma is usually insidious (but not always).

Management

Fibreoptic examination of the oesophagus, stomach and duodenum (OGD) should be performed as soon as possible. If unavailable a barium meal is performed.

Initial treatment

Take blood for grouping and cross-matching, liver function tests including the prothrombin time and full blood count with platelets. Treat shock if present with transfusion of blood and monitor progress by pulse and blood pressure recording. Conventionally, transfuse whole blood when the pulse is over 100/min, the systolic arterial blood pressure under 100 mmHg, and the haemoglobin under 10 g/dl if the trends are adverse. If bleeding is severe or continuous, a central venous pressure monitor should be inserted as a guide to further transfusion and rebleeding. A central venous pressure of +5 to +10 cm of saline should be maintained. Oxygen should be given.

NB Always attempt to have 4 units of blood available for further transfusions.

If blood is still supplied citrated (in bottles) give 10 ml 10% calcium gluconate for every 4 bottles to avoid hypocalcaemia and tetany.

After large transfusions of stored blood, deficiencies of clotting factors and platelets are best corrected by giving fresh frozen plasma and fresh platelets where indicated.

Sedate the patient if anxious. Diazepam probably causes less hypotension than morphine and heroin. The patient is usually allowed fluids and a light diet, unless awaiting surgery.

Vasopressin may stop haemorrhage from varices (page 256)

Fresh frozen plasma should be given if bleeding has occurred from varices.

The blood urea may rise to 15–25 mmol/litre due to absorption of protein from the gut. The serum creatinine is not increased unless renal disease is also present. Hepatic coma may be precipitated by protein in the gut.

If bleeding appears to have stopped (steady pulse, blood pressure and central venous pressure) assess progress with repeat haemoglobin and/or haematocrit.

Investigation (for site and cause of bleeding)

Within 24 h, as soon as the patient's condition allows fiberoscopy (or, if not available, barium swallow and meal) should be performed and shows the site of bleeding in up to 90% of cases. Selective angiography may show the site of active bleeding if not previously determined, particularly when angiodysplasia must be excluded. If bleeding is sufficiently fast (2 ml/min) a labelled red blood corpuscle isotope scan or selective angiography may help to locate bleeding, e.g. from a Meckel's diverticulum.

If bleeding continues or recurs, surgery may be necessary (see below). If bleeding has stopped the patient should be given oral iron and a normal diet. H_2 blockade is usually given and may reduce blood loss. Patients should be advised not to smoke.

Indications for surgery (in haemorrhage from peptic ulcer)

Although there are no clear-cut indications, surgery is usually indicated if bleeding does not stop spontaneously or the patient rebleeds in hospital (the central venous pressure may be the first indication of this, but slower continuous bleeds are indicated by a persistently low haemoglobin). The overall mortality is worse in older patients (10% in the over-sixties) than in the young (2% in the under-sixties). Bleeds from gastric ulcers (mortality up to 20% in the over-sixties) carry twice the mortality of bleeds from duodenal ulcers. Also the operative risk for gastric ulcer surgery is less than for duodenal ulcers.

Hence the tendency is to operate early in older patients, particularly if bleeding from a gastric ulcer. Supplies of compatible blood may be a controlling factor.

Lower gut

Acute loss occurs from haemorrhoids, fissures, ulcerative colitis and Crohn's disease, ischaemic colitis, colonic and caecal carcinoma and diverticular disease. Chronic and occult bleeding usually presents with lethargy and iron deficiency anaemia and is confirmed by positive faecal occult blood tests. Any of the causes of upper or lower gut bleeding given above may be responsible. Other very rare causes include polyps, and vascular abnormalities, such as arteriovenous malformations, angiodysplasia of the ascending colon, Peutz–Jeghers (small intestinal polyposis and blotchy pigmentation around the mouth) and Rendu–Osler–Weber syndromes. Meckel's diverticulum, polyps and endometriosis may also present with bleeding.

REFLUX OESOPHAGITIS

In the common type both stomach and oesophagus are present in the thorax. It occurs in midlife, in the fat and flabby, and during pregnancy.

It is often found if looked for by the radiologist but is symptomless unless there is a reflux oesophagitis from acid, pepsin and duodenal contents. Peptic oesophagitis is often seen on endoscopy.

Symptoms

These are heartburn with acid regurgitation on bending and pain, worse on lying down and in bed. Food may 'stick'. Bleeding may give positive occult blood tests and anaemia. Peptic oesophagitis may lead to ulceration and/or stricture.

Treatment

Sit up in bed with high pillows and a raised foot of the bed to stop slipping down. Lose weight and remove restrictive clothing. Avoid stooping when lifting load. Stop smoking and avoid foods which give symptoms.
Give antacids with or without alginate.
Metoclopramide may relieve nausea; treat anaemia with iron. High-dose H_2 blockade may occasionally be required for severe and persistent symptoms. Avoid surgery unless symptoms become intractable and dominate the patient's life.

ULCERATIVE COLITIS

Clinical presentation

The disease usually presents in the 20–40 year old group but may occur at any age. First presentation over 65 years is uncommon but carries a greater mortality. At presentation 30% have disease confined to the rectum and 20% have extensive disease. Intermittent diarrhoea with mucus and blood in the stool, associated with fever and remissions to near normal are the most frequent symptoms. Three patterns may be distinguished:
• The disease may occasionally present as a single short mild episode of diarrhoea which appears to settle rapidly but may at any time relapse
• Usually the history is of months or years of general ill health with continuous or intermittent diarrhoea. In these cases the disease is usually restricted to the rectum and descending colon, and then usually termed proctocolitis. General symptoms may be mild or severe. Secondary complications are frequent
• Approximately one-fifth of cases present with a severe acute episode of bloody diarrhoea with constitutional symptoms of fever and toxaemia and abdominal distension from toxic megacolon which may proceed to perforation

Diagnosis

This is suggested by the clinical picture and may be confirmed, except in the very ill, by sigmoidoscopy with biopsy and barium examination. The differential diagnosis includes:
• carcinoma of the colon which may present with bloody diarrhoea
• the acute case may resemble campylobacter enteritis or bacillary dysentery

and the chronic case amoebic colitis (these should be excluded by stool examination)
- Crohn's disease of the colon appears to be increasingly recognised and may resemble ulcerative colitis
- pseudomembranous (antibiotic-induced) colitis. On sigmoidoscopy, characteristically there are patchy yellowish areas of necrotic mucosa. Histology shows mucosal destruction with characteristic exudation of fibrin and inflammatory cells in the cross-sectional shape of a mushroom. Clostridium difficile and its toxin may be found in the faeces
- very rarely acute ischaemic colitis may occur and affect the rectosigmoid junction (but not the rectum)

Sigmoidoscopic appearances

These may be conveniently divided into three groups:
- Inactive: a granular mucosa with loss of normal vascular pattern
- Active: with pus and blood
- Very active: pus and blood with contact bleeding at the rim of the sigmoidoscope and visible ulceration

NB   The rectal mucosa is virtually always abnormal in ulcerative colitis, i.e. it is a distal disease with a variable extension proximally up the large bowel. Histology shows superficial inflammation with chronic inflammatory cells infiltrating the lamina propria with crypt abcesses, with little involvement of the muscularis mucosa and with reduction of goblet cells.

Radiology

Barium enema shows loss of normal haustral pattern with shortening of the large intestine. The bowel takes on the appearance of a smooth tube ('hosepipe appearance'). Undermined ulcers and pseudopolypi may be seen. The entire colon may be involved. Thickening of the oedematous colonic wall produces widening of the presacral space seen on lateral views of the sigmoid colon. Stricture formation or carcinoma produces fixed areas of narrowing.

Plain abdominal films will show acute dilatation when present, and bowel gas may outline mucosal ulceration. Barium enema examination in such circumstances may produce perforation.

Complications

General

Fever, anaemia, weight loss, iatrogenic steroid disease.

Colonic

Loss of protein with hypoalbuminaemia and oedema, loss of electrolytes (sodium and potassium) producing lethargy and contributing to intestinal dilatation. Pseudopolyps are common.

Carcinoma of the colon is more frequent if the entire colon is involved (total colitis), if the history is prolonged (10% after 10 years), if the first attack was severe, and if the first attack occurred at a young age.

Acute toxic dilatation of the colon with bleeding and perforation still has a high mortality.

Non-colonic

Skin rashes. Erythema nodosum (2%), pyoderma gangrenosum, leg ulcers (2%).

Arthropathy (15%). This usually involves the large joints, is symmetrical, and usually non-deforming. Sacroiliitis and ankylosing spondylitis are commoner in patients with ulcerative colitis.

Liver disease. Nearly all patients probably have some degree of liver involvement including fatty infiltration, chronic active hepatitis, or pericholangitis, and, less commonly, sclerosing cholangitis, ascending cholangitis and carcinoma of the bile duct. Some of these complications may result from a combination of malnutrition, portal pyaemia, and multiple blood transfusions. Secondary amyloidosis is uncommon but may follow prolonged chronic colitis.

Ocular. Iritis and episcleritis occur in about 5% of cases.

Venous thrombosis of the legs (5%).

Stomatitis (15%).

Management

High protein high fibre diet (150 g/day) is given often, with supplements of vitamins and potassium. Iron is given in the presence of anaemia and blood transfusion may be necessary to maintain the haemoglobin at not less than 11 g/100 ml, particularly in acute cases. Intravenous feeding is sometimes necessary.

Sulphasalazine (0.5 g bd–1 g qds) may be sufficient to control symptoms in mild cases and in remission. Mesalazine is commonly used for patients intolerant of sulphasalazine. Prednisolone phosphate retention enemas or hydrocortisone foam are added if symptoms persist. For more severe disease a course of prednisolone (40–60 mg daily) is required but maintenance oral steroids are not usually indicated.

Surgery is indicated if severe haemorrhage or perforation has occurred and in acute toxaemia with dilatation of the colon which fails to respond within 24–48 h to high dose steroids. Prophylactic colectomy should be performed if regular colonoscopy shows dysplasia. 'Continent' ileostomy and ileo-anal anastomosis is becoming the operation of choice.

Prognosis

The prognosis is best in those with disease confined to the rectum (ulcerative proctitis): only about 10% of these develop complications. About 70% of all cases remit with medical treatment in the first attack, 15% improve, and 15% come to surgery or die. The excess mortality is chiefly within the first year of presentation. In 10 years 30% have extensive disease, and 15% need surgery. Young patients do better than old patients, and subtotal colitis is less severe than total colitis in terms of both general health and the risk of colonic carcinoma. Surgery is therefore indicated early in patients who are older and have total colitis. The mortality from total colectomy when performed as a 'cold' procedure is 2–4% (in severely ill acute cases including toxic dilatation the mortality may be as high as 30–40%). However, 20% of these patients require further surgery usually to refashion the stoma or less commonly to divide obstructing adhesions. Impotence and loss of micturition control are serious complications of surgery, but should be rare because dissection is kept close to the bowel wall.

CROHN'S DISEASE (regional enteritis)

A granulomatous inflammatory disorder of the intestine, of unknown aetiology usually starting in the teens and early twenties. There is a second peak of colonic Crohn's disease in the elderly. Prevalence is 40–80/100 000. The terminal ileum is most frequently diseased but any part of the alimentary tract may be involved. The colon may be involved in up to 10–20% of cases. The process affects short lengths of the intestine leaving normal bowel between, i.e. 'skip lesions'. The wall is thickened and the lumen narrowed. Mucosal ulceration and regional lymphadenopathy are present. The characteristic microscopic features are of submucosal inflammation less marked than in ulcerative colitis. There are numerous fissures down to the submucosa with or without chronic granulation tissue consisting of noncaseating granulomata not unlike those found in sarcoid. It is a progressive chronic disease.

Clinical presentation

It usually presents (80–90%) as intermittent abdominal pain with diarrhoea and abdominal distension in a young thin person. There may be associated fever (30%), anaemia and weight loss in part secondary to malabsorption (50%), and rarely, fresh blood or melaena (40%), fistulae and perianal sepsis (15–20%). Intermittent intestinal obstruction may occur. Clubbing is fairly common (up to 50%). Occasionally uveitis (5%), arthritis (5%), and skin rashes (erythema nodosum and pyoderma) occur. Renal stones occur in 5–10%.

Less commonly it presents as an 'acute abdomen' with signs of acute appendicitis with or without a palpable mass in the right iliac fossa.

Radiology

The terminal ileum is most commonly involved and may produce incompetence of the ileocaecal valve. Mucosal ulceration may be deep and 'spikes' of barium may enter deep into the bowel wall ('rose thorn'). Lesions may be multiple with normal bowel between ('skip lesions'). Coarse cobblestone appearance of the mucosa appears early. Later in the disease fibrosis produces narrowing of the intestine ('string sign') with some proximal dilatation.

Diagnosis

This is usually made on the basis of the clinical picture and radiological findings. Characteristic Crohn's granulomata may occasionally be seen in jejunal biopsy specimens or in biopsy specimens taken at laparotomy for abdominal pain. In areas inaccessible to endoscopy, indium-labelled white cell scan may help to localise active disease.

Crohn's disease of the large bowel may resemble ulcerative colitis. The diagnosis of Crohn's disease is favoured by little blood loss, a normal rectal mucosa, the presence of perianal sepsis and the radiological differences. Irritable bowel syndrome (page 276) is in the differential diagnosis.

A mass in the right iliac fossa must be differentiated from a caecal carcinoma and an appendix abscess. Amoebic abscesses and ileocaecal tuberculosis are uncommon in Britain.

Prognosis and management

A few remit spontaneously. This is most frequent in the group presenting as acute appendicitis.

Long-term management for chronic recurrent disease requires:
• Bed rest during acute exacerbations
• High protein diet with vitamin and electrolyte supplements as required. Some physicians recommend a high fibre diet unless strictures are present
• Sulphasalazine or mesalazine may be used. Metronidazole is given to treat bacterial overgrowth producing steatorrhoea
• Steroids are sometimes effective in suppressing acute intestinal symptoms but less so than in ulcerative colitis. Low-dose steroids (prednisolone 10 mg daily) may improve health and decrease the frequency of recurrence in individual cases. Steroids may also be necessary for systemic complications. Immunosuppression (azathioprine) has been used successfully in a small number of cases over a short period of time. It appears to allow a reduction in steroid dosage with apparently little detrimental effect on well-being

Elemental diets are reported to be as effective as prednisolone but their universal use is not yet accepted. Surgery is retained for the relief of acute emergencies (obstruction), abscesses and fistulae. Surgery eventually becomes necessary in about 30% of cases. Resection of diseased intestine and bypass operations may become necessary for severe chronic ill health, but these are not curative and fistula formation may result and recurrence is the rule. Intestinal obstruction is best managed conservatively in the first instance with gastric aspiration and intravenous feeding to allow time for the acute inflammation to resolve.

STEATORRHOEA AND MALABSORPTION

Malabsorption signifies impaired ability to absorb one or more of the normally absorbed dietary constituents, including protein, carbohydrates, fats, minerals and vitamins.

Steatorrhoea signifies malabsorption of fat, and is defined as a faecal fat excretion of more than 18 mmol/day (6 g/day) on a normal fat intake (50–100 g). Apart from the occasions when the cause of steatorrhoea is obvious (such as obstructive jaundice) the diagnostic problem revolves around the differentiation between enteropathy (commonly gluten-induced) and other causes of steatorrhoea.

Diarrhoea is not necessarily a presenting symptom and malabsorption may present with one or more of its complications (e.g. anaemia, weight loss, osteomalacia).

Gluten-sensitive enteropathy (coeliac disease)

Aetiology

There is mucosal sensitivity to wheat gluten and to barley and rye, and occasionally oats (though not rice or maize). This may be due to the direct toxic effect of the polypeptide gliadin perhaps as a result of an immune disorder (a local deficiency of IgA or an antigen–antibody reaction at the mucosa). It is associated with HLA B8 and antibodies to reticulin may be present. There is an increased incidence in near relatives and there is a high incidence of gut lymphoma and carcinoma.

NB Virtually all patients with dermatitis herpetiformis have gluten-sensitive enteropathy.

Clinical presentation

There is usually a history of intermittent or chronic increased bowel frequency, classically with pale, bulky, offensive frothy greasy stools which flush only with difficulty. There may be a history of intermittent abdominal colic, flatus and abdominal distension. Depending on the severity and duration of the disease, there may be weakness and weight loss. If the malabsorption started in childhood, the patient may be short compared with his unaffected siblings, or parents. Children may present with irritability, failure to gain weight or 'failure to thrive'.

The malabsorption involves not only fat and the fat-soluble vitamins but also minerals and water-soluble vitamins (table 24).

Examination

In addition to the features mentioned above there may be:
- evidence of weight loss
- pigmented, scaly and bruised skin
- distended abdomen with increased bowel sounds

NB The anaemia has many causes including anorexia, blood loss, mucosal damage, folate deficiency, and bacterial overgrowth.

Table 24. Vitamin and mineral deficiency following malabsorption.

Vitamin B_{12}	To produce megaloblastic anaemia (page 357)
Iron (rare)	To produce iron deficiency anaemia (page 355)
Vitamin D and calcium	Resulting in osteomalacia with bone tenderness and muscle weakness. Tetany may occur. Children may develop rickets
Vitamin B group	Glossitis and angular stomatitis
Vitamin K	Deficient prothrombin formation to produce bruising and epistaxis
Associated impairment of amino acid absorption	May produce hypoproteinaemia and oedema
Potassium	May produce weakness

Clubbing may occur. Signs of subacute combined degeneration of the cord are very rare.

Other causes of malabsorption

Bile salt deficiency

Patients present with obstructive jaundice usually secondary to carcinoma of the head of the pancreas or to gallstones (which may sometimes be seen on plain abdominal X-ray) or, rarely, in primary biliary cirrhosis or bile duct stricture.

Pancreatic enzyme deficiency

Usually due to chronic pancreatitis or carcinoma affecting the pancreatic ducts (also rarely, fibrocystic disease, pancreatic calculi and benign pancreatic cystadenoma). The differentiation of these two diseases may be very difficult at presentation. Tests for malabsorption, glucose tolerance, serum bilirubin and barium meal are of little help. Tests of pancreatic secretion (secretin–pancreozymin–cholecystokinin stimulation) are said to give low volumes in carcinoma and low enzyme levels in chronic pancreatitis. More recent indirect tests of exocrine pancreatic function include the BT-PABA test (measure urinary excretion of para-amino benzoic acid specifically split from BT-PABA by pancreatic chymotrypsin) and the pancreolauryl test (measure urinary excretion of fluorescein specifically split from fluorescein dilaurate by pancreatic esterase in the presence of bile salts). Calcification of the pancreas on straight abdominal X-ray favours chronic pancreatitis. Similarly, duodenal fibreoscopy with cannulation of the pancreatic duct (ERCP) may help to distinguish between carcinoma of the pancreas and chronic pancreatitis. Carcino-embryonic antigen (CEA) studies are useful only for assessing completeness of resection of a CEA producing tumour. Symptoms of pancreatic malabsorption are improved by a low fat diet (40 g/day), replacing minerals and vitamins, and giving pancreatic supplements (e.g. Nutrizym, Creon, Pancrex V Forte) preferably with H_2 blockade. Avoid alcohol.

Other intestinal disease

Post-surgical. Incomplete food mixing may follow gastrectomy or gastroenterostomy and there may be a diminished area for absorption following small bowel resection.

Abnormal intestinal organisms. Bacterial overgrowth can be distinguished from ileal disease using the early (40 min) peak in breath hydrogen after lactulose (10 g) or glucose (50 g). The normal bacterial count in jejunal juice is $<10^3$–10^5 organisms/ml. The organisms (*E. coli* and bacteroides) break down dietary tryptophan to produce indoxylsulphate (indican) which is excreted in the urine. Overgrowth can be detected by urinary indican excretion of more than 80 mg/24 h. The aetiological role of the cultured organisms is difficult to prove but the steatorrhoea may respond to antibiotic therapy (tetracycline). There may be a close association between bacterial overgrowth and stasis from 'blind loops', diverticula and strictures. It may occur after gastrectomy due to reduced acid and pepsin.

Crohn's disease (page 269).

Rare causes

The following are very uncommon but well recognised:

• *Zollinger–Ellison syndrome* (page 263).

• *Disaccharidase deficiency*. Malabsorption of lactose, maltose and sucrose may occur in isolation due to primary enzyme deficiency, or as part of a general malabsorption picture in any disease which damages the intestinal brush border. The most important is isolated lactase deficiency which presents, usually in children, with milk intolerance and malabsorption. Patients have abdominal pain, diarrhoea, distension, and borborygmi (i.e. symptoms of bacterial fermentation of unabsorbed sugars) after 50 g lactose by mouth and the blood glucose rises by <1.1 mmol/litre over the following 2 h. The diagnosis is confirmed by the absence of lactase activity in the jejunal mucosa on biopsy. Management consits of withdrawal of milk and milk products from the diet.

• *Other intrinsic disease* of the intestinal wall due to tuberculosis Hodgkin's disease, lymphosarcoma, diffuse systemic sclerosis, amyloidosis, and Whipple's disease (intestinal lipodystrophy).

• *Tropical sprue* is a disorder which produces steatorrhoea and occurs almost exclusively in Europeans in or from the tropics, especially in India and the Far East. The aetiology is unknown. The most common associated deficiency is folic acid. The disease frequently remits spontaneously on return from the tropics. In some cases which do not remit a course of parenteral folic acid, metronidazole or oral tetracycline may be curative.

Very rarely, malabsorption is associated with diabetes, cardiac failure and giardiasis.

Investigation of malabsorption

In a patient with a characteristic history, the investigation with the greatest likelihood of achieving a diagnosis is jejunal biopsy.

However, tests of absorption may quantitate the degree of malabsorption and help with the differential diagnosis between pancreatic and intestinal steatorrhoea.

Using the hydrogen breath test, after an oral dose of lactose (2 g/kg up to 50 g, in 250 ml water), normal subjects show no rise in breath hydrogen over the following 3 h because they absorb the disaccharide completely. If, because it is not absorbed higher up the gut, the disaccharide reaches the colon, the anaerobic bacteria there ferment it so that hydrogen can be detected in the breath at about 90 min. The hydrogen breath test can also be used to assess small bowel transit time using lactulose.

NB Intestinal malabsorption tends to give a total malabsorption. Pancreatic malabsorption (page 272) is much less common and tends to affect the absorption only of fat and proteins and to leave the absorption of sugars, minerals, and water-soluble vitamins relatively unaffected.

Blood tests

Anaemia is common and may be 'iron deficient', megaloblastic or both (dimorphic).

Serum and red cell folate, iron and transferrin may be low.

Serum albumin may be reduced and the prothrombin time prolonged.

Serum calcium, phosphate and magnesium may be low and the serum alkaline phosphatase increased (osteomalacia pattern).

Tests of absorption

Faecal fat excretion. The diagnosis of steatorrhoea is made by measuring faecal fat excretion over 3–5 days on a normal diet (50–100 g of fat in 24 h). The upper limit of normal is 6 g/24 h (18 mmol/24 h).

Butter fat absorption test is a screening test that has replaced faecal fat collection. Change in plasma turbidity is measured following a standard fatty meal.

D-*xylose excretion.* More than 20% (5 g) of an oral load of 25 g is normally excreted in the urine in the 5 h after ingestion. Less than 4 g is excreted in intestinal malabsorption and also if there is renal dysfunction (and if the urine collection is incomplete). The 2-hour blood xylose level is normally 2.1–3.8 mmol/litre. The test is normal in pancreatic steatorrhoea but points to upper small bowel disease if abnormal.

NB Xylose was originally used because it was thought not to be metabolised (it is a little). It is absorbed mainly in the jejunum.

Glucose tolerance test. In intestinal malabsorption, the curve is usually flat. In chronic pancreatitis and pancreatic carcinoma the curve may be diabetic. In post-gastrectomy dumping, there may be a lag curve.

Other disaccharide (sucrose or lactose) absorption tests. The blood glucose should normally rise more than 20 mg/dl after a 50 g oral dose. Those with disaccharidase deficiency have a smaller rise and tend to develop abdominal colic and diarrhoea during the test.

Schilling test. Megaloblastic anaemia may be caused by vitamin B_{12} deficiency in malabsorption syndromes if the terminal ileum is involved (e.g. Crohn's disease). In this case the absorption of radio-cobalt-labelled B_{12} is not improved by the addition of intrinsic factor (unlike pernicious anaemia).

Radiology

A small intestinal barium meal with a flocculable contrast medium may show flocculation and segmentation of barium—evidence of excess mucus secretion. Of more significance are widening of the small intestinal calibre and increased distance between adjacent loops of bowel indicating thickening of the intestinal wall. All these changes are non-specific and the main purpose of barium meal is to detect diverticula, fistulae or Crohn's disease.

The bones may show evidence of osteomalacia and/or osteoporosis, and even of hyperparathyroidism (secondary or tertiary) if very severe and prolonged.

Jejunal biopsy

In gluten-induced enteropathy, dissecting microscopic examination usually reveals flattening of the mucosa, with partial or total villous atrophy. Endoscopy usually shows a reduced number of duodenal mucosal folds. If the mucosal appearance fails to respond to gluten withdrawal, other causes such as lymphoma should be considered.

Management of gluten-induced enteropathy

Gluten-free diet. In adults the response may take several months. Repeat biopsy is performed and the diagnosis is confirmed by a return of the appearances towards normal.

NB There may be a predisposition to malignancy—lymphomas and gut carcinoma (particularly oesophagus)—in gluten-induced enteropathy and there is some evidence that gluten-free diets may reduce the incidence of these. Hence the diet is continued for life.

Replace vitamins and minerals as indicated, and, if necessary, parenterally.

DIVERTICULAR DISEASE

Diverticula occur anywhere in the alimentary tract but chiefly in the colon—diverticulosis. They are due to a weakening of the colonic wall and increased intracolonic pressure. They affect chiefly the descending and sigmoid colon. It is a disorder of mid and late age (5% of the population over 50 years in Britain), more common in women than men and is usually discovered incidentally during barium enema performed to exclude colonic carcinoma.

Clinical features

Inflamed diverticula produce diverticulitis with:
* pain, discomfort and tenderness in the left iliac fossa (there may be a mass from pericolic abscess)—'appendicitis of the left side'
* change in bowel habit with constipation and/or diarrhoea sometimes alternating (NB exclude carcinoma)
* rectal bleeding which may be acute and sometimes massive and the first symptom
* subacute obstruction
* frequency of micturition and cystitis, due to vesicocolic fistula
* perforation with peritonitis or fistulae

Management

Acute diverticulitis may be extremely painful and require rest in bed, analgesia, local warmth and antibiotics (ampicillin or metronidazole or cotrimoxazole). Occasionally surgery is required, particularly colostomy and resection for obstruction.

Dietary fibre

Diverticulosis is rare in communities which take a fibre-rich diet. Such peoples also have far less carcinoma of the colon and appendicitis. A diet high in dietary fibre results in bulkier stools and rapid intestinal transit times. The soft stool prevents straining which may help to prevent diverticulosis. In the established disease added dietary fibre (2 teaspoonsful to 2 tablespoonsful daily) reduces symptoms in most patients. Fibre-rich diets also decrease serum cholesterol and increase faecal excretion of bile salts and their relative absence from Western diets has been suggested as a possible contributory factor in coronary artery atheroma and gallstones.

IRRITABLE BOWEL SYNDROME (irritable colon; spastic colon; nervous colon; mucous colitis)

Clinical presentation

One of the commonest bowel disorders which occurs in young adults, more often female than male, with colicky abdominal pain eased by bowel movement, often frequent and loose at onset of pain, altered bowel habit, bloating, and a sense of incomplete evacuation. Examination is normal though there may be tenderness in the left iliac fossa.

Investigation

Investigation is necessary to exclude more serious disease, i.e. ulcerative colitis, Crohn's disease, carcinoma of colon and malabsorption if diarrhoea is a feature. If the history is typical, the examination and sigmoidoscopy normal and three stools negative for occult blood, in the absence of other clinical pointers, serious alternative diagnoses are effectively excluded. If there are changes in bowel habit, barium enema can exclude carcinoma and demonstrate diverticula. Blood count, erythrocyte sedimentation rate, C-reactive protein, serum proteins and at least three faecal occult blood examinations should be normal.

Treatment

Bulking agents, e.g. bran (1–2 dessertspoonsful daily), usually help. Antispasmodics may be tried, e.g. hyoscine (Buscopan) 10–20 mg tds, or mebeverine (Colofac) 135 mg tds before meals. If a cause of anxiety can be identified and treated, symptoms may be markedly reduced. Occasionally specific foods may produce symptoms of irritable colon and these should be excluded from the diet.

ISCHAEMIC COLITIS

Clinical features

This is a disorder of middle and old age which often presents as an acute abdomen with the sudden onset of pain followed by bloody diarrhoea, sometimes copious.

Diagnosis

If subacute, it must be distinguished from the bleeding of diverticular disease and of ulcerative colitis. Any part of the colon can be affected, though, because it has the most precarious blood supply, the splenic flexure is usually involved. If the colon looks normal on sigmoidoscopy, ulcerative colitis is virtually excluded, though large bowel Crohn's disease or diverticular disease is not. Barium enema shows mucosal oedema with characteristic 'thumb-printing' as if a thumb had been pressed along the outside of the affected colon.

Prognosis

In mild cases there may be complete recovery but colonic strictures can develop later. In colonic gangrene, surgical resection is necessary. The differential diagnosis includes Campylobacter enteritis, and diverticular disease in which bleeding can be torrential. Pseudomembranous colitis does not usually cause bloody diarrhoea.

PANCREAS

Carcinoma

75% of tumours occur in the head.

Clinical presentation

Patients present with one or more of the following features:
- Anorexia and weight loss.
- Indigestion or epigastric pain often indistinguishable from duodenal or gastric ulceration. Back pain suggests pancreatic disease (and posterior ulcers).
- Obstructive jaundice. Intermittent jaundice suggests a gallstone in the bile duct (rarely carcinoma of the ampulla of Vater).
- About 20% of patients have diabetes usually of short duration and some present with it. In the elderly, sudden onset or worsening of diabetes may indicate malignancy

Investigation

Ultrasound or CT scan may show the tumour.
ERCP may confirm the diagnosis and allows palliative stenting of the obstructed common bile duct to relieve pruritus and jaundice.

Management

Ampullary carcinoma presents early with obstructive jaundice and can be resected.
Carcinoma of the head and body of the pancreas is usually fatal within 1 year.

Islet cell tumours

See Zollinger–Ellison syndrome and insulinoma (page 263).

Acute pancreatitis

Aetiology

About 90% are associated with gall bladder disease (especially gallstones) and alcoholism. It is uncommon after cholecystectomy.

Clinical presentation

There may be a previous history of cholecystitis as biliary colic associated with gallstones. Pancreatitis is more common in alcoholics and occurs occasionally in mumps.

Abdominal pain, often very severe, occurs suddenly, usually in the epigastrium or across the upper abdomen with radiation to the back or shoulder. It spreads to involve the entire abdomen which is tender with guarding and rebound tenderness. Hypotension with sweating and cyanosis occurs in severe attacks. There may be bruising around the umbilicus or in the flanks.

Differential diagnosis

It presents initially as an 'acute abdomen' and resembles
* cholecystitis
* acute myocardial infarction, dissecting aortic aneurysm, mesenteric vascular occlusion
* intestinal perforation, particularly duodenal ulcer (though shock is not often a feature of a perforated duodenal ulcer)

Investigation

The serum amylase is very high (over 1000 units/ml) within 24 h of onset. The level falls rapidly. Posterior duodenal ulcers can also cause very high amylase levels but not usually above 1000 units. Peritoneal fluid also has high amylase levels.

Straight abdominal X-ray may show gallstones, pancreatic calcification (indicating previous inflammation) and a distended loop of jejunum or transverse colon if they are close to the inflamed pancreas. Check serum calcium (which may fall due to the formation of calcium soaps). There is usually a leucocytosis.

Management

If the diagnosis is definite, conservative management is preferred by most clinicians.

Relieve pain with pentazocine or pethidine.

Gastric aspiration and intravenous rehydration.

Maintain the circulating volume.

Monitor the blood glucose.

If shock is present, give plasma expanders (e.g. dextran, plasma) whilst monitoring the central venous pressure, and give oxygen.

Other measures are of less certain value:

Propantheline 15–30 mg, 6-hourly to block the vagus and relax the sphincter of Oddi.

H_2 blockade.

Antibiotics to prevent infection.

Calcium if the serum level falls.

In very severe cases, peritoneal lavage, and parenteral nutrition may be tried.

Prognosis

Complete recovery occurs in over 95% of patients and recurrence is uncommon. Pancreatic abscess or pseudocyst may complicate acute pancreatitis. Patients should be investigated to exclude gallstones (<5%). Alcohol should be avoided if it is a possible cause.

Chronic pancreatitis

Clinical presentation

Recurrent though mild attacks resembling acute pancreatitis.
Malabsorption and steatorrhoea from pancreatic insufficiency (page 272).
Diabetes mellitus when the islet cells are involved.
Obstructive jaundice which may be intermittent.
In association with cystic fibrosis and haemochromatosis.

Investigation

Straight abdominal X-ray for pancreatic calcification and gallstones. There is a reduction in bicarbonate output in the duodenal juice in a response to secretin pancreozymin (secretin cholecystokinin) stimulation in most cases. CT san may show dilated ducts. ERCP shows duct anatomy (ectasia or stricture) and calculi. The serum amylase is valueless in chronic pancreatitis though sometimes slightly raised, and isotope scanning of the pancreas is of little value. Investigate for malabsorption (page 273), pancreatic exocrine function (page 272), diabetes mellitus (page 198) and obstructive jaundice (page 45) if relevant.

Treatment

There is no specific therapy for chronic pancreatitis.
Treat pancreatic malabsorption with low fat diet (45 g/day), fat-soluble vitamins, calcium, and pancreatic enzymes (e.g. Pancrex V, Creon) plus H_2 blockade.
Treat diabetes mellitus (page 202).
Remove gallstones if present.
Treat recurrent attacks and consider sphincterotomy or pancreatectomy.
Alcohol is forbidden.
Chronic severe pain is common and may lead to opiate addiction.

GALL BLADDER

Acute cholecystitis

Clinical features

The story is of fever, occasionally with rigors, abdominal pain, usually right subcostal with acute pain on palpation over the gall bladder region. The disease is more common in obese females over 50, but may occur in young adults. Gallstones are present in over 90% of cases. Occasionally, acute cholecystitis may be difficult to distinguish from a high appendix and right basal pneumonia and even perforated peptic ulcer, pancreatitis and myocardial infarction.

Management

The acute inflammation usually settles with bed rest, analgesia (pethidine) and antibiotics. Penicillin and cotrimoxazole are both secreted in the bile but a third of biliary coliforms are now ampicillin resistant. Cefotaxime is probably the antibiotic of choice. The gall bladder is removed 2–3 months later after the inflammation has settled, although some surgeons elect to operate within 48 h because this is technically easier.

Rarely, an empyema develops or the gall bladder perforates.

Chronic cholecystitis

Clinical presentation

Recurrent episodes of cholecystitis are usually associated with gallstones. The attacks are often less severe than classical acute cholecystitis, and may resemble peptic ulceration and peptic oesophagitis. Myocardial ischaemia may be confused if the site of the pain is high.

Gallstones

Twice as common in women as men. There is an increased incidence in women on the oral contraceptive. The incidence rises with age. Stones occur in 10% of women over 40, classically in the fair, fat, fertile, female of 40–50 on a low fibre diet. They are usually cholesterol or mixed. Rarely they are pigment stones associated with haemolytic anaemia.

Clinical features

Most stones produce no symptoms, but they may cause:

Flatulence upwards.

Biliary colic.

Acute cholecystitis.

Chronic cholecystitis.

Obstructive jaundice, which may be intermittent giving attacks of fever, jaundice and upper abdominal pain—Charcot's triad. Gall bladder empyema from bile duct obstruction is uncommon.

Gallstones are associated with acute and chronic pancreatitis and their presence indicates a higher risk of gall bladder carcinoma although this is still extremely rare.

Management

If causing symptoms, the gall bladder and stones should be removed. It is at this stage that pigment stones are detected and indicate investigation for haemolysis. In elderly patients or if surgery is contraindicated, sphincterotomy via ERCP may release the stones if they are in the common bile duct. Ursodeoxycholic acid (UDCA) may dissolve radiolucent stones if the stones are under 2 cm in diameter, and if the gall bladder is functioning. The stones may recur after treatment. Rowachol (a monoterpene mixture including menthol) is an adjuvant to bile acid therapy. Shockwave lithotripsy may be successful.

Investigation. Straight abdominal X-ray and ultrasonography with acoustic shadow will reveal many stones. Cholecystogram will confirm and reveal the rest but contrast medium will not concentrate in the gall bladder if the bilirubin is above 35 μmol/litre and intravenous cholangiography then becomes necessary, though it only shows stones in the biliary tree.

Although surgeons may explore the bile duct at surgery, stones are sometimes missed and may later produce symptoms. Operative cholangiography and/or fibreoptic examination of the bile duct make this less likely.

Respiratory disease

The commonest diseases are infections of the upper respiratory tract, e.g. the common cold. The commonest diseases of the lower respiratory tract are bronchitis (acute and chronic), asthma and carcinoma of the bronchus.

CHRONIC BRONCHITIS AND EMPHYSEMA

Definitions
Daily cough with sputum for at least 3 months a year for at least 2 consecutive years. This defines the hypersecretory form of chronic bronchitis. Airflow obstruction in small airways >2mm in diameter is more dangerous and is not necessarily associated with hypersecretion. It is a clinical definition and radiological, pathological and biochemical features are judged by this standard. The definition is chiefly of use epidemiologically: patients whose respiratory disease does not satisfy this definition may nevertheless have bronchitis. It causes about 30 000 deaths per annum in the UK.

'Emphysema' is a histological diagnosis and is therefore usually made with precision only post mortem. It is defined as enlargement of the air spaces distal to the terminal (smallest) bronchioles with destructive changes in the alveolar wall. In centrilobular emphysema, damage is limited to the central part of the lobule around the respiratory bronchiole, whereas in panacinar emphysema, there is destruction and distension of the whole lobule. If the air-spaces are >1 cm in diameter, they are called bullae.

Aetiological factors
*   *Tobacco smoking*. The increased mortality risk from bronchitis has an approximately straight-line relationship with numbers of cigarettes smoked per day (increased risk = ½ × cigarettes smoked per day)
*   *Atmospheric pollution*
*   There is a relationship to lower social class, industrial environment and to being British although mortality from chronic bronchitis has fallen progressively in the last 10 years in the UK. This is probably due not only to the general reduction in the number of cigarettes smoked, but also due to the considerable drop in tar and nicotine content. Other factors include control of air pollution, an increase in living standards and better working conditions
* α_1-*Antitrypsin deficiency* is a recessive disorder which accounts for about 5% of all patients with emphysema (and about 20% of neonatal cholestasis). Five per cent of homozygotes tend to develop emphysema by the age of 40 years and heterozygotes are at risk. The emphysema is predominantly of the lower zones and is much worse in smokers

282

Clinical presentation

Initially, the patient has productive morning cough and an increased frequency of lower respiratory tract infections producing purulent sputum. The organisms responsible are usually *Haemophilus influenzae, Streptococcus pneumoniae,* and the respiratory viruses. Over the years there is slowly progressive dyspnoea with wheezing, exacerbated in the acute infective episodes. There is clinical emphysema with hyperinflation of the lungs. Respiratory failure (page 289) or chronic right heart failure (cor pulmonale) may develop.

Investigation

Chest X-ray. This may be normal. Abnormalities correlate with the presence of emphysema and are due to:
- overinflation with a low, flat, poorly moving diaphragm and a large retrosternal window on lateral X-ray
- vascular changes with loss of peripheral vascular markings but enlarged hilar vessels. This heart is narrow until cor pulmonale develops
- bullae if present

The chest X-ray is an important investigation because it excludes other disease (carcinoma, tuberculosis, pneumonia, pneumothorax).

Ventilatory function tests. Spirometry shows a greater reduction in forced expiratory volume in 1 s (FEV_1) than in vital capacity (VC) (and their ratio, the FEV% is thus also reduced).

The peak expiratory flow rate (PEFR) is reduced. This airways obstruction is usually only partially reversible.

*Arterial blood gas estimations .*These may be normal. In later stages the Po_2 falls and the Pco_2 rises particularly with exacerbations.

ECG. This records the presence and progression of cor pulmonale (right atrial and ventricular hypertrophy).

Sputum for bacterial culture and sensitivity. This is useful in acute infective episodes when infections other than *H. influenzae* or *S. pneumoniae* may be present.

Haemoglobin estimation may show secondary polycythaemia.

Management

Stop smoking and control excess weight.

Treat acute bacterial exacerbations. Ampicillin (0.5–1.0 g qds) or trimethoprim (200 mg bd) are suitable. Change of therapy is directed by the clinical conditions. Bacterial sensitivities are useful if clinical improvement has not occurred.

Bronchodilators. The β_2 agonists, e.g. salbutamol (Ventolin), terbutaline (Bricanyl) or the anticholinergic ipratropium (Atrovent) are suitable and are given by metered aerosol or nebuliser.

Oral theophylline preparations may help.

Treat right heart failure with diuretics.

Secondary polycythaemia is sometimes managed by venesection at 3–6 month intervals if the haematocrit is over 0.52 down to 0.48 Supplementary iron should be given.

Physiotherapy—with emphasis on coughing and relaxation.

Home oxygen (controlled concentration and no smoking) is useful for hypoxic cor pulmonale and may reduce pulmonary hypertention.

Mucolytic agents are probably useless.

NB   Steroids are not usually indicated either orally or by aerosol. In severe refractory cases steroids may be given a short trial while ventilatory function is monitored. At least 25% improvement in FEV_1, or PEFR should be achieved. If not, steroids are not given long-term.

BRONCHIECTASIS

Bronchiectasis means dilation of the airways. It only becomes of clinical significance when infection and/or haemoptysis occurs within these dilated airways. Severe forms are now rare, especially in the young.

Aetiology

Following acute childhood respiratory infection, particularly measles and whooping cough and pneumonia.

Cystic fibrosis.

Bronchial obstruction predisposes to bronchiectasis (e.g. peanuts).

Tuberculosis has become less common as a cause.

Congenital (rare): the immotile cilia syndrome, e.g. Kartagener's syndrome.

Clinical features

Chronic cough, often postural.

Sputum often copious, especially with acute infections. Halitosis.

Febrile episodes.

Haemoptysis: may be the only symptom ('dry bronchiectasis') and is occasionally severe.

Dyspnoea, coarse basal crepitations and wheeze.

Cyanosis and clubbing.

Loss of weight and cor pulmonale in advanced cases.

Management

Stop smoking.

The object is to get rid of chronic sepsis. Twice daily postural drainage will help to empty dilated airways and decrease the frequency of further infections. Bronchodilators will often help to improve clearance of sputum. Antibiotics, as for chronic bronchitis, are given for acute infections and exacerbations. Treatment is unnecessary in the absence of symptoms.

Surgery is virtually never indicated unless there is uncontrolled bleeding because the disease is seldom limited to one or two lung segments. Patients with severe disease may develop respiratory failure.

CYSTIC FIBROSIS

A hereditary autosomal recessive disorder affecting 1/3000 births which occurs equally in males and females and usually presents in early childhood with repeated lower respiratory tract infections. These are secondary to bronchial obstruction from the viscid secretions of the bronchial mucosa. Secondary bronchiectasis or lung abscesses may result. Recurrent small haemoptyses and finger clubbing are common, and pneumothorax occurs. Neonates may present with meconium ileus. Persistent productive cough is associated initially with *Staph. pyogenes* (treat with flucloxacillin) and *Haemophilus influenzae* (treat with amoxycillin). Later, *Pseudomonas aeruginosa* (treat with ceftazidime or ciprofloxacin) is associated with a poor prognosis: this organism cannot be eradicated. Associated pancreatic malabsorption is common (80%) but symptoms (weight loss and steatorrhoea from inspissation of pancreatic secretions) are usually mild. A high sodium concentration in the sweat (above 70 mmol/litre) is characteristic, and exceptionally can lead to circulatory collapse from uncontrolled salt depletion during heatwaves.

Most males are sterile and women subfertile.

Haemoptysis or pneumothorax may occur in adolescents and adults. Management is with pancreatic enzymes (with H_2 blockade) and fat-soluble vitamins, postural drainage with bronchodilator therapy and antibiotics for episodes of deterioration. Death occurs in early adult life from respiratory failure with or without cor pulmonale. Lung or heart-lung transplantation may be indicated.

The social and emotional problems can be enormous and for this reason, as well as the complexity of clinical management, the condition should be supervised from specialist centres.

ASTHMA

Asthma is characterised by recurrent shortness of breath, wheeze or cough caused by variable or intermittent narrowing of the intrapulmonary airways. This is the result of airways hypersensitivity in response to many different stimuli such as cold air, smoke, exercise, emotion, as well as antigens. Wheeze is not an essential feature.

There are two common main clinical groups:

Extrinsic allergic asthma. It begins in childhood and there is usually a family history of other allergies (hayfever and eczema) and a family history of asthma. It is episodic and tends to improve in many patients.

Intrinsic asthma (late-onset asthma). It begins in adult life and there is usually no allergic or family history and no demonstrable skin sensitivities. Nasal polyps are common. Exacerbations are associated with infection and taking aspirin. Marked inspissation of sputum often occurs and attacks are less responsive to therapy than extrinsic asthma. Eosinophilia may be marked. It tends to be chronic and to get worse.

Aetiology

In the allergic type there is antigen release of histamine and other substances such as bradykinin, serotonin and leukotrienes from mast cells in lungs which have been sensitised with IgE antibody. The differential diagnosis of late-onset asthma includes chronic bronchitis and, far less likely, polyarteritis nodosa. Stridor from large airways obstruction may be confusing.

Pulmonary eosinophilia indicates the association of transient shadows on the chest X-ray with a high blood eosinophil count. When there is no asthma (Loeffler's syndrome), it is usually due either to various intestinal worms, especially *Ascaris*, or to drugs, especially nitrofurantoin. When there is asthma, allergic bronchopulmonary aspergillosis is the commonest cause but other antigens can be responsible. Filariasis in the tropics, polyarteritis nodosa and pulmonary embolism should also be considered.

Clinical features

Acute attacks

These may be fairly abrupt in onset and brief in duration (hours), or longer (a week or two), remittent and less severe. Longer severe attacks are called status asthmaticus (see below). In an attack the patient feels tightness in the chest and both inspiratory and expiratory difficulty. There may be a cough which is initially dry but later becomes productive, particularly if there is infection. The patient usually sits up with an over-inflated chest, an audible expiratory wheeze and a fixed shoulder girdle using the accessory muscles of respiration. The respiratory rate may be little altered but the pulse is invariably rapid. Acute attacks are precipitated by specific allergens (e.g. pollens or house dust mite), exertion, excitement, cold air, a respiratory infection or β-blockers.

Recurrent asthma

Mild asthmatics (particularly with extrinsic asthma) usually have normal respiratory function between attacks, but those with longstanding severe asthma tend to develop emphysema and some degree of dyspnoea and persistent airways obstruction between acute attacks.

Investigation

Investigation includes chest X-ray (for regional collapse, pneumonia, pneumothorax), haematology (eosinophilia and erythrocyte sedimentation rate—ESR), and measurement of ventilatory function (FEV_1 or PEFR, preferably at several times in a day on several days at home) and the response to bronchodilators. Variability through the day, especially with a 'morning dip' in PEFR, is characteristic. Skin hypersensitivity tests performed by pricking standard allergens into the skin can help the patient to recognise and avoid environmental precipitants. Bronchial reactivity may be more precise but should be tested only in carefully controlled conditions. Adrenaline (0.5 ml of 1:1000) must be available in case of acute anaphylactic reactions. (see *Acute anaphylaxis*, page 290).

Management

The patient should be asked about precipitant factors including the relationship of attacks to upper respiratory tract infection, season (grass pollen and fungal spores), cold, exercise, food, house dust (contains the mite dermatophagoides), smoke, emotion and drugs (e.g. aspirin, propranolol). New patients, and those being further investigated, should be given a peak flow meter to document waking and end-of-day values at home. Increasing morning dips can provide an early warning of deterioration in some patients.

Most patients and almost all extrinsic asthmatics respond to simple therapy and may be controlled by:
- removing known allergies, e.g. feather pillows and cats
- steroids by inhalation for adults
- β_2-agonists, e.g. salbutamol prn (with or without salmeterol bd) by inhaler
- disodium cromoglycate (Intal), 2–4 Spincaps daily or aerosol for children
- anticholinergic drug ipratropium by inhalation
- theophylline or aminophylline preparation by mouth. A slow release preparation at night can help nocturnal wheeze and cough especially in children
- hyposensitisation is of value in only a small number of patients who demonstrate specific allergies

NB When metered aerosols are used, always check inhaler technique. A number of simpler automatic inhalers are now available (disks, rotahalers, breath-actuated aerosols). A β_2 agonist delivered by nebuliser at home has helped many patients with severe recurrent asthma. In some patients the PEFR tends to fall for a few days before an acute attack and prophylactic therapy with steroids may then abate it. Such patients may be given a peak flow meter and prednisolone to use at home.

The increasing mortality of asthma may be due to over-reliance on inhaled β_2-agonists and a consequent failure to seek expert medical help early enough.

Systemic steroid therapy

In view of the serious side-effects, systemic steroids must be avoided whenever possible in the long-term maintenance of asthma. Steroid-responsiveness can be judged by an improvement in FEV_1 or PEFR of 25% or more after 10 days of prednisolone 20–30 mg daily orally. There is little place for steroids in those with a poor response. Few extrinsic asthmatics need steroids but many intrinsic asthmatics cannot be controlled without, although some may require as little as 1–2 mg prednisolone per day. Systemic steroids should only be considered after trying adequate doses of routine maintenance therapy with:
- β_2-agonists, e.g. salbutamol or terbutaline, orally or by inhalation
- aerosol steroids, e.g. beclomethasone, often in high dose
- oral theophylline derivatives

Severe asthma

Status asthmaticus is defined as an asthma attack of over 24 h duration. This is not a clinically useful definition since, of those who die in an acute asthma attack, half are dead within 24 h. Moreover, death is frequently sudden and sometimes unexpected as the patient may not appear severely ill. It is this lack of recognition of severity plus inadequate early treatment which is so dangerous. Most patients have some degree of respiratory failure at presentation.

Clinical presentation

Dyspnoea. Inability to speak or difficulty in maintaining speech is one criterion of severity. It also implies inability to drink and therefore dehydration. Hypoxaemia is usually then present, and wheeze frequently absent due to poor ventilation. Confusion and drowsiness are evidence of a perilous situation whatever the cause (abnormal blood gases, sedation or fatigue).

Cyanosis is also ominous and tends to occur at a lower Po_2 than in the chronic bronchitic (because the bronchitic tends to have polycythaemia).

Absence of wheeze may denote very severe airways obstruction. A severe attack may be suggested by tachycardia, a peak flow rate <30% of predicted values, a heart rate >110/min, pulsus paradoxus >10 mmHg, and arterial hypotension.

NB The clinical signs of drowsiness and cyanosis are those of a very severe attack and vigorous treatment is essential before they are apparent.

Investigation

A chest X-ray is mandatory to exclude a pneumothorax. Blood gases provide the most useful guide to the severity of the attack and to the success of treatment. Peak expiratory flow rates can usually not be obtained, though one should always try, and are less than a quarter of the predicted values.

Management

All asthma attacks which do not respond to treatment with standard bronchodilators (theophylline preparations and β_2-agonist drugs such as salbutamol) within a few hours should be regarded as severe. They usually merit admission to hospital. Sedation may depress respiration further and is contraindicated.

• *Continuous oxygen* should invariably be given in high concentration, e.g. by nasal cannula. It is not necessary to give controlled (28%) oxygen unless there is evidence of some chronic respiratory failure

• *Bronchodilators* β_2-agonists (e.g. salbutamol, terbutaline) by nebuliser or i.v. infusion.

Aminophylline bolus followed by ipratropium bromide by nebuliser.

NB Too rapid infusion may cause circulatory collapse. This can be dangerous in patients already on oral preparations including theophylline-containing cough-mixtures because of toxicity: check blood theophylline levels first. Children are particularly at risk.

• *Corticosteroids.* Hydrocortisone is given early and in large doses intravenously, e.g. 4 mg/kg immediately and 3 mg/kg 6-hourly if the patient cannot swallow. The patient is transferred to oral prednisolone (e.g. 10 mg tds) when he can swallow and this is subsequently withdrawn gradually.

• *Intravenous fluids* are required both to make up the initial dehydration and for as long as oral fluids are not taken. Monitor urine output.

• *Bacterial infection* is a rare trigger but *antibiotics* are given if it is present or strongly suspected. The usual organisms are *Strep. pneumoniae* or *Haemophilus influenzae*: amoxycillin or trimethoprim should be given.

- *Mechanical ventilation* may be necessary. Persistent or increasing elevation of arterial P_{CO_2}, especially with accompanying exhaustion suggests the need for artifical ventilation by an experienced anaesthetist.

NB   Check the chest X-ray for pneumothorax.

RESPIRATORY FAILURE

Respiratory failure can be defined as a reduction in arterial P_{O_2} below 8 kPa with or without an increase in arterial P_{CO_2} above 6.0 kPa.

In restrictive disorders, lung expansion is limited by:

1. Lung disease such as fibrosis collapse, oedema, consolidation.
2. Pleural disease such as fibrosis, effusion or mesothelioma.
3. Chest wall disease such as costospinal rigidity and deformity, or abdominal splinting by obesity, ascites, or pregnancy.
4. Neuromuscular disease such as muscular dystrophy, myasthenia, or phrenic nerve paralysis.

Sleep apnoea syndrome is defined as absence of airflow in periods of at least 10 s occurring not less than 30 times per night's sleep. It is called *obstructive* when respiratory efforts continue, and *central* when they do not.

NB   The mean P_{O_2} is about 13 kPa. Normally values of P_{O_2} are about 1.3 kPa (10 mmHg)—lower in the elderly.

The P_{O_2} may fall while the P_{CO_2} remains normal. This may occur with alveolar parenchymal lung disease: infiltrations, fibrosing alveolitis and 'pure' emphysema. Much more commonly, both arterial gas levels are abnormal. This occurs with ventilatory failure.

Acute

Patients with normal lungs, with upper airways obstruction (e.g. croup and acute anaphylaxis) or mechanical failure (e.g. flail chest, drug overdosage) or sleep apnoea.
Patients with abnormal lungs (e.g. asthma, chronic bronchitis).

Chronic

Usually in patients with abnormal lungs, especially chronic bronchitis. These patients are particularly likely to develop acute failure if infection occurs.

Acute on chronic respiratory failure

Usually chronic bronchitis.

Clinical presentation

Peripheral vasodilatation with headache, engorged veins in the fundi, warm hands and a bounding pulse, all due to CO_2 retention.
Varying degrees of agitated confusion, drowsiness and coma.
Increasing cyanosis.
Signs of right heart failure.
Flapping tremor of the outstretched hands and papilloedema are late signs.
NB   Unfortunately the physical signs are a poor guide to the presence of

respiratory failure and to its degree. It is therefore necessary to measure blood gases in all patients in whom the diagnosis is suspected.

Management

This consists of the measures used for chronic bronchitis as given above, with the addition of controlled oxygen therapy. The danger to life in this situation is hypoxia but paradoxically relief of hypoxia may make the situation worse because of the patient's reliance on hypoxic drive. Oxygen is given at 24% or 28% by Ventimask (or other controlled technique) if the arterial Po_2 is low. Oxygen is not required unless the Po_2 is <6.7 kPa (50 mmHg). It is given continuously until the acute situation (including infection and heart failure) has recovered. The Pco_2 is monitored either by the mixed venous rebreathing method or from the arterial blood. Intravenous aminophylline (10 ml) very slowly and doxapram infusion may be valuable. For chronic failure (Po_2 <7.3 kPa; Pco_2 >6 kPa; FEV_1 < 1.5 litre; FVC <2 litre), controlled oxygen can be given continuously at home usually from an oxygen concentrator for not less than 15 h in 24, over several months with improvement in symptoms and an increase in life expectancy.

NB   Sedatives are absolutely contraindicated.

Indications for mechanical ventilation

If the Pco_2 falls or rises only slightly (e.g. by 1.3 kPa (10 mmHg)) conservative therapy should be continued and reassessed periodically. If the Pco_2 rises, this indicates that the patient's ventilation is inadequate and is the prime indication for mechanical positive pressure ventilation. Patients should be ventilated before they become exhausted. The final decision to ventilate a patient is determined mainly on the basis of his respiratory function before the acute illness: if very poor, it may not now be possible to wean him off.

ACUTE ANAPHYLAXIS

This rare condition may occur in previously healthy people following drug therapy, e.g. penicillin, or insect stings. Patients with known previous hypersensitivity or allergy should not be given immune serum, live vaccine or known allergens.

Clinical features range from mild with flushing of the face, pruritus, and blotchy wheals, to severe with asthma which may proceed to respiratory obstruction from oedema of the larynx and to hypotension.

Immediate treatment is with adrenaline 0.5–1.0 ml of 1 : 1000 solution (1 mg/ml) given intramuscularly or subcutaneously and repeated every 15 min until improvement is observed to reverse the Type 1 acute reaction. Hydrocortisone takes 20–30 min to act and is not the immediate therapy of choice. It is given (after the first injection of adrenaline), in a dose of 200 mg i.v., with chlorpheniramine 10 mg slowly i.v. or i.m.

Hereditary angioedema due to C_1 esterase deficiency is a rare autosomal dominant condition and gives erythema but not wheals, patchy oedema and colicky abdominal pain. It responds to danazol prophylaxis and fresh frozen plasma in attacks.

PNEUMONIA

Bronchopneumonia

It may occur in previously normal lungs or be superimposed on underlying bronchitis or other respiratory disease, e.g. bronchiectasis or carcinoma. It is preceded by bronchial infection and is commonest in children (measles and whooping cough) and the elderly (chronic bronchitis and hypostatic pneumonia in debilitated patients in bed). In normal adults it may follow respiratory viral infections.

Clinical presentation

The history is initially often of acute bronchitis. Fever and malaise develop with a cough producing infected (yellow or green) sputum. On examination, coarse crepitations may be areas of consolidation with dullness to percussion, increased vocal resonance and bronchial breathing.

Investigation

The chest X-ray shows patchy consolidation. Blood cultures should be sent. Sputum should be sent for culture and Gram stain before starting antibiotics. These should not be withheld until sensitivities are available. Pneumococcal antigen in sputum, pleural fluid or urine may help with diagnosis even after antibiotics have been started.

Management

Streptococcus pneumoniae and *Mycoplasma pneumoniae* are the most common organisms but other bacteria (e.g. *Haemophilus influenzae, Legionella, Chlamydia psittaci, Klebsiella and Staphylococcus*) may be responsible. Initial therapy involves the use of:
- oxygen—28% in the presence of respiratory chronic failure
- antibiotics—erythromycin, covers the likely organisms in the first instance
- physiotherapy

Important predisposing causes should be considered including diabetes mellitus and carcinoma of the bronchus. Complications include lung abscess, pleural effusion and empyema.

Lobar pneumonia

This condition, usually caused by *Streptococcus pneumoniae*, has become less common possibly due to early administration of penicillins.

Clinical presentation

The onset is sudden with cough, rusty sputum, marked fever and rigors classically in the young (aged <30 years). There are signs of consolidation if a large area of lung is involved. Vesicles of herpes simplex occur around the lips. Chest X-ray shows consolidation in lobar distribution. Cerebral abscess is a rare complication. The pneumococcus is particularly dangerous to the splenectomised patient. (Give pneumococcal vaccine before splenectomy where possible).

Management

The organism most frequently cultured from sputum and blood is *S. pneumoniae* (pneumococcus) and this responds to i.v. crystalline penicillin (1–2 million units 6-hourly) which is the drug of first choice.

NB   Lobar consolidation, particularly with loss of volume on chest X-ray, may indicate an underlying bronchial obstruction, e.g. neoplasm, foreign body.

Other bacterial pneumonias

Staphylococcal pneumonia

This produces widespread infection with abscess formation. It occurs in patients with underlying disease which prevents normal response to infection, e.g. chronic leukaemia, Hodgkin's disease, cystic fibrosis, and patients on steroid therapy. It may complicate influenzal pneumonia and this makes it relatively common during epidemics of influenza. The organism may not be penicillin-sensitive, so flucloxacillin and fusidic acid are the drugs of choice. Lung abscess, empyema and subsequent bronchiectasis are relatively common complications.

Legionnaire's disease

This was first described in a group of American army veterans (legionnaires). The organism flourishes in the cooling waters of air conditioners and may colonise hot water tanks kept at <60° C. It begins as an influenzal-like illness with fever, malaise and myalgia and proceeds with cough (little sputum), dyspnoea and sometimes severe anoxia, marked confusion and coma. Diarrhoea and vomiting are common and renal failure may develop. Examination shows consolidation which usually affects one or both lung bases. Radiological changes may persist for more than 2 months after the acute illness.

The bacterium is the Gram-negative bacillus *Legionella pneumophila* and the diagnosis confirmed by a rising antibody titre.

Erythromycin or tetracycline are the antibiotics of choice but the mortality remains high (20%).

NB   Legionnaire's disease (and *Mycoplasma pneumoniae* or psittacosis) should be suspected in all patients who develop 'atypical pneumonia' which does not respond to standard antibiotics.

Recurrent bacterial pneumonia

In the absence of chronic bronchitis, recurrent pneumonia arouses the suspicion of:

• bronchial carcinoma preventing drainage of infected areas of the lung
• bronchiectasis (including cystic fibrosis)
• achalasia of the cardia, 25% of which present as chest disease, pharyngeal pouch and neuromuscular disease of the oesophagus, e.g. bulbar palsy
• hypogammaglobulinaemia and myeloma

Viral pneumonia

The most common virus producing pneumonia in children in the UK and the USA is the respiratory syncytial virus (RSV)— so called as it is a respiratory virus which produces syncytium formation when grown in tissue culture. The agent is not responsive to antibiotics and it may be indistinguishable from acute bacterial bronchitis or bronchiolitis in children and infants. The presence of an associated skin rash supports the likelihood of RSV infection.

Acute virus pneumonia in adults is very rare and occurs during epidemics of influenza A (Asian 'flu). The picture is of rapid and progressive dyspnoea and death may occur within hours from acute haemorrhagic disease of the lungs. The most common cause of pneumonia during epidemics of influenza results from secondary bacterial infection, the most serious being staphylococcal pneumonia. The viruses of measles, chickenpox, and herpes zoster may directly affect the lung. The diagnosis is confirmed by a rise in specific antibody titre.

Mycoplasma pneumonia

This is caused by *Mycoplasma pneumoniae*, the only mycoplasma definitely pathogenic to man. The clinical picture resembles bacterial pneumonia although cough and sputum are absent in one-third of cases.

Respiratory symptoms and signs and X-ray changes (patchy consolidation with small effusions) are usually preceded by several days of 'flu-like symptoms. Polyarthritis occurs and may persist for months. Malaise and fatigue may persist long after the acute illness is over. The diagnosis is confirmed by a rise of specific antibody titre, the presence of cold agglutinins and/or isolation of the organism. Tetracycline (0.5–1.0 g qds) is the antibiotic choice. Psittacosis and ornithosis (Chlamydiae), may cause a similar picture and also respond to tetracycline, though diarrhoea is commoner.

Opportunistic infection of the lungs

This is seen in immunosuppressed patients with AIDS, (page 384) or those on steroids, azathioprine, or cytotoxic agents following transplantation or for leukaemia or lymphoma. The range of organisms found is very wide and includes bacteria (*Pseudomonas, M. tuberculosis, E. coli*), fungi (*Aspergillus, Monilia, Cryptococcus*), viruses (Cytomegalovirus, Herpes zoster) and *Pneumocystis carinii* in the immunocompromised (page 384). It is important to attempt to isolate the organism from the sputum, and to carry out blood culture, endobronchial brush biopsy, and/or percutaneous lung biopsy. Treatment should not be delayed, because the prognosis is very poor.

Aspiration pneumonia

There are two main varieties differentiated from each other by the type of fluid aspirated and the circumstances in which it occurs.

Aspiration of gastric contents may produce a severe chemical pneumonitis with considerable pulmonary oedema and bronchospasm (Mendelson's syndrome). The acute respiratory distress and shock can be rapidly fatal and very difficult to treat. It tends to occur in states of reduced consciousness such as general anaesthesia, drunks, and when gastric lavage (for drug overdose) has been performed inexpertly.

Aspiration of bacteria from the oropharynx may follow dental anaethesia and can occur in bulbar palsies. The bacteria, apart from bacteroides, are nearly all penicillin-sensitive and crystalline penicillin with metronidazole are the antibiotics of choice initially until sensitivities are known. Recurrent episodes occur in some oesophageal diseases including hiatus hernia, stricture, achalasia of the cardia, and in patients with diverticula or pharyngeal pouch.

It is not possible to wait for bacteriology before treating acute severe pneumonia. When the organism is uncertain, erythromycin will cover most common pathogens. (*H. influenzae*, Pneumococcus, Legionella, Psittacosis, Mycoplasma). In the very sick, particularly the elderly, add cefotaxime to cover Gram-negative organisms as well.

Lung abscess

Aetiology

Aspiration (*see above*)

Bronchial obstruction usually by carcinoma or a foreign body (espically peanuts and teeth).

Pneumonia partially resolved or treated, particularly when caused by the *Staphylococcus*, *Klebsiella* or *Pneumococcus* organisms.

Clinical features

There is a swinging fever and the patient is very ill. The sputum is foul and purulent and there is a high polymorph cell count. Clubbing may develop.

Investigation

Sputum is sent for Gram stain and culture, and blood for culture. Chest X-ray shows round lesions which usually have a fluid level, and serial X-rays monitor progress. It may be necessary to proceed to bronchoscopy to exclude obstruction and to obtain a biopsy and sputum trap specimen.

Treatment

Antibiotic therapy is given according to sensitivities and continued until healing is complete. Repeated postural drainage is started. In resistant cases, repeated aspiration, antibiotic instillation and even surgical excision may be required.

CARCINOMA OF THE BRONCHUS

Incidence

This causes about 40 000 deaths per year in the UK, half of them under 65 years of age. About 40% are squamous cell (epidermoid) and 25% oat-cell (anaplastic small-cell). They are 2–3 times commoner in men than women. Twenty per cent are undifferentiated large cell tumours and about 15% are adenocarcinoma. Alveolar cell carcinoma is very rare.

Aetiological factors

Cigarette smoking. The increased mortality risk of carcinoma of the bronchus (squamous and oat-cell) has an approximately straight-line relationship with numbers of cigarettes smoked per day (increased risk of death = cigarettes smoked per day, numerically). Stopping smoking decreases the risk by about one-half in 5 years, and to only twice that of life-long non-smokers in 15 years. Other atmospheric pollution (coal smoke and diesel fumes) may prove to be aetiologically relevant, but quantitatively small compared with cigarettes.

Exposure to chromium, arsenic, radioactive materials or asbestos (which in addition produces interstitial fibrosis and mesotheliomata) is associated with a higher incidence of bronchial carcinoma.

Clinical presentation

The patient is usually, or has been until the onset of his symptoms, a cigarette smoker. Cough or the accentuation of an existing cough is the commonest early symptom, and haemoptysis the next. Dyspnoea, central chest ache or pleuritic pain, or slowly resolving chest infection are common early manifestations. The patient may present with metastic deposits involving brain, bone, liver, skin, kidney, adrenal glands or other site, or symptoms from local extension (superior vena cava obstruction, Horner's syndrome, Pancoast syndrome, hoarseness, cervical lymph glands, dysphagia, cardiac arrhythmia or pleural effusion). Occasionally patients are identified following a routine chest X-ray.

The presence of systemic and non-specific symptoms (anorexia, weight loss and fatigue) usually, but not always, implies late and possibly inoperable disease.

Blood and marrow

Anaemia (often normochromic or normocytic). Polycythaemia is uncommon. Marrow infiltration is common in small cell carcinoma.

Neuromuscular

Dementia (due to cerebral secondaries or rarely cortical atrophy), cerebellar syndrome, mixed sensorimotor peripheral neuropathy, proximal myopathy, polymyositis (page 151) and the myasthenic syndrome (page 153).

Skin, connective tissue, bone

Clubbing, hypertrophic pulmonary osteoarthropathy, dermatomyositis and acanthosis nigricans.

Endocrine

Syndromes due to ectopic hormone production, the pituitary-like ones (adreno-corticotrophic hormone—ACTH, antidiuretic hormone—ADH, prolactin) usually from oat-cell tumours, and parathyroid hormone from squamous cell tumours. Hypercalcaemia is usually due to bone secondaries.

Cardiovascular

Atrial fibrillation (local extension) and migratory thrombophlebitis. Pericarditis.

Diagnosis

Chest X-ray:

- the tumour may be visible often as a unilaterally enlarged hilum or peripheral circular opacity occasionally cavitated
- collapse/consolidation due to bronchial obstruction by the tumour
- effusion, raised hemidiaphragm of phrenic paralysis, and bone erosion suggest local extension

CT scan or tomography may show the tumour position better and demonstrate bronchial narrowing and mediastinal involvement. Exfoliative cytology may be diagnostic.

Fibreoptic bronchoscopy with biospy is performed if possible to establish diagnosis and assess operability. This may provide a histological diagnosis. The site of the tumour is a guide to operability (not less than 2 cm from the carina).

Treatment

Surgery offers the only 'cure': 15–20% of all cases are resectable and only 30% of these survive 5 years. Surgery is contraindicated by metastasis (present in 60% at the time of presentation— in bone and liver) local spread and inadequate respiratory function.

Radiotherapy is valuable for relief of distressing symptoms (major airway narrowing, haemoptysis, mediastinal compression, pancoast syndrome and relief of pain produced by bony secondaries). Cancer chemotherapy may also relieve symptoms, especially of mediastinal obstruction and effusions with small cell carcinoma.

BRONCHIAL ADENOMA

This rare tumour is usually benign but locally invasive. Ninety per cent are histologically 'carcinoid' tumours but only a few cases present with the carcinoid syndrome (page 206). They usually present with cough and haemoptysis. The tumour may either occur: (*a*) anywhere within the thoracic cavity and appear as well circumscribed peripheral mass on chest X-ray, or more often (*b*) in the major bronchi and appear as a pedunculated intrabronchial mass seen bronchoscopically. The tumours are removed in view of the risk of neoplastic change.

SARCOIDOSIS

This is a disease of unknown aetiology. It appears to be a systemic granulomatous reaction to various stimuli which may involve any tissue. It most commonly affects the lungs, mediastinal lymph nodes and skin.

Clinical presentation

Pulmonary sarcoid (90%)

Most commonly it presents a subacute syndrome in young people (20–40 years, and in females five times more commonly than males) with fever, malaise and lassitude, erythema nodosum (sarcoid is the most common cause in the UK), polyarthralgia, usually of the ankles and knees, and mediastinal hilar lymphad-enopathy. Dyspnoea is not usually a feature of this acute form which is self-limiting (2 months–2 years).

Less commonly and more seriously it may present as a chronic insidious disease with respiratory symptoms of cough and progressive dyspnoea. There may be malaise and fever. Progressive pulmonary fibrosis may develop.

Non-pulmonary sarcoid

Apart from erythema nodosum, this is relatively uncommon, and causes with approximate frequency of clinical manifestation:
- Skin (70%). Erythema nodosum (not sarcoid tissue) in the acute syndrome; infiltration of scars: lupus pernio
- Hypercalcaemia: occurs in about 10% of patients with sarcoidosis and may be the presenting abnormality (page 223). Hypercalciuria is even more common. This is probably due to an excessive sensitivity to vitamin D and responds to steroids
- Eyes (15%). Uveitis and keratoconjunctivitis sicca. Blindness may result
- Parotitis (5%)
- Hepatosplenomegaly (12%)
- Generalised lymphadenopathy (30%)
- Bone and joints, producing cystic lesions most commonly in the phalanges (4%)
- Nervous system, causing isolated cranial nerve lesions and peripheral neuropathy (3%)
- Endocrine, producing diabetes insipidus from pituitary involvement (very rare)

Investigation

Chest X-ray usually shows symmetrical lobulated bilateral hilar gland enlarge-ment (interbronchial rather than tracheobronchial) (80%), or less commonly (40%) parenchymal mottling or diffuse fibrosis. CT scan will help distinguish gland enlargement from prominent pulmonary artery shadows.

Biopsy to show non-caseating epithelioid cell granulomata—biopsy of mediasti-nal glands at mediastinoscopy may confirm the diagnosis. Liver biopsy may be diagnostically valuable if the liver is enlarged. 'Blind' transbronchial lung biopsy at bronchoscopy is positive in most cases.

The Mantoux test is usually negative (70%): a positive test is thus not uncommon but a strongly positive test very unusual.

Kveim test (intradermal inoculation with 0.1 ml splenic homogenate from a previous case of sarcoid). The skin becomes indurated and biospy of the papule at 4–6 weeks shows characteristic sarcoid granulomata. False negative reactions occur in up to 25%, depending partly on the quality of the antigen.

Hypercalcaemia (10%) may be present and if so this returns to normal with steroids.

Polyclonal increase in γ-globulins is non-specific but common.

Management

The differential diagnosis of bilateral hilar lymph node enlargement is from Hodgkin's disease (and other reticuloses), and any deviation of the patient's syndrome from the usual pattern makes a definite diagnosis by biopsy imperative. Treatment, other than simple analgesics and non-steroidal anti-inflammatory agents is usually unnecessary.

Indications for corticosteroids in sarcoidosis (e.g. prednisolone 20 mg daily reducing after 1 month to the minimum dose necessary to suppress activity for 1 year) include:

- Progressive lung disease, to try to prevent fibrosis. The indication is progressive pulmonary shadowing or increasing breathlessness. The effect of therapy is monitored by symptoms, chest X-rays and lung function tests including carbon monoxide transfer factor, $T_{L}CO$
- Hypercalcaemia
- When vital organs are threatened, e.g. eyes, nervous system, kidneys and heart

Prognosis (of pulmonary sarcoid)

The chest X-ray remains abnormal in about half of all cases (table 25). Clinical disability due to the disease is much less common and is related to:

- age—the younger, the better
- presence of erythema nodosum where over 95% recover by 1 year
- extent of extrapulmonary involvement. Bone or chronic skin lesions indicate chronicity and the more widespread it is the worse the prognosis
- extent of intrathoracic involvement

NB In systemic sarcoidosis, the activity and clinical course of the disease in any one tissue (e.g. skin, eyes) is a guide to the activity in any tissue less easily observed (e.g. lungs).

Table 25. Prognosis of pulmonary sarcoid.

Chest X-ray appearance	Stage	Recovery X-ray	Recovery Clinical
Bilateral hilar lymphadenopathy alone	I	75%	90%
Bilateral hilar lymphadenopathy with fine pulmonary reticular–nodular shadowing	II	50%	60%
Coarse reticular–nodular shadowing or fibrosis	III	30%	30%

TUBERCULOSIS

Infection with the acid alcohol fast bacillus (AAFB) of *Mycobacterium tuberculosis* affects predominantly the lungs, lymph nodes and gut. Some features of the disease vary with the patient's sensitivity to tuberculin.

Primary tuberculosis

This is the syndrome produced by infection with *M. tuberculosis* in non-sensitive patients, i.e. in those who have not previously been infected. There is a mild inflammatory response at the site of infection (subpleural in the mid-zones of the lungs, in the pharynx, or in the terminal ileum), followed by spread to the regional lymph nodes (hilar, cervical and mesenteric respectively)—the primary complex. One to two weeks following infection, with the onset of tuberculin sensitivity, the tissue reaction changes at both the focus and in the nodes, to the charateristic caseating granuloma. The combination of a focus with regional lymph node involvement is called the 'primary complex'. Patients are usually symptomless. The complex heals with fibrosis and, frequently, calcifies without therapy. The enlarged lymph node may, however, be obvious in the neck or cause obstruction to a bronchus with consequent collapse-consolidation. Blood dissemination of the organisms may occur rarely from the primary complex to cause widespread miliary disease especially in infants.

Post-primary tuberculosis

This is the syndrome produced by infection with *M. tuberulosis* in the previously infected and therefore tuberculin-sensitive patient. Reactivation (or reinfection) is thus followed by an immediate brisk granulomatous response which tends to localise the disease and regional lymph node involvement is uncommon. As with primary tuberculosis, the lesion may:
- heal with fibrosis (and calcification)
- rupture into a bronchus giving tuberculous bronchopneumonia
- spread via the blood to produce miliary tuberculosis of liver, spleen, lungs, choroid, bone and/or meninges.

Presenting features

Symptoms occur relatively late and therefore in established disease. The earliest are non-specific such as malaise fatigue, anorexia and weight loss. Of more specific symptoms, the most common is cough often with mucoid sputum. Other symptoms include repeated small haemoptysis, pleural pain, slight fever or occasionally exertional dyspnoea. Frequently the diagnosis is made presymptomatically on routine chest radiography. Signs also occur late in the disease and are not very specific, e.g. crepitations (usually apical) and, later, signs of consolidation, pleural effusion or cavitation.

Diagnosis

Diagnosis depends, in part, on clinical suspicion which should be particularly high in high-risk groups, for instance:
- the hostel-dwelling 'down-and-out', and the alcoholic
- Pakistani, Indian and Irish immigrant (lymph node tuberculosis is common in Indian and Pakistani patients)
- diabetics
- patients with AIDS

- patients on immunosuppressive therapy (steroids or cytotoxic drugs)
- occupations at risk—doctors and nurses

Ideally the diagnosis is made by repeated examination for AAFB in sputum and bronchial washing on direct smear, by culture on Lowenstein–Jensen medium or by guinea-pig inoculation. Six to twelve specimens (or more) may be required. Sometimes the diagnosis can only be made radiologically and activity is suggested by:

- changing 'soft' shadows
- progression of apical lesions
- cavitation
- strongly positive Heaf test

It may be necessary to treat on clinical grounds alone and response to specific therapy (e.g. isonicotinic acid hydrazide—INAH) in 2 weeks is taken as proof of diagnosis.

NB   AAFB on smear may not be pathogenic mycobacteria, particularly in urine specimens.

Management

Isolate patients who are sputum-positive for the first fortnight of treatment (this is standard practice in Britain but the Madras trials suggest that this may not be necessary). It is notifiable in the UK.

Investigate family and social contacts for infection (or via the local Community Physician) by chest X-ray and tuberculin sensitivity (Mantoux or Heaf) immediately and 6 weeks later. Then:

- if both tests are negative, give BCG, check for conversion and follow up for 2 years
- if the initial test is negative and the 6-week test positive this indicates recent infection. These patients are treated with two antituberculous drugs (ethambutol and isoniazid) for 12–18 months unless primary resistance is discovered in the contact.
- if the initial tuberculin test is positive, give isoniazid for 1 year to children under 7 years not previously inoculated with BCG, and follow up all other patients for 2 years and then annually for 3 years.

Start therapy if AAFB are detected in sputum. If the clinical suspicion of tuberculosis is high but the sputum smear is negative, collect sputa for culture and start therapy with three of the first-line drugs:

Rifampicin 450–600 mg.
Isoniazid 300 mg (with pyridoxine 10 mg).
Ethambutol 15 mg/kg.
Streptomycin 1 g.
Pyrazinamide 1.5–2.0 g.

Therapy should be started with a warning about possible adverse effects and early clinic review. Continue triple therapy until sensitivities are reported (6–8 weeks). If the organism is sensitive to all three drugs, stop ethambutol and continue rifampicin and isoniazid for 9 months with 3-monthly follow-up, radiographic and clinical. The patient's sputum is tested regularly to detect relapse (failure to take drugs is the most common reason).

For TB meningitis see page 143.

Common drug complications

Rifampicin	Abnormal liver function tests. Colours the urine pink.
INAH	Peripheral neuropathy and encephalopathy—these are extremely rare, occur in slow acetylators and respond to pyridoxine, often given prophylactically
Ethambutol	Optic neuritis with colour vision and acuity reduced
Streptomycin	Vertigo and nerve deafness. In the elderly and in the presence of raised blood urea, the dose is reduced to 0.75 g or 0.5 g daily to maintain blood levels of 1–2 μg/ml

Second-line drug complications

Ethionamide	Nausea and vomiting; hepatotoxic
Pyrazinamide	Hepatotoxic (rare but severe)
Cycloserine	Neurotoxicity with confusion and depression
PAS	Nausea, vomiting and skin rash

NB Twice-weekly treatment with streptomycin and high-dose isoniazid or rifampicin with isoniazid have been shown to be effective. Other combinations of 2, 3, and 4 antituberculous drugs given for shorter periods are under trial.

Corticosteroids

May be used in miliary tuberculosis; severely ill tuberculous patients at the onset of chemotherapy; tuberculous meningitis, to try to prevent fibrosis. The value of steroids other than when life is immediately threatened, remains unproven and they probably do not effect long-term morbidity.

OCCUPATIONAL LUNG DISEASES

Dust diseases

These include the pneumoconioses, asthma, allergic alveolitis and the effects of irritant gases:

- coal pneumoconiosis
- silicosis in rock drilling and crushing but also occurs in coalminers
- asbestosis in insulation workers; this can produce fibrosis, carcinoma, and pleural mesothelioma
- benign (no fibrosis).

These are radiographic diagnoses made in the light of the patient's known occupational hazards, the shadows are due to the metals themselves, e.g. siderosis (iron) and stannosis (tin). All are rare.

Clinical features

In the early stages there are no symptoms but X-ray changes occur; later there is dyspnoea on exertion, cough, sputum and attacks of bronchitis. In coal miners, progressive massive fibrosis may occur and Caplan's syndrome occurs in association with rhematoid arthritis. The patients may eventually develop cor pulmonale.

Asthma

Occupational asthma can occur in response to precipitants of animal, vegetable, bacteriological or chemical origin. Some of the commoner occupations are: animal laboratory workers (urinary proteins), grain and flour workers (mites and flour), sawmill operatives and carpenters (hardwoods), those who manufacture 'biological' detergents (inhalation of *Bacillus subtilis* proteolytic enzymes), in the electronics industry (colophony in solder flux), paint sprayers and polyurethane workers (isocyanates), and workers with epoxy resins or platinum salts, and in the pharmaceutical industry. All these are recognised for compensation under industrial injuries legislation in the UK.

Extrinsic allergic alveolitis

Inhalation of organic dusts may given a diffuse allergic (type III precipitin-mediated) reaction in the alveoli and bronchioles.

Aetiology

Exposure to mouldy hay (*Micropolyspora faeni*) causes farmer's lung, to mouldy sugar cane causes bagassosis, to mushroom dust causes mushroom picker's lung, to bird droppings (containing avian serum proteins) causes bird fancier's lung, to contaminated malting barley (*Aspergillus clavatus*) causes malt worker's lung and to pituitary snuff (containing foreign serum protein) causes pituitary snuff-taker's lung. Precipitating antibodies against the offending antigen can be found in the patient's blood.

Clinical features

Acute (i.e. 4–6 h after exposure). Dyspnoea, dry cough, malaise, fever and limb pains occur, and examination shows fine inspiratory crepitations with little wheeze. The symptoms subside in 2–3 days.
Chronic. After repeated acute attacks fibrosis occurs with persistent inspiratory crepitations, respiratory failure and cor pulmonale.

Investigation

Chest X-ray shows a diffuse haze initially and later micronodular shadowing develops, progressing to honeycombing. Ventilatory function tests initially show a reversible restrictive defect with low CO transfer (TLCO) during the acute attacks. This becomes permanent as the chronic disorder develops. There is little or no obstruction. The Po_2 falls and Pco_2 is normal or reduced by the hyperventilation. There is no eosinophilia.

Treatment

Separate the patient and the allergen. Masks are of little use and positive pressure helmets should be worn. High dose steroids are tried in serious cases and should be continued only if there has been a measured response in lung function.

Irritant gases

May give acute pulmonary oedema.

PULMONARY EMBOLISM

Emboli usually arise in the veins of the pelvis or legs and rarely from the right atrium. They occur more frequently:

- following surgery (classically though not always after about 10 days (40–75%)
- in congestive heart failure
- following myocardial infarction (20–37%)
- following a stroke (40–75%)
- in disseminated malignancy
- in prolonged bed rest associated with illness
- following trauma, especially to the pelvis and legs (including Caesarian section)

The risk may increase if other factors also present:

- postphlebitic leg
- varicose veins
- obesity
- advancing age
- postpartum
- oral contraception
- past history of deep venous thrombosis
- possibly blood group A
- pregnancy

About 50% of those who die from pulmonary embolism have had premonitory signs and symptoms of small emboli (unexplained little breathless attacks) or venous thrombosis in the preceding week. A deep vein thrombosis should be regarded as a potential pulmonary embolus and must be suspected, diagnosed and treated early.

Diagnosis of deep vein thrombosis is made on one or more of the following findings:

Tenderness between the heads of the gastrocnemius where the thrombosed vein may be palpable.

Stiffness of the calf muscles (increased tugor).

Delayed cooling of the involved limb on exposure.

There may be tenderness at the saphenous opening.

Oedema, cyanosis and engorged superficial veins are late signs.

Homans' sign is neither specific nor sensitive.

NB Diagnosis is confirmed by Doppler ultrasound with vein compression or venography. Thromboses which extend above the knee are more likely to produce clinically recognisable pulmonary emboli.

Swelling of the calf occurs also in rupture of a Baker's cyst behind the knee. An effusion into the knee makes this most likely. The cyst can often be shown on ultrasound.

Clinical presentation

This depends upon the size of the embolus. Multiple small acute emboli ma remain undetected until up to 50% of the vascular bed is involved and presen with effort dyspnoea:

- *Small.* Transient faints and dyspnoea, with slight pyrexia
- *Medium.* Usually result in infarction and produce, in addition, haemoptysis pleurisy and occasionally a pleural effusion
- *Large.* (Affecting over 60% of the pulmonary bed). Acute cor pulmonale with sudden dyspnoea and shock. There is a small-volume rapid pulse, with hypotension, cyanosis, peripheral vasoconstriction and a raised jugular venous pressure. There may be a gallop rhythm

Investigation

Chest X-ray to demonstrate:
- pulmonary oligaemia of the affected segment (usually present but difficult to diagnose except in retrospect)
- the corresponding pulmonary artery is sometimes dilated at the hilum
- small areas of horizontal linear collapse, usually at the bases, with a raised diaphragm
- a small pleural effusion

With larger emboli, the heart enlarges acutely and the superior vena cava distends

ECG changes usually occur only with larger emboli but are then common. The characteristic changes are (see also page 82):
- tachycardia
- right ventricular 'strain' pattern (inverted T waves in leads V_{1-4})
- acute, often transient, right bundle branch block pattern
- S_1, Q_3, T_3 pattern
- transient arrhythmias, e.g. atrial fibrillation

Arterial blood gases. With larger emboli, a fall in P_{CO_2} is common.

Lung perfusion scan is a useful non-traumatic investigation in doubtful cases and may show underperfusion of one or more parts of the lung which are radiologically normal (and ventilated normally on ventilation scan).

Combined ventilation and perfusion scans may be helpful in pre-existent lung disease in which ventilation and perfusion defects are usually matched. A normal scan virtually excludes pulmonary embolism.

Pulmonary angiography is the most precise for cases presenting difficulty in diagnosis.

Treatment

Prophylaxis pre- and postoperatively, especially lower abdomen and lower limb, and in patients confined to bed or with predisposing disorders (e.g. cardiac failure) with regular leg exercises. Low-dose subcutaneous heparin may reduce the incidence of deep venous thrombosis following major surgery.

For established deep vein thrombosis or pulmonary embolism, anticoagulate with heparin initially, followed by warfarin—for 6–12 weeks in the first instance depending upon whether a non-recurring cause for the deep vein thrombosis (e.g. surgery) was present or not.

In massive pulmonary embolism, cardiac massage and correction of acidosis plus urgent intravenous heparin may improve survival. With large emboli, oxygen in high concentration and thrombolytic therapy with urokinase or streptokinase may be valuable. Morphine may be necessary. The operative removal of large emboli with bypass surgery may be lifesaving.

PNEUMOTHORAX

Aetiology

Spontaneous. This is the most common type and usually occurs in normal thin young men following rupture of a small subpleural bulla. The history is of the sudden onset of one-sided pleuritic pain and/or dyspnoea. Dyspnoea rapidly increases in tension pneumothorax and the patient becomes cyanosed. The classical signs are of diminished movement on the affected side with deviation of the trachea to the other side. There is hyperresonance to percussion and reduced pulmonary sounds (breath sounds, tactile fremitus and vocal resonance). All pneumothoraces are best diagnosed by seeing a lung edge on X-ray which is clearest on an expiratory film. Conditions predisposing to pneumothorax include:

Emphysematous bullae.
Tuberculosis—often with a small effusion.
Bronchial asthma.
Other rare causes include staphylococcal pneumonia, carcinoma, occupational lung disease and connective tissue disorders e.g. Marfan's and Ehlers–Danlos syndrome.

Management (of spontaneous pneumothorax)

Often no therapy is required if the pneumothorax is small. Spontaneous recovery occurs in 3–4 weeks. Indications for aspiration of air are:
- tension pneumothorax (an acute emergency)
- severe dyspnoea
- collapse of more than 50% of the total lung field on chest X-ray

Insert an intercostal tube with a valve or water seal. When the lung is re-expanded, X-ray the chest. If the lung remains expanded for 24 h the tube may be removed and if not, suction should be applied to the tube.

Rarely, a continuing air leak persists from the lung into the pleural space (bronchopleural fistula). Pleurodesis with defibrinated blood, camphor in oil or surgical pleurectomy may be required.

HYPERVENTILATION SYNDROME

Breathlessness in the absence of abnormal clinical signs and increased by emotion (e.g. clinical examination and ward rounds) should never be described as psychogenic until the following diagnoses have been excluded:
- early pulmonary congestion of left ventricular failure
- 'silent' multiple pulmonary emboli (lung scan may be diagnostic)

- lymphangitis carcinomatosa
- interstitial fibrotic pulmonary infiltrations
- metabolic acidosis (e.g. uraemia, diabetic ketosis)
- respiratory muscle weakness

The chest X-ray may appear normal in all of these at the time of presentation.

The hyperventilation syndrome may be the presenting symptom of psychiatric disease and the patient should be asked about symptoms of depression and enquiries made about his pre-morbid personality. The breathlessness is usually episodic and not directly related in degree to exertion (often even occurring at rest). It is often described as an inability to take a deep breath or shortage of oxygen. There are associated symptoms of hypocapnia (tingling in the fingers, dizziness, headache, heaviness in the chest, cramp). Frank tetany may occur with carpopedal spasm. Spirometry usually gives a disorganised trace but the FEV_1 and forced vital capacity (FVC) are usually normal when obtained.

FIBROSING ALVEOLITIS (diffuse interstitial pulmonary fibrosis)

Clinical features

The disease begins in middle age and presents with progressive dyspnoea and dry cough usually without wheeze or sputum. The typical signs are clubbing, cyanosis and crepitations in the mid and lower lung fields. Polyarthritis is common. There is an association with the collagen diseases, particularly rheumatoid arthritis. The disease usually progresses slowly, but occasionally is very rapid (Hamman–Rich syndrome).

Investigation

The arterial Po_2 is reduced and hyperventilation may cause a reduction in Pco_2. Spirometry (page 61) demonstrates a restrictive pattern, i.e. a grossly reduced FVC with rapid initial exhalation of this small volume, thus giving a normal or high FEV_1/FVC. The transfer factor is reduced.

Chest X-ray shows diffuse bilateral basal nodular/reticular shadowing which extends upwards as the disease progresses. The differential diagnosis of the chest X-ray includes other causes of diffuse pulmonary fibrosis and infiltration: occupational dust lung diseases, sarcoidosis, scleroderma, lymphangitis carcinomatosa, collagen diseases, miliary tuberculosis, radiation pneumonitis, drugs (busulphan and other cytotoxic drugs, nitrofurantoin, paraquat), histoplasmosis, coccidioidomycosis, and histiocytosis X. Clinically the problem is less difficult. Lung biopsy, either open by thoracotomy or transbronchial via a bronchoscope, may be diagnostic. Bronchoalveolar lavage may predominantly show lymphocytes in sarcoidosis and neutrophils in fibrosing alveolitis.

Management

The disease is progressive and, though steroids are usually given, response is variable. Improvement sometimes appears to occur. The patient eventually dies with severe hypoxia.

ADULT RESPIRATORY DISTRESS SYNDROME
(ARDs, shock lung)

This refers to the acute progressive respiratory failure starting several hours to 2 days following severe trauma such as road traffic accidents or septicaemia. Characteristic features include a 'white' lung on chest X-ray, stiff lungs and progressively severe hypoxaemia. The pulmonary oedema is due to capillary leakage rather than the elevated left atrial pressure of heart disease. The aetiology is probably a combination of various factors including aspiration pneumonia, pulmonary oedema, fat embolism, disseminated intravascular coagulation and substances released as a consequence of the injury (activated complement, histamine, kinins and superoxides). Treatment requires intermittent positive pressure ventilation using a volume-cycled ventilator with positive end-expiratory pressure (PEEP). Though high inspired oxygen pressures may be required, they should not be so constant that they produce direct pulmonary oxygen toxicity. The mortality is 60–70%.

Cardiovascular disease

The commonest diseases are atherosclerosis and hypertension, which cause ischaemic heart disease and heart failure. Chronic rheumatic valve disease is becoming less common in practice but is still seen frequently in exams. Congenital heart disease is relatively rare but important because half can be cured surgically.

Sudden death can be due to unheralded cardiac arrest from cardiac arrhythmia in an otherwise fit man as the first (and last) symptom of coronary artery disease. Other associated and predisposing conditions include mitral leaflet prolapse, cardiomyopathy, hypertension, other valvular disease, myocarditis, long QT syndromes, and drug and electrolyte disturbances.

ISCHAEMIC HEART DISEASE (IHD)

The disease is usually inferred from a history of cardiac pain (angina of effort) or of myocardial infarction. Less commonly it may present as an arrhythmia or a defect of conduction.

Myocardial ischaemia in the UK is normally due to atherosclerosis but cardiac pain can also be produced by:
- aortic valve disease (page 324)
- paroxysmal tachycardias
- severe anaemia, coronary embolism, cardiomyopathy and polyarteritis nodosa, are all rare causes.

Factors associated with coronary atherosclerosis
- *Sex*. Men more than women, particularly before the menopause
- *Age*. Steady increase with age
- *Heredity*. Important especially in the relatively young and probably mediated by hyperlipoproteinaemia and hypertension
- *Diet*. Epidemiological studies suggest that a high consumption of saturated fats is important. Too much salt or too little dietary fibre may be relevant
- *Occupation*. Emotional stress and possibly lack of exercise may predispose. Social classes IV and V have a greater incidence than I and II
- *Medical conditions*. Recognised risk factors are hypertension, obesity, hyperlipoproteinaemia and cigarette smoking

The excess risk of death for smokers is 2–3 times that of non-smokers. However, ischaemic heart disease is so common compared with bronchitis and lung cancer that about 50% of all excess deaths attributable to cigarette smoking are due to ischaemic heart disease

- Diabetes mellitus and gout are associated
- In the UK, place of residence for middle-aged men; low in the south, high in Scotland

Angina

Diagnosis

This is a clinical diagnosis. There should be the characteristic four-feature history—site, character, radiation and precipitation/relief (NB: effort, food, emotion and cold). In the diagnosis of chest pain, angina is more likely if the pain is precipitated during exertion, persists until the exertion stops and is then relieved within 5 min. Large meals and cold weather reduce the amount of exertion necessary to precipitate pain. A non-cardiac cause is favoured by continuation for several days, precipitation by changes in posture and by deep breathing, the ability to continue normal activities and the fact that rest does not consistently relieve the pain. Relief within 5 min by subligual or buccal glyceryl trinitrate makes angina more likely. There are no specific characteristic physical signs. The commoner alternatives in the differential diagnosis are oesophageal pain, musculoskeletal pain and the left precordial stabbing pain of cardiac neurosis.

Unstable angina (crescendo angina) describes a rapid increase in the frequency, severity or length of anginal attacks. There may be a sudden decrease in exercise tolerance or the onset of anginal pain at rest. Patients who present with a short and sometimes severe story of angina on effort, many of whom think they have acute indigestion, may also have unstable angina. This clinical situation includes the pre-infarction syndrome, crescendo angina, acute coronary insufficiency, decubitus (lying flat) angina, and variant angina (Prinzmetal's angina). By definition, myocardial death has not occurred even though it is imminent, and can be avoided with effective and immediate specific therapy. The prognosis is then that of the underlying heart disease. Parenteral nitrates such as isosorbide dinitrate, plus β-blockade plus aspirin and heparin are used, and finally the calcium channel blockers. Early thrombolysis may be used using streptokinase, alteplase (rt-PA) and aspirin.

Variant angina (Prinzmetal) refers to cardiac pain occurring at rest and characterised by transient ST elevation (instead of the classical plane ST depression of exertional angina). It may be due to coronary artery spasm and the therapeutic implication is that vasodilators (GTN, isosorbide, nifedipine) may be more useful in relieving symptoms and reducing mortality than β-blockade which may worsen it.

Investigations are used to confirm or deny a doubtful or difficult clinical diagnosis. A treadmill exercise ECG adds little to the risk and may be diagnostic with transient ST segment changes associated with symptoms. A negative test indicates a very good prognosis. Coronary arteriography has a small morbidity and mortality which varies from centre to centre. It may supply unequivocal evidence of arterial narrowing and define its site so that revascularisation procedures may be undertaken. Up to 10% of anginal patients may have normal coronary arteries or no critical lesions. Radionuclide and echocardiographic studies can give additional information (page 90).

Management

The patient needs considerable reassurance about symptoms and their implications. He should stop smoking, lose weight and take regular non-strenuous exercise. Specific hyperlipidaemic syndromes should be treated (page 209).

Anaemia should be investigated and treated. Sublingual glyceryl trinitrate (0.5 mg) remains the mainstay of therapy. The major side-effect is headache and as many tablets as necessary may be taken. It should be taken for pain and prophylactically before known precipitating events. If attacks are frequent, vasodilation therapy with oral isosorbide or percutaneous GTN may be added. Long-term therapy with β-blocking drugs and/or a calcium antagonist drug such as nifedipine usually prevent attacks.

NB Hypertension should be treated as the mortality from strokes and renal failure is thereby reduced. The incidence of myocardial infarction is possibly not affected.

Unstable angina may develop into VT. Treat with triple therapy: β-blockade, nitrates (given intravenously) and calcium blockers, with the possible addition of anticoagulants and antiplatelet agents. Proceed to surgery immediately if this is unsuccessful and to exercise testing as above if the response is satisfactory. Coronary angioplasty is indicated for localised left anterior descending disease not responding to medical therapy. The right coronary artery vessels are also suitable but not the left main stem.

Where available, radionuclide imaging (with radio thallium) of the myocardium is used to detect areas of reversible myocardial ischaemia before coronary artery bypass grafting. It can also demonstrate ventricular function (radio technetium) and graft patency after surgery.

Coronary arteriography with a view to aortocoronary saphenous vein bypass grafting or internal mammary artery anastomosis is indicated in angina uncontrolled by full medical therapy or if there is induced pain, particularly with ST changes on the ECG and a blood pressure fall on formal exercise testing.

Stable angina and angina in failed medical therapy can be identified in angiograph responders who have a positive exercise test at slope 1 or 3 (not slope 3 or later). Use surgery on: (a) triple vessel disease, (b) left main stem artery disease, or (c) double vessel disease including proximal left anterior descending disease especially where there is demonstrable impairment of left ventricular function. The prognosis is then improved. The mortality rate is 1–2%.

Surgery is indicated particularly in left main stem coronary artery stenosis (figure 49, page 314) for prognostic reasons. It gives no prognostic improvement in mild angina regardless of the disease distribution.

Myocardial infarction (page 68)

The predisposing and precipitating factors are those of atherosclerosis. Infarction may also occur during hypotension (including surgery). The immediate mortality (within 4 weeks) is 30–40% chiefly in the first 2 h. There is sudden death in 25% mainly from dysrhythmias. After recovery from the acute attack, 90% survive 1 year, 70% survive 5 years, and 40% survive 10 years.

Management

Bed rest

The optimum duration of bed rest remains undetermined. There is an increasing tendency to mobilise uncomplicated cases early (4–5 days) to prevent venous thrombosis and progressive physical weakness. It seems sensible to keep patients in bed for longer if complications are present or fever (usually due to pericarditis) prolonged. (see Clinical features page 337). In the elderly, bed rest is seldom indicated.

Pain relief and sedation

Morphine and diamorphine are the drugs of choice. Both may produce hypotension. Morphine causes vomiting and diamorphine is preferred for this reason. The dose required is the minimum which will relieve pain (i.e. start with diamorphine 5 mg). Diazepam (5 mg tds) is a suitable sedative.

Oxygen therapy

High concentration oxygen is given in pulmonary oedema or shock (except in chronic respiratory failure, page 289).

Long term β-blockade

There is evidence that β-blockade for 1–2 years reduces reinfarction and late mortality. Probably all β-blockers are equally effective.

Anticoagulants

Short-term (until mobile). Full anticoagulation is commonly used to reduce the incidence of deep venous and mural thrombosis, but there remains conflicting evidence that mortality is reduced. It seems reasonable to give low dose subcutaneous heparin and full anticoagulation in cases complicated by cardiac failure, arrhythmias, obesity and after severe infarcts when prolonged bed rest will be necessary unless thrombolysed.

Long-term. The MRC trial showed a marginal benefit in reduced mortality and reinfarction over 2 years, but only in men under the age of 55. Most of the advantage occurred in the first 6 months and some physicians would give anticoagulants for this period of time in young men. This decision is strongly influenced by the accuracy of anticoagulant control available since poor control has a considerable morbidity and mortality.

Thrombolytic therapy

It is imperative to use thrombolytic therapy as soon as possible because most of the benefit occurs within the first 4 h ('time is muscle'). The objective is to remove the thrombus as quickly and completely as possible to minimise the size of the infarct and maintain myocardial function. Various combinations of the following drugs have been shown to reduce mortality in trials: streptokinase (150 000 units), aspirin (600 mg), actiplase (tissue plasminogen activator— t-PA), and anistreplase (anisoylated plasminogen-streptokinase activator complex—APSAC).

The roles of immediate thrombolytic therapy with streptokinase and of coronary artery dilation (percutaneous angioplasty) are being studied.

Contraindications to streptokinase therapy are:
- Very severe hypertension
- Bleeding disorder
- Less than 10 days since surgery, 2 months of cerebrovascular accident (1 year DU/GU)
- Diabetes and new vessels in eyes
- Streptokinase use between 5 days and 6 months previously.

Early complications

Shock (10% of hospital admissions)

The patient is hypotensive, pale, cold, sweaty and cyanosed. Oxygen is given and dysrhythmias treated. A central venous pressure line and left pulmonary artery flotation catheter (Swan–Ganz) (page 90) will guide possible fluid replacement if hypovolaemia is present. Slow infusion of dobutamine (or dopamine) may raise blood pressure without decreasing renal or cerebral perfusion.

Cardiac failure

Treatment is with:
- Sixty per cent oxygen (unless chronic obstructive airway disease is present)
- Diuretics. Frusemide is given for left pulmonary oedema but it tends to reduce cardiac output by reducing ventricular filling pressure.
- morphine for acute pulmonary oedema to reduce preload and relieve anxiety

Continuing, for severe or persistent failure, to:
- hydralazine, to reduce afterload
- inotropes (dopamine, dobutamine) or nitrates

The overall mortality is over 70%.

Arrhythmias

Ninety per cent of patients develop 'warning' arrhythmias, but treatment is not usually indicated unless there is evidence of reduced cardiac performance.

Sinus tachycardia. If there is no evidence of heart failure or hypotension the arrhythmia itself requires no specific treatment. It may be a sign of early cardiac failure.

Supraventricular extrasystoles. Treatment is only required if they are frequent enough to cause hypotension of heart failure. Consider digitalisation and β-blockade—with care in heart failure.

Supraventricular tachycardia (SVT). Firstly try procedures such as carotid massage (unilateral), and the Valsalva manoeuvre. β-blockade possibly with the addition of digoxin, is frequently effective, and may be used orally if a rapid response is not required. Verapamil given slowly intravenously may be effective, but must be used with care in patients who have recently been on β-blockers. DC cardioversion is used when rapid results are required (e.g. acute heart failure), and following the other procedures mentioned (though preferably not if the patient has been digitalised). Disopyramide or amiodarome are useful in resistant SVT. If all else has failed, 'over-pacing' can be attempted with a pacing catheter.

NB   Ninety-five per cent of broad complex tachycardias in the 'ischaemic' age group are ventricular tachycardia (see cardiac resuscitation, page 69).

Atrial flutter and atrial fibrillation. Usually oral digoxin is adequate to slow the ventricular rate. Verapamil will also slow the ventricular rate (but do not use it with β-blockade). Consider DC cardioversion.

NB   Supraventricular arrhythmias may be caused by digitalis toxicity (serum levels are helpful) particularly if there is hypokalaemia. In this situation, stop the digitalis, give potassium if indicated, and follow with parenteral β-blocker. Continue with oral β-blocker. Avoid DC shock because it may produce resistant ventricular fibrillation in digitalis intoxication.

Sinus or nodal bradycardia. This may be due to heavy sedation particularly with morphine or diamorphine. If the rate is <50/min and the patient is hypotensive, give atropine 0.6 mg i.v. and repeat twice if necessary. If unsuccessful, consider cardiac pacing. Ventricular extrasystoles may be due to the bradycardia and should not themselves be treated unless they persist after the bradycardia has been corrected.

Heart block. All degrees of heart block are more serious if they complicate anterior rather than inferior infarcts:
- First degree: no immediate therapy is required but the patient must be closely monitored
- Second degree (page 77): monitor and consider atropine. Many physicians would insert a pacing catheter for 'on-demand' pacing for Möbitz 2 with anterior infarcts
- Third degree: complete heart block (CHB). Atropine and isoprenaline may be helpful while awaiting insertion of a pacing catheter

NB   CHB is commoner in inferior myocardial infarctions because the AV nodal artery is a branch of the right coronary artery (figure 49, page 314); CHB complicating anterior infarction is an ominous situation since it implies a very large muscle infarction.

Permanent pacing should be considered in patients who have had Stokes–Adams attacks, low output states secondary to the bradycardia, and those with extensive damage to the conduction systems.

Ventricular ectopic beats. If they are multifocal, close to the T waves, in pairs or short runs or >12/min and causing circulatory disturbance, give lignocaine 50 mg bolus i.v. and repeat up to twice at 5-min intervals if necessary. If successful continue with a slow lignocaine infusion at 1–2 mg/min. (**NB**   2 g lignocaine per 24 h is about 1.5 mg/min). Boluses of lignocaine can be added to this

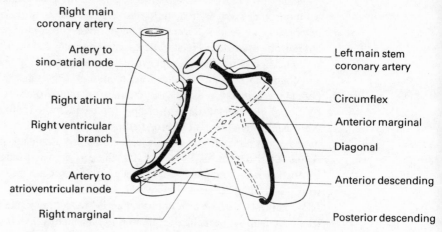

Right main coronary artery

Artery to sino-atrial node

Right atrium

Right ventricular branch

Artery to atrioventricular node

Right marginal

Left main stem coronary artery

Circumflex

Anterior marginal

Diagonal

Anterior descending

Posterior descending

Figure 49. The coronary arteries.

periodically if full control is not obtained. Check the serum potassium and give KCl if it is low.

Ventricular tachycardia. Try lignocaine as above, then DC cardioversion under short-acting general anaesthetic.

Ventricular fibrillation. This is frequently within 6 h of infarction. External cardiac massage with artifical ventilation followed by DC cardioversion and intravenous adrenaline 1 mg (page 70). Follow with a lignocaine drip for 24–48 h.

Asystole (page 70). Blows on the chest may be sufficient stimulus to provoke repeated systole, but if an arterial pulse is not definitely detected, external cardiac massage and artifical ventilation are essential. One milligram of adrenaline (1 ml of 1/1000) may result in ventricular tachycardia which may then respond to cardioversion. External pacing may be successful but a transvenous pacing catheter should be inserted as soon as possible. Asystole may recur. Permanent pacing may be necessary.

Electromechanical dissociation (QRS without palpable pulse). Give adrenaline 1 mg i.v. and consider calcium chloride (10ml of 10%) i.v. for hyperkalaemia, hypocalcaemia and adverse effects of calcium antagonists. Treat hypovolaemia, pneumothorax, cardiac tamponade and pulmonary embolism.

Later complications of myocardial infarction

- Papillary muscle dysfunction or rupture may either produce no symptoms or various degrees of cardiac failure. There is a pansystolic or late systolic mitral regurgitant murmur. Echocardiography confirms the valvular dysfunction and also gives an index of ventricular myocardial function. Surgery may be indicated.
- Cardiac aneurysm. This is more common than is usually supposed. The features, which may be intermittent, are severe heart failure, recurrent arrhythmias, recurrent emboli from thrombi within the aneurysm, angina and considerable cardiac enlargement, and abnormal cardiac pulsation (e.g. an impulse at

the sternal border). Its presence may be suggested by persistent ST elevation in convalescence. X-ray screening may show abnormal pulsation and an abnormal cardiac contour. Left ventriculography may confirm these findings and operation is indicated for the features mentioned above

- Ruptured ventricular septum is rare. Patients usually present with sudden severe pulmonary oedema and urgent surgery may be required
- Myocardial rupture with consequent tamponade

Discharge from hospital

An early coronary rehabilitation programme is preceded, for safety and assessment of suitability, by an exercise stress test, and consists of graded exercises supervised by trained staff. Dietary and health education is also given to promote physical and psychological fitness.

The uncomplicated case may be discharged without excess risk at 7–10 days. The patient should be encouraged to increase activity gradually over about 2 months with regular walks after 1 month (1 mile per day if this is within his exercise tolerance), and can then return to work. If possible the job should not be too physically demanding. A formal treadmill ECG test will give guidance if necessary. An optimistic attitude to the future coupled with an active involvement in his own rehabilitation should be encouraged. The patient and his family should try to reduce all 'risk factors' (page 308). Various prophylactic regimes are under trial. It is not yet shown definitely that aspirin, sulphinpyrazone or dipyridamole reduce the incidence of reinfarction. β-blockade probably does at 1 year follow up.

Ischaemic heart disease and driving

Patients should not drive (and must inform the licencing authorities) within 2 months of a myocardial infarction, if angina is easily provoked by driving or emotion, or when medication or arrhythmia has caused faintness, vertigo, fatigue, or lack of alertness. Unexplained syncope and heart block also debar driving unless a satisfactory permanent pacemaker established for not less than 1 month has corrected the problem. The regulations applying to drivers of HGV or PSV (ambulance, fire, police, taxi and hire car drivers) vehicles are complicated and are to be interpreted by the authorities. An annual expert examination of the cardiovascular system is required.

HEART FAILURE (page 67)

Congestive heart failure affects about 1% of the population with an annual incidence of about 3/1000. The annual mortality of NYHA functional class IV is over 50%.

Heart failure results in diminished blood flow to the tissues (forward failure) and congestion in the pulmonary bed or peripheral tissues (backward failure). It is caused either by a diseased myocardium (low output failure with a cold cyanosed periphery) or by an excessive workload, e.g. in anaemia, Paget's disease, thyrotoxicosis or aortic regurgitation (high output failure with a warm periphery).

In *left ventricular failure* (LVF) the pressure in the left ventricle is increased (increased left ventricular end-diastolic pressure—LVEDP). Lung compliance is reduced due to pulmonary oedema, causing dyspnoea, orthopnoea, paroxysmal nocturnal dyspnoea, and fatigue. It occurs in systemic arterial hypertension, aortic valve disease, mitral regurgitation and following myocardial infarction and is often accompanied by right ventricular failure.

In *right ventricular failure* (RVF) the pressure in the right ventricle is increased. The jugular venous pressure rises (pages 63–5), peripheral dependent oedema develops and the liver becomes congested and tender. It occurs in pulmonary valve disease, pulmonary embolism, pulmonary hypertension especially following lung diseases such as chronic bronchitis and emphysema (cor pulmonale). It also follows both large left to right shunts in atrioseptal defect, and left ventricular failure.

Preload refers to the ventricular filling pressure or left ventricular diastolic stretch on the myocardium. The Starling curve shows that, in the normal situation—up to the peak of the curve—the greater the stretch, the greater the cardiac output. Over the peak of the curve any further increase in stretch, resulting from preload, reduces cardiac output. This is the rationale for reducing preload in heart failure, by reducing salt and water with diuretics and altering venous tone with drugs.

Afterload refers to the systemic vascular resistance against which the heart is beating. Increase in afterload occurs in arterial hypertension and in peripheral arteriolar constriction due to increased sympathetic tone—such as may occur secondary to heart failure.

Aetiology

In a patient with heart failure, it is important to identify the cause.
- Hypertension
- Primary pump failure (ischaemic heart disease and cardiomyopathy)
- Heart valve disorders (aortic stenosis, bicuspid aortic valve, mitral regurgitation)
- Secondary to cor pulmonale
- Congenital heart disease (atrial septal defect, ventricular septal defect)
- Pericardial disease (constrictive)
- Metabolic (hyperthyroidism, phaeochromocytoma, severe Paget's disease)
- Other (trauma, neoplasm)

There may also be precipitating factors.
- Anaemia
- Fluid retention (non-steroidal drugs, stopping diuretic therapy, excess drinking)
- Infection (especially of the lungs, with fever and PO_2 reduced, and bacterial endocarditis)
- Increased cardiac work (pregnancy, obesity, excess exercise, hyperthyroidism)
- Pulmonary emboli (large, or multiple small)
- Drugs with negative inotropism (β-blockers, most anti-arrhythmic drugs—except digoxin and amiodarone)

The New York Heart Association (NYHA) functional classification of chronic heart failure is as follows:

Class I: no limitation of ordinary physical acitivity.
Class II: slight limitation of ordinary physical activity.
Class III: marked limitation of ordinary physical activity.
Class IV: inability to perform physical activity without discomfort.

Treatment

ACE inhibitors, in particular enalapril, have been shown to reduce mortality. The combination of isosorbide dinitrate with hydrazaline is less effective. Hypotension and deteriorating renal function are complications of therapy.

Treatment is given in the following order:

1   Reduce preload with a diuretic such as frusemide and with venodilators such as the nitrates (glyceryl trinitrite, isosorbide) and, for pulmonary oedema, morphine which also reduces anxiety.

2   Reduce afterload with ACE inhibition or with arterial vasodilators such as hydralazine or nifedipine.

3   Directly increase the force of the heart with inotropic drugs such as digoxin, dobutamine, dopamine and enoximone.

4   Consider transplantation in the young if other therapy fails.

In mild heart failure, if frusemide 80 mg plus amiloride is insufficient, try ACE inhibition with captopril in small doses (6.25 mg) whilst monitoring the blood pressure for the next 4–6 h. Progressively build up the dose as necessary while monitoring the blood pressure and electrolytes. Amiloride (and potassium-containing drugs) should be stopped.

HYPERTENSION

There is no 'normal' blood pressure except in the statistical sense of those which fall within a certain distance of the mean of a 'normal' population. However, even within this 'normal' range (down to 100/60 mmHg) the complications normally regarded as characteristic of hypertension have an incidence related to the height of the diastolic pressure.

About 20% of the adult population of the UK have blood pressures above 160/95 mmHg.

Hypertension is the most significant risk factor in strokes and heart failure, and in ischaemic heart disease it is as important as smoking, obesity or hypercholesterolaemia.

Those with a regular intake of alcohol may achieve significant falls in blood pressure if they abstain.

Since treatment for hypertension is lifelong, it is important to have the diagnosis firmly established. The blood pressure should be taken at rest and measured three times on at least three separate occasions and until three successive readings are essentially the same. If the arm circumference is over 33 cm, as it may be in 10%, a larger cuff should be used. The reading must be checked in both arms and, if different and consistent, the higher value taken.

Phase V diastolic (disappearance) is used, and when values are recorded the patient's posture and the arm used should also be noted.

Aetiology

'Essential': 95% of all cases and diagnosed as such by elimination of the following:

Renal disease: chronic glomerulonephritis, chronic pyelonephritis, renal artery stenosis, polycystic disease, polyarteritis nodosa.
Endocrine disease: Cushing's syndrome, Conn's syndrome, phaeochromocytoma, acromegaly.
Contraceptive pill
Eclampsia and pre-eclamptic toxaemia.
Coarctation of the aorta.

Symptoms

The patients are usually symptom-free. There may be a family history of hypertension in essential hypertension.

Signs

There may be no abnormal signs other than the raised blood pressure.

In the heart there may be left ventricular hypertrophy with an aortic ejection murmur and a loud aortic second sound. There may be also signs of coarctation of the aorta with radial-femoral delay .

The optic fundi may show retinopathy. This is often graded for convenience but it is better to describe the changes seen. Grades I and II indicate atherosclerosis.

Grade I: arterial narrowing.
Grade II: arteriovenous nipping.
Grade III: haemorrhages and exudates.
Grade IV: (malignant hypertension): grades I–III plus papilloedema.

In the abdomen there may be the enlarged kidneys of polycystic disease and a bruit from renal artery stenosis.

Complications

Pulmonary oedema (left ventricular failure).
Strokes and hypertensive encephalopathy.
Renal failure.
Myocardial infarction.
Retinopathy.
Complications of treatment (postural hypotension, hypokalaemia).

Investigation

- The degree to which a doctor investigates a patient with hypertension varies with the facilities available, and the patient's age and the degree of hypertension. Any factors pointing to the aetiology will determine some special investigations (e.g. endocrine disease). For instance, when glycosuria occurs with hypertension, investigations for Cushing's syndrome, acromegaly, and phaeochromocytoma are indicated. The association is most commonly due to none of these but only to the coincidence of these two common diseases (with the hyperglycaemia possibly increased by thiazide diuretics). Otherwise routine investigations are aimed at detecting treatable renal disease, and assessing cardiac and renal function. Repeated measurements of blood pressure are necessary except in severe cases: few physicians will treat a single moderately raised pressure reading

- All patients require chest X-ray and ECG to assess the size of the left ventricle
- MSU × 2–3 (for cells, casts, proteinuria and evidence of infection)
- Blood urea and electrolytes for the hypokalaemic alkalosis of Conn's or Cushing's syndromes or from diuretic therapy. If there is renal damage:
- 24-h urine sample for creatinine clearance, protein output (if proteinuria has been found) and Vanillymandelic acid (VMA) or 4-hydroxy-3-methoxymandelic acid (HMMA) output (Phaeochromocytoma, page 196). Check serum calcium
- Ultrasound to define renal size and IVU to detect structural abnormalities in patients who are young and with considerably raised pressures, those who do not respond to drug therapy and those with evidence of renal disease.
- Radioactive renography and scan where available is a simple technique which may give evidence of renal artery stenosis or of outflow obstruction
- Renal arteriography is indicated if surgery or angioplasty might be performed e.g. in patients with evidence of unilateral renal disease aged under 35 years
- Blood renin and aldosterone levels where indicated

Management

Non-pharmacological management

Diet. Four aspects of diet should be considered:
- Salt intake should be under 100 mmol (2.3 g)/day, and preferably under 75 mmol (1.75 g). The usual British daily intake is 200–250 mmol, i.e. up to about 6 g
- Energy intake should be reduced in most people to maintain a normal weight. A drop of about 1 mmHg per kg loss may be achieved
- Saturated fat and cholesterol intake will need attention apart from energy intake *per se*
- Alcohol intake should be limited to no more than the usually accepted maximal weekly intake of 21 units for men and 14 units for women (page 253)

Though change in dietary habits is difficult to achieve long-term, all patients can train their palates to be satisfied with less salt and sweet things.

Stress reduction and change in life style can be important and might even reduce blood pressure in some, though it is difficult to achieve.

Secondary hypertension

Direct treatment of the underlying condition may sometimes be indicated:
- endocrine disease and coarctation surgically
- renal artery stenosis is not often successfully corrected surgically, but this or angioplasty should be considered in patients under 35–40 years of age, particularly if control of the hypertension is difficult
- stop the contraceptive pill

Primary (essential) hypertension

Men develop more hypertensive complications than women. In uncomplicated hypertension, most physicians would always start therapy when repeated diastolic readings are above 100 mmHg in men and 105 mmHg in women. Many would start at 95 mmHg and 100 mmHg respectively. There may be no net benefit in treating uncomplicated diastolic hypertension of <100 mmHg. Diastolic blood pressures of up to 115 mmHg may settle with a few weeks observation. There may even be an increased incidence of coronary heart disease if diastolic blood pressures are reduced to levels below 87 mmHg—the J-shaped curve, since coronary heart disease (CHD) increases each side of this point.

Higher values are acceptable in the elderly chiefly because of the high incidence of side-effects of drug therapy, and less potential benefit. Systolic hypertension in the elderly (due to a rigid arterial tree) should not be treated per se.

Treatment may be indicated at lower pressures in the presence of ECG and radiological evidence of left ventricular hypertrophy, or in the presence of other complications.

Hypotensive drugs. It is usual to start with a β-blocker if no contraindication exists (chiefly bronchospasm and heart failure) and to follow with a thiazide diuretic, e.g. bendrofluazide 2.5–5 mg daily, if necessary. In simple hypertension treated with thiazide diuretics, potassium supplements are probably not necessary. Salt restriction ('no added salt') seems logical in these circumstances and a more severe restriction may be necessary in unresponsive hypertension. If a third drug is necessary, use either a calcium channel blocker such as nifedipine, or an angiotensin converting enzyme inhibitor such as captopril or enalapril. ACE inhibitors are now often used as first-line therapy especially in diabetes mellitus where thiazides and β-blockade are relatively contra-indicated. Vasodilators such as prazosin or hydralazine are kept in reserve as are the centrally acting drugs, methyldopa and clonidine. In hypertension resistant to conventional therapy, the vasodilator minoxidil coupled with β-blockade, frusemide, and a potassium preparation may be successful.

While paying attention to the treatment of hypertension to reduce the risks of cardiovascular disease, it should not be forgotten that there are a number of other risk factors. These include cigarette smoking, glucose intolerance, obesity, and blood lipids.

Malignant hypertension and hypertensive encephalopathy

Very rapid reduction of blood pressure (within minutes) is seldom inidicated. Beta-blockers, nifedepine, and methyldopa (0.5 g) orally or intramuscularly will work within 1–3 h. Rapid reduction (i.e. in the presence of fits or a rapidly rising blood pressure) may be achieved with labetalol or diazoxide (150 mg i.v. rapidly repeated up to 600 mg if necessary), or hydralazine (10–20 mg i.v.), or sodium nitroprusside (0.5–8 µg/kg/min infusion adjusted by results). It is best to become familiar with one or two standard drugs. The patient should be monitored in an intensive care unit. The blood pressure is best monitored using an arterial line.

Prognosis. Mortality from strokes and uraemia is decreased if hypertension is treated. The incidence of myocardial infarction is possibly unaffected. It is better in women than men.

VALVULAR HEART DISEASE
See also pages 65–7.

Mitral stenosis
Occurs in 60% of patients following acute rheumatic fever and is four times as common as mitral regurgitation (MR) and twice as common as mitral stenosis and mitral regurgitation combined. Thirty per cent of patients with mitral stenosis given no history of rheumatic fever. It is four times more common in women than men. It may occur 2–20 years after the acute episode of rheumatic fever.

Symptoms
Dyspnoea on exertion and paroxysmal nocturnal dyspnoea of pulmonary oedema.
Palpitations or emboli from atrial fibrillation.
Haemoptysis (bronchial vein rupture, bronchitis, left ventricular failure, pulmonary embolism).
Recurrent bronchitis.
Fatigue and cold extremities from a low cardiac output. Angina may occur rarely.

Signs
Mitral facies (malar flush).
Arterial pulse: there is a small volume pulse (obstruction to flow at the mitral valve).
Apex: the apex beat is tapping (a palpable first sound).
There may be a left parasternal heave of right ventricular hypertrophy. There may be a diastolic thrill in severe disease.

Auscultation
The mitral first sound is loud because the mitral valve is held wide open by high atrial pressure until ventricular systole slams it shut.
The length of the murmur is proportional to the degree of the stenosis. The murmur starts when blood starts to flow through the mitral valve, i.e. when atrial pressure exceeds ventricular pressure. The tighter the stenosis, the higher the

atrial pressure and the longer the murmur. In mild cases, exercise tachycardia may bring out the murmur and the patient should lie on his left side. The presence of an opening snap and loud first sound denotes a pliable valve. If the valve is already rigid this cannot occur. Presystolic accentuation is due to the increased flow through the valve produced by atrial systole and it is, therefore, absent in atrial fibrillation (AF).

NB Some of the signs and symptoms of mitral stenosis can be given by the Austin Flint murmur associated with aortic regurgitation (and very rarely by a left atrial myxoma).

Assessment

The *degree of stenosis* is assessed from the severity of the dyspnoea, the duration of the murmur and evidence of the degree of left atrial enlargement on chest X-ray and ECG. The tighter the stenosis the longer the murmur and the closer the opening snap to the second sound.

The *mobility of the valve* is denoted by the presence of an opening snap and a loud mitral first sound (and absence of valve calcification on the chest X-ray). *Pulmonary hypertension.* Fatigue, symptoms of right heart failure and a reduction in dyspnoea indicate raised pulmonary vascular resistance. The development of pulmonary hypertension is indicated by a dominant 'a' wave in the jugular venous pulse (unless in atrial fibrillation), a loud pulmonary second sound, right ventricular hypertrophy, rarely pulmonary incompetence, and a low volume peripheral arterial pulse volume (mnemonic: 'APRIL').

Presence of other lesions, e.g. mitral regurgitation and other valve lesions must be noted and assessed, particularly if symptoms indicate surgical intervention. AF may suggest a greater degree of myocardial disease, which is always present to some degree.

ECG. Atrial fibrillation may be present or, if not, the P mitrale of left atrial hypertropy. Right ventricular hypertrophy may be present.

Chest X-ray. Left atrial enlargement. Upper lobe venous congestion with septal lines (Kerley B) just above the costophrenic angles may be present with enlargement of the pulmonary arteries. The mitral valve may be calcified. Absence of calcification in pure mitral stenosis suggests that closed valvotomy may be attempted. Haemosiderosis in the lung fields is rare.

Echocardiogram. This allows measurement of the reduced diastolic closure rate of the mitral valve—it also demonstrates valve thickening and calcification, an gives an assessment of ventricular function (page 87). 2-D echocardiography can measure the valve orifice.

Complications

Pulmonary oedema (acute).
Right heart failure.
Atrial fibrillation (40%).
Systemic embolism (10%).
Subacute infective endocarditis.

Management

Prophylactic parenteral penicillins are given half an hour before dental treatment, cystoscopy, etc. They should be bactericidal drugs other than pencillins if the patient is already on them (page 336).

No other treatment is indicated in the absence of respiratory symptoms, evidence of enlargement of the left atrium, pulmonary hypertension (normal 25/8 mmHg) or systemic embolism.

Anticoagulation is indicated when atrial fibrillation develops or following systemic embolism. Some physicians anticoagulate all patients with proven mitral stenosis prophylactically and nearly all will if there is a large left atrium or atrial appendage, recent onset of fibrillation or paroxysmal fibrillation, and a low cardiac output.

Ventricular rate in atrial fibrillation is controlled by digitalisation.

Valvotomy or balloon valvuloplasty is usually indicated for effort dyspnoea. The operative risk is small (2–5%). Re-stenosis tends to occur in 5–10 years and may require re-valvotomy or mitral valve replacement. Mitral regurgitation may result from closed valvotomy.

Mitral stenosis in pregnancy. Fluid retention in pregnancy may produce a 30% increase in blood volume during the last trimester and may precipitate heart failure in the presence of underlying mitral stenosis. Valvotomy may be performed *at any time* during pregnancy if indicated by the above criteria. If possible this is best deferred until the last trimester to ensure viability of the fetus. However, the cardiac output falls in the last 2 months of pregnancy and most patients who can manage at that time can go to term. Antibiotics should be given through labour to cover the organisms of the genital tract if there are obstetric complications.

Mitral regurgitation

Aetiology

Floppy (prolapsing) mitral valve leaflets.

Ischaemic papillary muscle dysfunction, particularly after inferior myocardial infarction.

Severe left ventricular failure with dilatation of the mitral ring.

Rheumatic carditis.

Rarely, cardiomyopathy, congenital malformation (Marfan's syndrome), infective endocarditis and rupture of the chordae tendineae.

Symptoms

Progressive dyspnoea develops as a result of pulmonary congestion and this is followed by right heart failure. Angina and haemoptysis are uncommon compared with mitral stenosis. Fatigue and palpitation are common.

Signs

Left ventricular hypertrophy and systolic thrill. A parasternal heave may be present and due to systolic expansion of the left atrium (rather than from right ventricular hypertrophy).

Auscultation. There is an apical pansystolic murmur, radiating to the left axilla, sometimes with a thrill. The mitral first sound is soft. There may be a third sound (of rapid ventricular filling). A short mid-diastolic flow murmur in severe mitral regurgitation does not necessarily indicate valve stenosis.

Mitral valve prolapse may produce a late systolic click and murmur which is late because the posterior leaflet of the valve only starts to leak when the ventricular pressure is at its highest. It occurs in two clinical situations. In the middle-aged and elderly it is associated with disorder of the leaflet (wear and tear), chordae or papillary muscle (postmyocardial infarction). In the young (floppy valve) it occurs particularly in slender females (about 15% under 30 years by echocardiogram) and has been associated with tachyarrhythmia, syncope, atypical chest pain, transient ischaemic attacks and bacterial endocarditis. It seems sensible to advise prophylactic antibacterial drugs.

Assessment ECG: left ventricular hypertrophy. P mitrale of left atrial hypertrophy. Atrial fibrillation is less common than in mitral stenosis.

Chest X-ray: the left atrium and ventricle are enlarged, the former sometimes being enormous.

Echocardiography will help distinguish between the various causes of regurgitation and help assess left ventricular function.

Assessment: dominance of lesions in combined mitral stenosis/mitral regurgitation

Mitral stenosis is more likely to be the dominant lesion if the pulse volume is small (in the absence of failure) and if there is no left ventricular hypertrophy. The final decision is made if necessary by catheterisation.

Complications

As with mitral stenosis except that infective endocarditis is more common and embolism less common.

Management

Prophylactic antibiotics for dental treatment (page 336). Valve replacement is indicated if symptoms are severe and uncontrolled by medical therapy or pulmonary hypertension develops.

Indications for anticoagulation are systemic embolism and prosthetic valves. Some authorities recommend anticoagulation for all patients with atrial fibrillation.

Aortic stenosis

Aetiology (of valvular stenosis)

Under 60 years: rheumatic or congenital.

60–75 years: calcified congenital bicuspid valve, more common in men.

Over 75 years: degenerative calcification, more common in women.

NB Supravalvar stenosis (associated with 'fish-face' and infantile hypercalcae-mia) and subaortic stenosis (obstructive cardiomyopathy) are both very rare.

Symptoms

There may be no symptoms. They usually occur late. The symptoms are angina, syncope (which may be due to the low cardiac output) and dyspnoea. Sudden death is relatively common probably due to ventricular dysrhythmia, and left ventricular failure may occur.

Signs

Slow rising, slow falling, regular pulse ('plateau').

Small pulse pressure (e.g. blood pressure 105/90 mmHg).

Left ventricular hypertrophy (sustained and heaving apex beat).

An aortic thrill in systole radiating to the carotid arteries favours stenosis.

Auscultation. An aortic systolic ejection murmur maximal in the right second intercostal space radiating to the neck with a quiet delayed or absent aortic second sound. An ejection click may be present and indicates valvar stenosis. The murmur becomes less marked when the stenosis is very tight because the flow falls as the pump fails.

NB Non-valvar aortic stenosis: neither supravalvar nor subvalvar has an ejection click, and a poststenotic dilatation is uncommon in subvalvar stenosis (*see* Cardiomyopathy page 339).

Assessment ECG: left ventricular hypertrophy and sometimes left atrial hyper-trophy. Severe stenosis in adults is unlikely if left ventricular hypertrophy is not present.

Chest X-ray: left ventricular enlargement may not be present even in the presence of a prominent apex beat. The aorta is small and may be dilated distal to the valve (poststenotic dilatation). The aortic valve may be calcified (best seen on lateral chest X-ray).

Echocardiography can help determine the size of the orifice and degree of calcification. Left ventricular function and hypertrophy can also be assessed.

Complications

Left ventricular failure.

Infective endocarditis (10% of all cases).

Management

Observe if symptom-free.

Digitalis and diuretics for heart failure.

Valve replacement is indicated for asymptomatic severe stenosis (because of the risk of sudden death) or for symptomatic deterioration including syncope, a rapidly enlarging heart and 'strain' on ECG, as soon as failure has occurred. Catheter studies and angiography are performed to determine the site of the obstruction, the state of the coronary arteries and the systolic gradient across the valve (surgery considered if more than 50 mmHg). Operative mortality is about 3%. Antibiotic prophylaxis, see page 336).

Aortic regurgitation

Aetiology

Congenital bicuspid valve and infective endocarditis are the most common identifiable causes. Rheumatic carditis is now a rare cause. Even less common causes include seronegative rheumatoid syndromes (ankylosing spondylitis, Reiter's syndrome, colitic and psoriatic arthropathy), congenital lesions (e.g. Marfan's syndrome, coarctation of the aorta), syphilis and traumatic rupture.

Atherosclerosis and severe hypertension are of disputed importance.

Symptoms

There are usually none until dyspnoea occurs. Angina is not common.

Signs

The pulse has a 'sharp rise and fall' ('waterhammer' or 'collapsing') and there is a wide pulse pressure. The carotid pulsation in the neck may be marked. The left ventricle is enlarged and the apex displaced laterally.

There is an early blowing diastolic murmur at the left sternal edge maximal in the left third and fourth intercostal spaces, heard best with patient leaning forwards with the breath held in expiration. The second sound is quiet. There is usually also a systolic flow murmur which does not necessarily indicate associated stenosis. There may be a diastolic murmur at the apex (Austin Flint) which sounds like mitral stenosis.

Assessment ECG: left ventricular hypertrophy.

Chest X-ray shows cardiac enlargement

Echocardiography will demonstrate dilatation of the aortic root and the separation of the cusps. Left ventricular function and dimensions can also be assessed. The mitral valve can be affected with fluttering of the anterior leaflet and premature closure, if the regurgitation is severe.

Prognosis

Death occurs within 2–3 years after the onset of left ventricular failure with conservative treatment.

Management

Digoxin and diuretics for heart failure. Treat underlying endocarditis or syphilis. Valve replacement should be considered for symptomatic deterioration if the heart size increases rapidly or if the left ventricular internal diameter is >55 mm on echocardiographs in a young patient even when asymptomatic. Antibiotic prophylaxis, see page 336.

Dominance of lesions in combined rheumatic aortic stenosis/aortic regurgitation

Aortic regurgitation is dominant if the pulse volume is high and the pulse pressure collapsing. The left ventricle is enlarged and displaced. Aortic stenosis is dominant if the pulse is of small volume (plateau pulse) and the pulse pressure low. The ventricular apex, though hypertrophied, is not necessarily displaced.

Tricuspid regurgitation

Rheumatic. Invariably associated with disease of mitral and/or aortic valves (rare).

Functional in congestive heart failure (usually when the jugular venous pressure is over 10 cm) and following pulmonary hypertension in mitral stenosis or in atrial septal defect.

Endocarditis in drug addicts.

Signs

Clinically there is right ventricular enlargement with a pansystolic murmur at the bottom of the sterum. Giant 'cv' waves are present in the jugular venous pulse with systolic pulsation of an enlarged liver, and there may be jaundice from hepatic congestion (page 63).

Pulmonary stenosis

Congenital. Five per cent of all congenital heart disease and may follow maternal rubella

$\left.\begin{array}{l}\textit{Rheumatic} \\ \textit{Carcinoid}\end{array}\right\}$ very rare

Symptoms

Fatigue and syncope occur if stenosis is severe.

Signs

Peripheral cyanosis, low volume pulse and a large 'a' wave in the jugular venous pressure. The heart may show right ventricular hypertrophy. There is a systolic thrill and murmur in the pulmonary area (second left intercostal space) and an ejection click. The pulmonary component of the second sound is quiet and late.

Atrial myxoma

Atrial myxoma is excessively rare. It presents with features usually of mitral stenosis, systemic emboli and constitutional upset with fever. Thus it can mimic bacterial endocarditis and systemic lupus erythematosus (SLE). It is best diagnosed by echocardiography where the tumour produces characteristic wavy echoes as it moves between the mitral valve leaflets in diastole and in the atrium in systole. It is fatal unless removed surgically.

CONGENITAL HEART DISEASE

Congenital heart disease may present as an isolated cardiac abnormality or as part of a systemic syndrome.

Maternal rubella

It is dangerous in the first 3 months of pregnancy (particularly the first month—50% of fetuses are affected). The cardiac lesions are in three groups:

- patent ductus arteriosus
- septal defects: atrial septal defect (ASD), ventricular septal defect (VSD), Fallot's tetralogy
- right-sided outflow obstruction: pulmonary valve, artery or branch stenoses

The systemic syndrome includes cataract, nerve deafness and mental retardation.

All children are offered rubella vaccine at the age of 12 years. Fertile women given vaccine must not become pregnant in the immediate future.

If a pregnant woman is in contact with rubella, she should be given γ-globulin and serum taken for antibody levels to rubella. If raised, this is evidence of previous infection and there is little or no risk to the fetus. If the titre is not raised, a repeat sample is measured 3–4 weeks later (or if symptoms appear in the mother) and if the titre has risen significantly, this is evidence of recent infection. The earlier the pregnancy, the greater the risk to the fetus. Some elect for termination pregnancy.

Down's syndrome (usually 21-trisomy)

Associated with septal defects, particularly ventricular.

Turner's syndrome (XO)

Associated with coarctation of the aorta.

Marfan's syndrome (arachnodactyly)

An autosomal dominant connective tissue disorder which affects the aortic media, eyes and limb skeleton.

Incidence: 5000 in UK (5% of cases are a 'new' mutation). 10% are seriously affected.

It is characterised by a disproportionate length of the long bones which results in span exceeding height and long fingers and toes. There is frequently a high arched palate, pectus excavatum, scoliosis, little subcutaneous fat and lens dislocation with myopia. The aortic media is weak with a tendency to dilatation of the ascending aorta and aortic valve ring, resulting in aortic valve regurgitation and dissection of the aorta. Mitral regurgitation may develop. Joints tend to be hyperextensible.

Working classification

An asterisk denotes the most frequent.

Stenosis

Semilunar valves: aortic stenosis (supra- and sub-valvar and valve stenoses), pulmonary stenosis.

Atrioventricular valves: mitral stenosis, tricuspid stenosis.

Major arteries: coarctation of aorta*, pulmonary artery stenosis.

Regurgitation

Semilunar valves: aortic regurgitation, pulmonary regurgitation (very rare).

Atrioventricular valves: mitral regurgitation, tricuspid regurgitation, Ebstein's anomaly.

Shunts

Left to right: ASD*, VSD*, patent ductus arteriosus (PDA)*, aorto-pulmonary window.

Right to left (cyanotic: transposition of the great vessels (frequent but die at birth), Fallot's tetralogy*, Eisenmenger's syndrome.

Atrial septal defect (ASD)

Ten per cent of congenital heart disease. Occasionally in Marfan's syndrome.

Ostium secundum (70% of ASDs) is usually uncomplicated. Compared with congenital heart defects, there is a high (late) incidence of atrial fibrillation (20%) and an extremely low incidence of endocarditis.

Ostium primum (30% of ASDs) is often complicated because it tends to involve the atrioventricular valves and produces mitral and tricuspid regurgitation and even an associated VSD. In most respects (embryology, cardiodynamics, complications and prognosis) it is quite different from ostium secundum ASD.

Symptoms

In simple lesions there are usually no symptoms though dyspnoea occurs in 10% of cases. Symptoms usually occur for the first time in middle age. It is usually detected at routine chest X-ray.

Signs

Characteristically there is a fixed wide split of the second sound. Flow through the defect does not itself produce a murmur but increased right heart output may give a pulmonary flow murmur and large shunts may produce a tricuspid diastolic flow murmur. In ostium primum there may be a signs of the associated lesions, and mitral regurgitation (tricuspid). The precordium may be deformed. The pulse volume may be small. There may be a left parasternal lift of right ventricular hypertrophy.

Assessment ECG

Ostium secundum: partial right bundle branch block with right axis deviation and right ventricular hypertrophy. Atrial fibrillation may occur.

Ostium primum: there is usually left axis deviation with evidence of right ventricular hypertrophy. Conduction defects and junctional dysrhythmias may occur.

Chest X-ray

Enlargement of the right atrium and ventricle with enlarged pulmonary arteries and plethoric lung fields (evidence of increased right-sided. flow). The aorta appears small (evidence of decreased left-sided blood flow).

Complications

Pulmonary hypertension may lead to flow reversal through the defect (Eisenmenger's syndrome).

Atrial fibrillation.

Tricuspid regurgitation (from right ventricular enlargement).
Infective endocarditis occurs in ostium primum defects.

Management

Ostium secundum: operate if pulmonary–systemic flow ratio is more than 2 : 1.
Ostium primum: operate for symptoms or for cardiac enlargement with mitral
regurgitation.
NB Eisenmenger's syndrome precludes surgery.

Patent ductus arteriosus (PDA)

Fifteen per cent of all congenital heart disease. It is associated with the rubella
syndrome. It is commoner in females.

Symptoms

Usually there are none. Bronchitis and dyspnoea on exertion occur with severe
lesions.

Signs

The pulse may be collapsing (waterhammer). The left ventricle may be
hypertrophied. There is a continuous (machinery) murmur with systolic accentuation maximal in the second left intercostal space and posteriorly. This
continuous murmur must be distinguished from other causes, i.e. jugular venous
hum, mitral regurgitation plus aortic regurgitation, VSD plus aortic regurgitation, pulmonary arteriovenous fistulae.
Assessment ECG: normal or there may be left ventricular hypertrophy.
Chest X-ray: aorta and left ventricle may be enlarged. The pulmonary artery is
enlarged and there is pulmonary plethora.

Complications

'Endocarditis' (of the ductus).
Heart failure (Eisenmenger's syndrome following pulmonary hypertension and
shunt reversal).

Management

Indomethacin, if given within 1–3 weeks of birth may close the duct possibly by
blocking prostaglandin-E production in the duct muscle. If this is unsuccessful,
surgical ligation (1–5 years) is required or possibly an umbrella occlusion device.
Cyanosis contraindicates surgery. Antibiotic prophylaxis (page 336).

Ventricular septal defect (VSD)

Twenty-five per cent of congenital heart disease.
Small defect. Maladie de Roger, i.e. a loud murmur with a normal sized heart,
chest X-ray and ECG.
Large defect. The clinical importance depends on pulmonary vascular resistance
which determines how much shunting is present and its direction of flow.

Symptoms

None unless the VSD is large when there may be dyspnoea and bronchitis.

Signs

There may be a small volume pulse. Left ventricular hypertrophy may be present (and right ventricular hypertrophy if there is pulmonary hypertension). A pansystolic murmur (and thrill) is present in the fourth left intercostal space. A mitral diastolic flow murmur may be present and implies a large shunt.

Assessment ECG: left ventricular hypertrophy.

Chest X-ray: enlargement of the left atrium and ventricle may be present. The pulmonary arteries may be enlarged in pulmonary hypertension.

Complications

Endocarditis in 20–30% with emboli into the pulmonary circulation.

Eisenmenger's syndrome.

Management

Chemoprophylaxis to prevent endocarditis (page 336).

Small VSD: these may close spontaneously. Surgery is not indicated for the endocarditis risk alone.

Large VSD: surgery is indicated in most cases to prevent the development of irreversible pulmonary vascular damage developing. It is contraindicated once Eisenmenger's syndrome has developed.

Fallot's tetralogy

Ten per cent of congenital heart disease and 50% of cyanotic congenital heart disease.

There is a VSD in which the shunt is from right to left because of pulmonary stenosis (infundibular or valvar). The load on the right ventricle results in right ventricular hypertrophy. There is associated dextraposition of the aorta so that it sits over the septum in the defect.

Symptoms

Syncope (20%).

Squatting (this may help to decrease the right to left shunt by increasing systemic resistance).

Dyspnoea.

Retardation of growth.

Signs

Cyanosis and finger clubbing.

The typical murmur is of pulmonary stenosis. P_2 is quiet or inaudible. There is no VSD murmur.

Assessment ECG: usually moderate right atrial and ventricular hypertrophy.

Chest X-ray: there is a normal-sized, but boot-shaped heart and a large aorta with a small pulmonary artery and pulmonary oligaemia.
Polycythaemia is common.

Complications

Cyanotic and syncopal attacks (sometimes fatal).
Cerebral abscesses (10%).
Endocarditis (10%)
Paradoxical emboli.
Strokes (thrombotic—polycythaemia).
Epilepsy is commoner than in the general population
NB　Only 1 in 10 reach 21 years if untreated.

Management

Total correction on cardiopulmonary bypass.
Blalock shunt (not performed now), i.e. anastomosis of the left subclavian to the left pulmonary artery to increase pulmonary blood flow.

Pulmonary stenosis

Five per cent of congenital heart disease. It is usually acyanotic unless it is part of a Fallot's tetralogy (central cyanosis) or is very severe (peripheral cyanosis). The stenosis is usually valvar but may be subvalvar (infundibular). It may occur late in the carcinoid syndrome (page 206).

Symptoms

Even with considerable stenosis there may be no symptoms. Severe stenosis may give dyspnoea, fatigue, angina and syncope.

Signs

The characteristic sign is a pulmonary systolic murmur with or without a thrill. An ejection click implies a valvar stenosis. Classically its intensity increases with deep inspiration. Moderately severe stenosis produces a large 'a' wave in the jugular venous pulse, signs of right ventricular hypertropy and a wide split of the second sound (the delay in P_2 is due to raised right ventricular (RV) pressure—the greater the delay, the tighter the stenosis). Severe stenosis results in a reduced cardiac output with a small volume arterial pulse, peripheral vasoconstriction (with peripheral cyanosis) and P_2 becomes soft or absent if very severe.
Chest X-ray: poststenotic dilatation of the pulmonary artery with pulmonary oligaemia when the stenosis is moderately severe or worse.
Assessment ECG: degrees of right atrial hypertrophy (P pulmonale) and right ventricular hypertrophy (with 'strain pattern') corresponding to the degree of stenosis (a better guide than the symptoms).

Complications

Endocarditis.
Right heart failure.

Management

If mild or moderate (right ventricular systolic pressure <70 mmHg) observe: if more severe, balloon valvuloplasty or valvotomy (or infundibular resection) is indicated.

Coarctation of the aorta

Five per cent of congenital heart disease. It is associated with berry aneurysms, Marfan's and Turner's syndromes. Ninety-eight per cent are distal to the origin of the left subclavian artery.

Symptoms

Sixty per cent have none. Forty per cent have symptoms including stroke, endocarditis, occasionally intermittent claudication and those secondary to hypertension.

Signs

There may be radiofemoral delay with a small volume femoral pulse. Blood pressure may be raised in the arms especially on exercise, and may be different on the two sides and low in the legs. Asymmetry of radial pulses may be present. Visible and/or palpable scapular collaterals.
Left ventricular hypertrophy may be present.
The following murmurs may be heard:
- a systolic murmur at front and back of the left upper thorax
- collateral murmurs over the scapulae
- an aortic systolic murmur (of an associated bicuspid valve in 70% of cases) is usually obscured by the coarctation murmur.
Assessment ECG: 50% have left ventricular hypertrophy.
Chest X-ray: double aortic knuckle due to stenosis and poststenotic dilatation, rib notching (and at the scapular margin), and normal or large cardiac shadow.

Associations

Bicuspid aortic valve, cerebral artery aneurysms (berry aneurysms), and patent ductus arteriosus.

Prognosis

Ninety per cent die by the age of 40 years from endocarditis, heart failure or cerebrovascular haemorrhage.

Management

Surgical resection. The operative mortality is 5%. Antibiotic prophylaxis (page 336).

Eisenmenger's syndrome

This refers to the situation in which there is a reversal of a left to right shunt (e.g. VSD, ASD, PDA) due to pulmonary hypertension. With left to right shunts there is a pulmonary circulatory overload and an increase in pulmonary vascular resistance may follow with the development of pulmonary hypertension. When the pressure on the right side of the shunt exceeds that on the left side, the shunt flow reverses. The patient becomes cyanosed and deteriorates rapidly with symptoms of dyspnoea, syncope and angina. The lesion must be surgically corrected before this stage is reached.

INFECTIVE ENDOCARDITIS

Acute

This is a rare disease in which the heart valves are infected as part of an acute septicaemia of which the features are swinging fever, rigors, delirium and shock. Healthy valves may be affected (50% of cases). This may follow infection with staphylococcus usually from primary infection of the lungs or skin. *Streptococcus pneumoniae*, *Haemophilus influenzae*, gonococcus and meningococcus may be responsible.

The prognosis is that of the generalised septicaemia unless valve destruction leads in addition to acute intractable cardiac failure.

Subacute

This is usually bacterial and subacute in onset (SBE).

Predisposing abnormalities

Congenital. Ventricular septal defect, patent ductus arteriosus, coarctation of the aorta and bicuspid aortic valves may be infected.

NB Atrial septal defect of the secundum (common) variety does not develop endocarditis although the rare primum lesion where the mitral valve is also involved may become infected.

Acquired. Any rheumatic valve may be affected, the mitral more than the aortic and mitral regurgitation more frequently than mitral stenosis but chronic rheumatic heart disease now accounts for less than a quarter of all UK cases. Syphilitic aortic regurgitation and calcified aortic stenosis predispose to endocarditis. It may occur postoperatively following cardiac catheterisation or surgery and often on prosthetic valves which are always at risk. The normal tricuspid valve may become involved in mainlining drug addicts.

Organisms

Streptococcus viridans (non-haemolytic) is still the commonest in Britain (45%) and the most usual source is the teeth.

Staphylococcus aureus and *albus* (25%).

Streptococcus faecalis (7%) especially in young women (abortion) and old men (genito-urinary surgery and catheterisation). Other bacteria include gonococcus, brucella and proteus.

Coxiella burneti (Q fever).

Fungi (monilia, aspergillus, histoplasma).

The origin of infection varies with the infecting organisms and includes the teeth and tonsils (*Strep. viridans*), urinary tract (*Strep. faecalis*), cardiac catheterisation (staphylococcus), and the skin (staphylococcus).

Clinical features

The disease classically used to affect young adults (20–30 years) with rheumatic valve or congenital heart disease, but is now more commonly recognised in the over-sixties (30%).

The symptoms and signs may be considered in three groups:

1   *Signs of general infection.* Lethargy, malaise, anaemia and low-grade fever are frequent but not invariable (fever exists at presentation in 70% but is occasionally intermittent or persistently absent). Clubbing of the fingers (20% of cases) and splenomegaly (40%) are fairly late signs (6–8 weeks). There may be transient myalgia and/or arthralgia (25%). 'Cafe au lait' complexion is now exceedingly rare since it occurs only in the neglected late stage. The white cell count may be raised, normal or low.

2   *Signs of underlying cardiac lesions* must be sought though not present in 50% of patients. New lesions and changing murmurs are highly suggestive and the patient must be examined for these daily.

3   *Embolic phenomena.* Large emboli (30%) may travel to the brain (15%) and viscera or cause occlusion of peripheral arteries. Emboli from left to right shunts (VSD and PDA) and on the right-sided heart valves (tricuspid regurgitation and pulmonary stenosis) go to the lungs giving pleurisy and lung abscesses.

Immune complex phenomena ('small emboli') occur in up to 50% and include microscopic haematuria (30%)—usually in streptococcal infection, and splinter haemorrhages in the nail bed. Osler's nodes in the finger pulp are pathognomonic but rare. Roth spots in the eye may also occur very rarely.

The renal lesions in SBE appear to be of two kinds:

• A diffuse acute proliferative glomerulonephritis. The changes are not necessarily associated with streptococcal SBE and also not specifically diagnostic of SBE

• A focal 'embolic' glomerulonephritis in which only a part of the glomerulus is involved. The tissue is sterile on culture

Both the above may be due to precipitation of immune complexes: antigen/antibody complexes are present in the serum and complement levels are reduced. Rheumatoid factor and latex fixation may be positive.

Diagnosis

The diagnosis should be considered in any patient with a predisposing cardiac lesion who becomes ill. It may have to be made on the basis of the clinical picture even when unconfirmed by the isolation of the organism from blood culture. The most efficient way to make the diagnosis is:

• repeated examination particularly for changing heart murmurs
• blood culture (six samples)
• mid-stream urine examination for microscopic haematuria
• antigen–antibody complexes in serum
• echocardiogram for vegetarians

• latex fixation test may be positive

NB   Endocarditis may present with atrial fibrillation in the elderly.

Prognosis

The mortality is 95% in untreated cases. It is still over 30% even with modern therapy. Adverse features include the presence of congestive heart failure, advanced age or of peripheral emboli. Death is often from the heart failure of valve destruction or from major (e.g. cerebral) emboli.

Management

Prophylaxis. When valves are abnormal antibiotics must be given during intercurrent infections and before any surgical procedures in the mouth, genitourinary tract or gastrointestinal tract in those at risk.

Dentistry. For adults not allergic to penicillins, amoxycillin 3 g orally 1 h before surgery. For those who are receiving or have recently received a penicillin, give erythromycin stearate 1–5 g orally 1 h before surgery and 0.5 g 1 h later. Vancomycin is an alternative. Good dental hygiene is essential. Prophylactic dental extraction is not indicated in the absence of dental disease.

Urinary tract. Amoxycillin 1 g i.m. plus gentamicin 120 mg i.m. immediately before the procedure and 0.5 g amoxycillin 1 h later. It is not usually needed for simple catheterisation.

Obstetrics, and gynaecology and gastrointestinal surgery (including endoscopy and enemas).

Chemotherapy. It is essential to obtain blood cultures before starting chemotherapy but it should not be delayed in the presence of good clinical evidence even if cultures are negative. Penicillin G, 10–20 megaunits (6–12 g) parenterally is the drug of first choice. Since 30% of infecting organisms are now penicillin resistant most physicians would also add an aminoglyoside (e.g. gentamicin). When the results of bacterial sensitivities are available, therapy is guided by this, an attempt being made to achieve serum levels of the antibiotic at least three times the minimal inhibitory concentration (MIC) of the organism. Therapy should be continued for 8 weeks (intravenously for the first 2 weeks), if effective blood levels can be achieved. The patient should be carefully followed for recurrence. Emboli may occur for up to 1–2 months after 'cure'.

Indications for surgery

Surgery must be considered early for valve rupture, intractable cardiac failure, resistant infection particularly of a valve prosthesis, and if the organisms are drug resistant.

'Culture-negative endocarditis'

This diagnosis is considered after 6 successive negative cultures when culture technique is known to be good. The following should be considered:

• unsuspected organisms, e.g. *Coxiella burneti* (Q fever)—especially if the aortic valve is diseased. The diagnosis is dependent upon finding a rise in antibody titre. Bacteroides—anaerobic culture is required (and kept for up to 3

weeks). Fungi—monilia, aspergillus, histoplasma
- partly-treated bacterial cases
- right-sided endocarditis
- polyarteritis nodosa, SLE and atrial myxoma
- non-bacterial thrombotic endocarditis associated with carcinoma

ACUTE PERICARDITIS

Aetiology

Pericarditis is common within the first week of acute myocardial infarction. Dressler's syndrome is uncommon and occurs 2 weeks–2 months after myocardial infarction or cardiac surgery. It is characterised by fever, pleurisy, pericarditis and the presence of antibodies to heart muscle.

Infective pericarditis is usually a complication of chest infection. 'Acute benign pericarditis' affects young men, often follows a respiratory infection and is probably viral. A rising antibody titre to Coxsackie B virus is sometimes found. Suppurative pericarditis is rare. It results from infection with the staphylococcus or occasionally haemolytic streptococcus. Tuberculous pericarditis is very rare and non-suppurative.

Pericarditis may be part of a systemic syndrome: rheumatic fever, severe uraemia, local extension of carcinoma of the bronchus and following trauma. It may be the first indication of SLE.

Clinical features

There is central, poorly localised tightness in the chest which varies with movement, posture and respiration. There may be pain referred to the left shoulder if the diaphragm is affected. A pericardial rub is usually present which varies with time, position and respiration.

Pericardial effusion may develop and produce toxaemia (if it is purulent) or cardiac tamponade. The signs of pericardial effusion, without tamponade are an 'absent' apex beat, a 'silent' heart, and disappearance of the rub.

Tamponade, which is rare, produces:
- pulsus paradoxus. The pulse volume decreases in the normal person on inspiration. This is more marked with tamponade and is then known as pulsus paradoxus. The paradox which Kussmaul noted was that the heart continued to beat strongly whilst the peripheral arterial pulse virtually disappeared during inspiration.
- a rise in the jugular venous pressure on inspiration (Kussmaul's sign).

Both may be the result of descreased cardiac filling on inspiration due to the descending diaphragm stretching the pericardium and increasing the intraperi-cardial pressure.

Assessment ECG: there is raised concave elevation of the ST segment in most leads (especially II and V_{3-4}) and there may be T wave inversion. The voltage is low in the present of effusion.

Chest X-ray: it is unchanged in the absence of effusion. Effusion classically produces an enlarged pear-shaped cardiac shadow with loss of normal contours.

Echocardiography is the most sensitive way of demonstrating pericardial fluid with free space between the heart and percardium both in front and behind.

Management

Aspirate for tamponade (if the systolic arterial blood pressure falls below 90–100 mmHg). Treat the underlying condition. Steroids are used for lupus erythematosus and in acute benign pericarditis if it is severe or prolonged. Recurrent effusion with tamponade is treated by insertion of a drain or creation of a pericardial window.

CONSTRICTIVE PERICARDITIS

It is now very rare in Britain.

Aetiology

Some are due to tuberculosis following spread from the pleura or mediastinal lymph glands. Others follow acute viral or pyogenic pericarditis. Haemopericardium, irradiation and carcinoma account for most of the rest. It never follows acute rheumatic fever. It may be simulated by restrictive cardiomyopathy (page 341).

Clinical features

Symptoms appear from a few weeks to 30 years after a primary tuberculous infection. They result from cardiac constriction with decreased filling and a low cardiac output. Fatigue and ascites with little or no ankle swelling are characteristic, but dyspnoea and ankle swelling may occur later. Pulmonary oedema and paroxysmal nocturnal dyspnoea are rare.

Examination

The pulse is rapid and the volume is small and there may be arterial paradox (pulsus paradoxus) as with acute pericarditis. Atrial fibrillation is present in 30% of cases. The jugular venous pressure is raised and rises further on inspiration (Kussmaul's sign). There is diastolic collapse of the jugular venous pressure (steep 'y' descent). The liver is enlarged and ascites may be present. Ventricular contraction may caused localised indrawing of the chest wall at the apex. The heart sounds may be normal though quiet. A third sound due to an abrupt end to ventricular filling may be present. There is no rub.

Assessment ECG: there may be widespread ST changes with low voltage complexes.

Chest X-ray: there is calcification of the pericardium (sometimes seen only in the lateral film) in 50% of the cases which are secondary to tuberculosis.

Management

No action is needed if the patient is symptom-free and the tuberculosis inactive. Pericardiectomy may be required if severe constriction is present. Diuretics and salt restriction are given for ascites and oedema.

SYPHILITIC AORTITIS AND CARDITIS

It is now very rare in Britain. Acquired syphilis affects the aorta, the aortic ring to produce dilatation or aneurysm, and aortic regurgitation and the coronary artery orifices to cause angina.

NB Congenital syphilis does not produce aortitis.

Pathology

Endarteritis and occlusion of the vasa vasorum of the aortic muscle wall which becomes degenerate and fibrotic. Atheromatous plaques form over the damaged areas.

Aortic regurgitation

The symptoms are similar to those of rheumatic aortic regurgitation (page 326 for differential diagnosis). It is often gross with no haemodynamic stenosis (though there may be a systolic murmur).

Syphilitic angina

Fifty per cent of patients with syphilitic aortitis are affected. The angina is severe, attacks are long, often nocturnal, and respond poorly to glyceryl trinitrate.

Syphilitic aneurysms

Ascending aorta. This is the 'aneurysm of signs' with evidence of gross aortic regurgitation, local pulsation and systolic bruit and thrill in the second or third right interspace, marked carotid pulsation in the neck, signs of superior vena cava obstruction if the aneurysm is sufficiently large, and dilatation and calcification of the ascending aorta.

Arch of aorta. This is the 'aneurysm of symptoms' as it compresses the trachea and recurrent laryngeal nerve to produce cough, the left bronchus to produce collapse of the left lower lobe, the vertebrae producing erosion and pain, and occasionally the oesophagus causing dysphagia. Horner's syndrome may result from compression of the sympathetic trunk, and the left radial pulse may be absent due to compression of the left subclavian artery.

Abdomen. These are usually atheromatous and rarely due to syphilis. They present as pulsating abdominal masses.

CARDIOMYOPATHY

This word means 'disorder of heart muscle'. It is usually restricted to cardiomyopathies 'of unknown cause or association'. They are classified into three major groups depending upon the clinical effects of the abnormality of the function of the left ventricle which may be: (a) hypertrophied, (b) dilated or (c) restricted.

Hypertrophic cardiomyopathy

Also known as HCM. It is usually familial. It results in asymmetrical left ventricular hypertrophy associated with:

- loss of left ventricular distensibility which leads to symptoms of dyspnoea, pulmonary oedema and syncope. Some patients develop angina

• hypertrophy particularly of the left ventricle and septum with mitral regurgitation. In some patients this may disappear with progression of the disease as the heart muscle fails

Signs

There is a steep-rising jerky pulse (unlike the slow-rising plateau pulse of aortic valve stenosis), cardiac hypertrophy, a palpable atrial beat followed by a late systolic aortic ejection murmur, usually heard best in the left third and fourth intercostal spaces. There may be associated signs of mitral regurgitation. Complications include atrial fibrillation (10%), systemic embolism, congestive heart failure and sudden death.

Investigation

Echocardiography usually confirms the diagnosis showing asymmetrical septal hypertrophy, systolic anterior movement of the mitral valve and a narrow left ventricular cavity with hypertrophied trabeculae and papillary muscles. A 24-hour ECG record may identify those most at risk from sudden death from dysrhythmias.

Management

Beta-adrenergic blockade may be effective in reducing symptoms probably by increasing left ventricular compliance or reducing the incidence of dysrhythmias and angina. The response is variable. If the patient develops atrial fibrillation, anticoagulants and digoxin or verapamil may be added. Serious arrhythmias may be best treated prophylactically with amiodarone. Surgery is seldom indicated. Patients are at risk from endocarditis. Treat for cardiac failure and if medical therapy fails consider transplantation.

Dilated (congestive) cardiomyopathy

This is very rarely familial.

The label 'congestive cardiomyopathy' covers a large group of aetiologically unrelated disorders which tend to present as low-output congestive heart failure. By convention the more common and more easily diagnosed myocardial disorders are excluded, i.e. ischaemic, hypertensive and rheumatic heart diseases.

Angina (10%), systemic and pulmonary infarcts, conduction defects and arrhythmias occur.

Aetiology

Unknown (idiopathic): this is determined by the elimination of the following causes:

Alcoholism and thiamine deficiency (beri-beri).
Infections: viruses, e.g. influenza A_2, Coxsackie B, toxoplasma, diphtheria.
Infiltrations: sarcoidosis, amyloidosis (primary and secondary to myeloma), haemochromatosis.

Collagen disease: SLE, polyartertis nodosa, diffuse systemic sclerosis.
Muscular dystrophies and Friedreich's ataxia.
Endocrine: hyper- and hypothyroidism.
Postpartum.

Management

Bed rest, diuretics and ACE inhibitors form the basis of treatment of the cardiac failure. Anticoagulants are given because of the risks of embolism. Any underlying pathology (e.g. thyroid disease, collagen disease) should be treated appropriately.

Restrictive cardiomyopathy

The efficiency of the ventricles as pumps are restricted by endocardial fibrosis or granulation tissue—respectively EMF (endomyocardial fibrosis of equatorial Africa) and Loeffler's endomyocardial disease. In the UK, amyloidosis is the commonest cause of this rare condition, and is best diagnosed (or excluded) by endomyocardial biopsy.

PERIPHERAL ARTERIAL DISEASE

There are four common clinical syndromes:

Intermittent claudication

Ninety per cent are males over 50 years of age. The disorder is associated with smoking and diabetes mellitus, very occasionally with hyperlipidaemia and occasionally precipitated by anaemia. Obstruction may be femoro-popliteal (80%) aortoiliac (15%), or distal (5%).

Diagnosis

The history is of pain in the calf on effort with rapid relief by rest. The Leriche syndrome is buttock claudication with impotence. The major peripheral arterial pulses are reduced or absent. There may be arterial bruits over the aorta, iliac or femoral arteries. The tissues of the leg atrophy (muscle bulk is reduced) and hair loss is common. There may be cyanosis, pallor or redness, oedema, ulcers or gangrene.

Doppler ultrasound is useful to exclude obstruction in doubtful cases. Arteriography is required if surgery is contemplated.

Prognosis

The symptom indicates generalised vascular disease and 80% die from cardiovascular or cerebrovascular disease. Life expectancy is similar to a healthy population 10 years older. Diabetes mellitus and persistent smoking are associated with a worse prognosis. Age, cerebrovascular disease and ischaemic heart disease are poor prognostic features. Leg gangrene is uncommon.

Management

Stop smoking.

Exercise within the effort tolerance to help to develop collateral vessels. Treat obesity, hypertension, hyperuricaemia and hyperlipidaemia, despite the lack of firm evidence that this affects the prognosis: a positive attitude to therapy is itself reassuring.

Check for diabetes, polycythaemia and anaemia and treat if necessary.

Keep the body and arms warm, and the legs cool.

Attend carefully to foot hygiene.

Surgery. Endarterectomy is indicated if there is a high block with good distal blood flow on angiography. Bypass (prosthetic or vein graft) surgery may be indicated if angiography shows the vessels to be satisfactory distal to the block. Dilatation of narrowed arteries using balloon catheter angioplasty is used successfully in some centres. Sympathectomy is rarely successful in relieving symptoms of muscle ischaemia.

Acute obstruction

This may be due to thrombosis or to embolism (usually blood clot in atrial fibrillation). Ninety per cent are in the legs.

Diagnosis

Pain (usually severe) is associated with numbness, paraesthesiae and paresis. There is pallor and coldness of the limb below the obstruction followed by cyanosis. The limb becomes anaesthetic and the arterial pulses weak or absent.

Management

Maintain the limb at room temperature or below to decrease local cell metabolism and therefore its oxygen demand.

Assess early for surgical disobliteration which is the treatment of choice, even if shocked. The embolus is sent to the laboratory for histology and culture. The muscles are probably viable if firm and tender and resist movement. The skin is probably not viable if it is densely cyanosed and anaesthetic.

Hyperbaric oxygen, if available, may be helpful. Heparin and low molecular weight dextrans are used while awaiting surgery and, in addition, thrombolytic agents and vasodilators may be tried if surgery is contraindicated or delayed.

Ischaemic foot

This is caused by chronic arterial obstruction distal to the knees. It is most commonly seen in diabetes, and is associated with neuropathy and local infection.

Symptoms

Areas of necrosis and ulceration.

Pain in the foot (often not present in diabetics because of associated peripheral neuropathy).

Intermittent claudication.

Signs

If the large arteries are narrowed there are pallor and/or cyanosis, empty veins in the feet with trophic changes in nails and absence of hair. The feet are cold and pulses diminished or absent.

In diabetes, it is often chiefly the small vessels which are affected and the foot pulses can be present despite severe ischaemia of the toes.

Management

Foot hygiene is especially important in diabetes. Pain may be severe and require morphine. Sympathectomy may improve skin blood supply and reduce pain. Endarterectomy or vascular grafting are seldom technically feasible and angiography therefore seldom indicated. If amputation is required it is frequently above-knee. Conservative management includes stopping smoking and various drugs which are not fully evaluated. These include agents to reduce platelet stickness (aspirin, dipyridamole), reduce blood viscosity (oxpentifylline), dilate arteries (isoxsuprine and naftidrofuryl) and alter tissue metabolism (nicofuranose). None is very effective.

Raynaud's phenomenon

Definition

Intermittent, cold-precipitated, symmetrical attacks of pallor and/or cyanosis of the digits without evidence of arterial obstructive disease (page 341). The digits become white (arterial spasm), then blue (cyanosis) and finally red (reactive arterial dilatation).

Aetiology

Idiopathic and familial usually in young women (Raynaud's disease).
Collagen disease, especially systemic lupus erythematosus and scleroderma.
Arterial obstruction, e.g. cervical rib.
Trauma, usually in occupations involving vibrating tools.
Drugs including β-blockers, the contraceptive pill and ergot derivatives.

Management

Treatment is disappointing. The hands and feet should be kept warm and free from infection. The patient is reassured about the long-term prognosis (usually good) and advised to stop smoking. Electrically heated gloves can be very helpful. Reserpine, griseofulvin and thyroxine are of unproven value as is α-blockade with, for example, thymoxamine. More recently, calcium antagonists (e.g. nifedipine) and local glyceryl trinitrate have been tried. Sympathectomy is sometimes successful as a last resort particularly in the presence of recurring skin sepsis.

Dermatology

The commonest diseases are dermatitis, psoriasis, acne vulgaris, drug eruptions, athlete's foot, warts and basal cell carcinoma.

PRIMARY SKIN DISORDERS

Psoriasis

This affects about 1–2% of the population and may be inapparent, cosmetically debilitating or chronic. Rarely it may be acute and life-threatening. Partial remissions are characteristic.

Psoriasis may present acutely with multiple small round silver-scaly lesions on an erythematous base on the body, limbs and scalp (guttate psoriasis). Removal of the scales leaves small bleeding points. This tends to remit spontaneously over 2–4 months, but some patients subsequently develop chronic psoriasis.

Similar chronic skin lesions occur mainly on the extensor surfaces (back, elbows, knees) and scalp, but any area of skin may be affected and symmetry is a feature. Thimble-pitting of the nail-plate is common. In flexures it looks different with smooth, confluent red areas and pruritus is then fairly common, though not necessarily in the flexural parts.

Psoriatic arthropathy occurs in 5–10% and resembles sero-negative rheumatoid arthritis and is associated with thimble-pitting in the nail plate (page 174).

Treatment

Dithranol in Lassar's paste, preceded by a tar bath and followed by exposure to UVB light may be very effective, but is time-consuming and unaesthetic (because of the brown-staining dithranol). Photochemotherapy with PUVA (psoralens and ultraviolet A) therapy is successful in clearing and delaying recurrence in chronic psoriasis. There is a very slightly increased risk of skin cancer.

Etretinate (Tigason), vitamin A derivative, and the folate antagonist methotrexate are used to treat severe psoriasis unresponsive to other therapy. Both PUVA and methotrexate should only be used in otherwise resistant psoriasis under expert supervision. Hydroxyurea, colchicine, and cyclosporin can be held in reserve.

Lichen planus

An uncommon disorder, usually of the middle-aged, who present with an irritating rash affecting the flexures of the wrist and forearms, the trunk and the ankles. About 10% have nail involvement. The rash consists of discrete purple, shiny polygonal papules with fine white lines passing through them (Wickham's

344

striae), often occurring in scratch marks and other sites of injury (Koebner's phenomenon). The lesions may be widespread or confined to one or two papules. Lesions may occur on the buccal mucosa with a white lacy network or in the nails without other lesions on the skin.

The disorder usually resolves within 6 months but recurrences may occur. The cause is unknown but many drugs may produce an identical eruption, e.g. gold, antimalarials, and antituberculous drugs. The dermis is infiltrated with T-cells. Only 50% resolve in 9 months (85% in 18 months).

Treatment

Topical steroids may be sufficient to suppress symptoms until resolution has occurred. Systemic steroids may be required to suppress the pruritus of widespread lichen planus, especially planter and palmor lesions.

Pityriasis rosea

The rash is preceded by a 'herald patch'—a solitary red, scaly oval lesion on the abdomen or over the scapular area. This is followed after 1–2 weeks by a mildly itching macular rash which may cover the entire trunk, the upper thighs and upper arms. The macules tend to be oval and aligned along the natural skin creases with peripheral scales. The disorder occurs in small outbreaks in schools and families and may be caused by a virus.

The disorder is self-limiting usually within 6 weeks.

Treatment

Mild sedation can help. Mild to moderate topical steroids may be needed.

Dermatitis and eczema

Dermatitis is often used to refer only to skin inflammation due to an exogenous agent. The term is, however, synonymous with eczema, a term used colloquially for endogenous dermatitis i.e. atopic dermatitis. It affects 10% of the population.

Clinical features

Clinically the term describes a patchy diffuse irritating and sometimes painful lesion, often with vesicles which rupture to leave a raw weeping surface. Itching may be the dominant symptom. Secondary infection is common. In chronic lesions scaling may be present and the skin may become thickened (lichenification). Healed lesions do not scar but may pigment.

Histologically the initial abnormality is oedema of the epidermis and this finally results in vesicle formation. Vesicles or oedema dominate depending upon the thickness of the horny layer, i.e. in eczema of the face and genitalia oedema is marked, but on the palms and soles vesicles are more prominent.

Contact dermatitis

There are two groups: irritant and allergic.

1 *Irritant* contact dermatitis follows prolonged or repeated exposure to physical or chemical trauma and may occur in anyone exposed. It is a common problem in certain occupations such as hairdressers and engineers.

2 *Allergic* contact dermatitis requires previous sensitisation and may subsequently be provoked by very small quantities of the allergen. The rash is usually confined to the sites of exposure. A careful history is often necessary to discover possible sensitisers. Patch tests should be performed on all suspected cases. Chromates, nickel, rubber, dyes, perfumes, antibiotics (topical), some plants and antiseptics are frequent sensitisers.

Seborrhoeic dermatitis

A red, itchy, inflamed and scaly remittent dermatitis which appears on oily areas of the skin especially around the head including the scalp, eyebrows and creases of the nose and ears. It also occurs in flexures (axillae, infra-mammary and perineal), as intertrigo and, with ammonia from urine, as nappy rash.

Atopic dermatitis

Atopy refers to a hereditary tendency to develop allergic responses to various allergens and is usually shown by asthma, rhinitis and conjunctivitis as well as dermatitis. About a quarter of the UK population is atopic. Atopic dermatitis usually presents in infancy in an individual (and from a family) with other atopic manifestations. Prick tests to common allergens are usually positive and serum IgE levels often raised, though this does not help management. There is itching and inflammation, usually flexural, and lichenification is common.

Treatment

The local irritant or sensitiser must be removed if possible and practicable. Dietary manipulation and hyposensitisation have only a minor role in routine management. Commercial soaps may contain such irritants, and it is best, therefore, to wash with water only or use soap substitutes. If the lesion is weeping, local soaks (e.g. 1/8000 potassium permanganate will aid healing, and then apply topical mild to moderate steroids. If dry, an emollient such as aqueous cream may be sufficient, but topical steroids may also be required. Sedative antihistamines by mouth may relieve pruritus and allow sleep. If secondary infection occurs in the skin, systemic antibiotics may be needed.

Acne vulgaris

A disease chiefly of puberty (but onset can be up to 40 years) in which androgens cause increased sebaceous gland activity. Plugging of hair follicles by keratin causes retention of sebum producing the characteristic comedo ('blackhead'). These may become secondarily infected with skin bacteria. The comedos are distributed on the face, the shoulders and upper thorax. The skin is usually greasy. It usually disappears in early adult life often with residual scarring. Acne is seen in Cushing's syndrome (page 191).

Treatment

Frequent washing with soap and water or local detergents (e.g. cetrimide) to degrease the skin.

Topical benzoyl peroxide cream or lotion (2.5–10%) or antibiotics (clindamycin or erythromycin) usually helps, often with oral antibiotics.

Oral antibiotics such as oxytetracyline (or erythromycin) 1 g daily are given for 6 months or longer and are usually effective for mild to moderate disease, though results may take 3 months to appear.

Isotretinoin (Roaccutane) is a vitamin A derivative taken orally for severe disease when topical therapy and oral antibiotics have failed. Side effects are common including facial erythema, dry skin, myalgia, and a rise in plasma lipids and abnormal liver function tests.

Rosacea

A disorder, more common in women, beginning usually after 30 years of age, with the erythema, papules, pustules and telangiectasia over the cheeks, nose, chin and forehead.

Treatment

Avoid precipitating factors (e.g. hot drinks, sunlight, alcohol and topical steroid preparations).

Oxytetracycline (500 mg bd) may be effective when given long-term intermittently, two months at a time with or without topical metronidazole.

FUNGUS INFECTIONS

Candidiasis (monilia, thrush)

In general medical practice this yeast infection, though common in fit people, should raise the suspicion of underlying diabetes mellitus (and the rare hypoparathyroidism), or other factors which suppress normal immune mechanisms, e.g. leukaemia, Hodgkin's disease, steroid therapy, AIDS when overwhelming systemic infection may occur.

The nail folds are commonly involved, sometimes producing obvious paronychia. Thrush occurs frequently in the vagina, on the penis, and on the oral mucosa especially in users of inhaled steroids. It may spread to affect the entire gastrointestinal tract especially after antibiotics.

NB Oesophageal moniliasis has a characteristic radiological appearance with barium adhering to the patches of monilia.

Treatment

Nystatin orally (500 000 units 6-hourly). Imidazole creams (e.g. clotrimazole) are the drugs of choice but may be ineffective if the underlying disorder does not respond to specific therapy. Itraconazole is used orally if necessary but may be hepatotoxic. Griseofulvin is ineffective.

Pityriasis versicolor

This is a yeast infection with *Pityrosporum orbiculare (Malassezia furfur)* usually of the trunk which causes brownish scaly lesions of varying size which may coalesce. Depigmentation, which may last many months after effective treatment, may resemble vitiligo because only the unaffected skin pigments in sunbathers. Diagnosis is made by skin scrapings. An application of 2.5% selenium sulphide repeated after a week may be sufficient. Topical imidazole for several weeks may be used. Griseofulvin is not effective.

Ringworm (tinea)

The ringworm fungi are a group of related organisms (Trichophyton, Microsporum, Epidermophyton) which live in the keratin layer of the skin. The disorders produced are described after their site on the body, viz, tinea pedis, tinea cruris and tinea capitis. Diagnosis is confirmed either by observing fungal hyphae in skin scrapings treated with potassium hydroxide or by culture. Ringworm is commonly misdiagnosed and treated inappropriately.

Tinea pedis (athlete's foot)

The most common of the group affecting the interdigital skin usually between the fourth and fifth toes. The nails may be involved. The lesion is irritating and the skin appears white and macerated. It may provide an entry for bacterial infection (streptococcal cellulitis). The infection tends to be recurrent or chronic. The disorder must be distinguished from simple skin maceration, atopic dermatitis, psoriasis and footwear (contact) dermatitis.

Tinea cruris

This may result from spread of infection from the feet. The lesion affects the upper inner thighs and has a slightly raised, well defined, spreading scaly margin. In contrast, monilia is symmetrical, with ill-defined edges and small satellite lesions. Tinea gives pruritus.

Tinea capitis

A disease of prepubertal children who present with an area of baldness with scaly skin and stumps of broken hair. Some infections show characteristic fluorescence when viewed under Wood's light. The underlying scalp is scaly and may become secondarily infected.

Treatment of dermatophytes in general

Topical imidazole (e.g. clotrimazole, miconazole), treatment is usually effective for localised areas, but if the infection is severe, widespread or if there is nail and hair involvement, systemic therapy may be needed. Griseofulvin (0.5–1 g daily) is given for 6 weeks for simple scalp infections and for up to 2 years for toenail involvement. They should only be started after laboratory confirmation of the diagnosis.

DRUG ERUPTIONS

Many drugs can produce eruptions which may be erythematous, maculopapular, urticarial or purpuric. The pattern for any one drug may not always be the same and most drugs may at times produce one or other type of reaction, i.e. virtually any drug can produce any eruption—an overstatement but necessary to consider in any patient with a rash. The commonest now are the thiazides, allopurinol, captopril, and penicillamine. Topical antibiotics, particularly the penicillins and the neomycin group frequently produce skin eruptions. The common drug rash of ampicillin is maculopapular and may be specific to it and not to all penicillins. (It is almost universal in patients with infectious mononucleosis.)

Urticarial reactions

The penicillins are probably the most common group of drugs which produce urticaria. Of all patients receiving a penicillin, 1–2% have adverse reactions, and many of them (if asked) give a history of previous sensitivity. Reactions are more frequent in adults, probably a measure of previous exposure. Sensitivity to one penicillin may mean sensivity to all, and cephalosporin sensivity in about 1 in 10 patients. The urticarial eruption usually occurs 3–7 days after therapy is started. Rarely, an acute hypersensivity reaction occurs within minutes and is associated with serum-sickness-like features of fever, wheezing, arthralgia and hypotension. Chronic cases should avoid dairy produce as antibiotics are generously used in farming.

Other drugs which produce urticarial reactions include barbiturates, salicylates, streptomycin, sulphonamides, tetracyclines, phenothiazines and chloramphenicol.

Purpura

This may be a feature of any severe drug reaction and results from capillary damage. Bone marrow suppression by gold, carbimazole, or phenylbutazone may cause thrombocytopenic purpura (page 99).

Other disorders

Light sensitivity (sulphonamides, tetracyclines, thiazides, chlorpropamide, tolbutamide, griseofulvin, chlorpromazine).

Fixed drug eruption. This describes an eruption which has the same character and occurs in the same site when the causative drug is taken. Phenolphthalein, used in some laxatives, is frequently incriminated. Other drugs include penicillin, phenylbutazone, aspirin and sulphonamides.

Lichen planus (gold, phenylbutazone, quinidine) (page 344).

Exfoliative dermatitis (gold, barbiturates, phenytoin, chlorpropamide).

Erythema multiforme (page 353).

Lupus erythematosus (page 161).

Management

Stop all drugs.

Oral antihistamines for urticaria.

Mild topical steroids may help itching.

Adrenaline may be life saving in acute hypersensivity reactions including shock and angioneurotic oedema (page 290), and systemic steroids may be required in severe but less acute cases.

SKIN MANIFESTATIONS OF SYSTEMIC DISEASE

Erythema nodosum

Clinical presentation

Tender, red, raised lesions usually on the shins and less frequently the thighs and upper limbs. The lesions pass through the colour changes of a bruise. It is five times commoner in females and occurs usually between 20 and 50 years of age. Arthropathy, especially in the legs, occurs in 50% and bilateral hilar lymph gland enlargement is usually seen on chest X-ray in sarcoidosis (page 296).

Aetiology

Sarcoidosis is probably the most common cause in this country (35%). Streptococcal infection and hence rheumatic fever.
Tuberculosis.
Drugs (particularly sulphonamides and including penicillin and salicylates).
Other causes include ulcerative colitis. Crohn's disease, Behçet's disease and fungal infections (e.g. Histoplasma). Erythema nodosum occasionally occurs as an isolated, sometimes recurrent, disorder.

Lyme disease (Erythema chronicum migrans—ECM)

Borrelia burgdorferi is a spirochaete spread by ioxdid ticks from deer and rodents to man. The infection may produce clinical features in the skin (ECM), joints, central nervous system and heart.
•   Erythema chronicum migrans begins as an indistinct red macule, from around the tick bite, which enlarges progressively
There may be other features of infection with fever, malaise, myalgia and lymphadenopathy plus:
• migratory arthralgia, usually of large joints
• neurological features including aseptic meningitis and cranial nerve lesions (especially seventh nerve)
• Cardiac disease with AV block and myocarditis
The diagnosis is confirmed serologically by the presence of a high titre of antibodies to *B. burgdorferi*, and treatment is with tetracycline, penicillin, or a third generation cephalosporin (e.g. cefotaxime).

Haemolytic streptococcal infection

Skin lesions frequently occur as a sign of streptococcal sensivity and present as erythema nodosum, erythema marginatum (very rare but virtually diagnostic of rheumatic fever), and erythema multiforme (also occurs in rheumatic fever). Skin infections produce cellulitis or erysipelas (slightly raised, well circumscribed, acutely painful bright red lesions of half to one hand's-breadth in diameter). The elderly are more commonly affected and the legs and face the most common sites. There may be generalised symptoms of headache, fever and vomiting. Response to parenteral penicillin is usually rapid. Transient skin rashes are common with streptococcal infection but the classical endotoxic rash of scarlet fever is now rarely seen.

Malignancy

Generalised pruritus is associated with tumours of the reticuloendothelial system such as Hodgkin's disease (also renal and hepatic failure, and old age).

Herpes zoster ('shingles')

Although it usually occurs in isolation, herpes zoster may occur in any debilitating disease and particularly with Hodgkin's disease, the leukaemias and patients on steroids. The lesion consists of groups of vesicles on an inflamed base. Pain precedes the lesions in nerve root distributions. Postherpetic neuralgia may be severe and intractable. The virus (*Varicella zoster*) is identical with the virus of chickenpox and denotes earlier clinical or subclinical infection in childhood. The virus remains latent within dorsal root ganglia until diminished resistance allows reactivation. Patients should be isolated from the non-immune and immunocompromised population until the lesions are crusted, otherwise chicken pox, may develop. Topical idoxuridine or acyclovir may help if given early, and parenteral acyclovir is usually required in the immunosuppressed.

Dermatomyositis (see page 164)

Twenty per cent of adult cases occur in association with carcinoma, leukaemia or lymphoma.

Acanthosis nigricans

Brown pigmented warts or plaques most marked in the axilla are associated with underlying carcinoma particularly of the bronchus, gastrointestinal tract, prostate, breast and uterus. It is very rare. Benign forms occur, especially in the obese.

Other manifestations

These include acquired ichthyosis (Hodgkin's disease), chronic myeloid leukaemia skin infiltration, secondary skin metastases, migratory thrombophlebitis, and exfoliative dermatitis.

Xanthomatosis

Tendon xanthomata, usually most easily felt in the Achilles tendon and in the finger extensors on the dorsum of the hand, are chacteristic of familial hypercholesterolaemia and associated with premature cardiac death. Xanthelasmata are dull yellow plaques commonly in the inner angles of the eyelids. They may, though not always, indicate hyperlipidaemia with raised serum cholesterol and are associated with myxoedema, diabetes and primary biliary cirrhosis. Eruptive xanthomata may occur with greatly elevated serum lipid levels.

Other rare manifestations

The following conditions are well recognised:

* Necrobiosis lipoidica in diabetes mellitus
* Pretibial myxoedema in thyrotoxicosis
* Lupus pernio (a purple eruption) in sarcoid
* Lupus vulgaris and erythema induratum (Bazin's disease) in tuberculosis
* 'Café au lait' spots and multiple neurofibromata of neurofibromatosis (von Recklinghausen's disease)
* Light sensitivity and blistering in porphyria (page 207)
* Erythema chronicum migrans in Lyme disease

MUCOSAL ULCERATION

This may be localised to the buccal mucosa or associated with generalised disease. Causes include aphthous ulcers, herpes simplex ulceration, herpangina (Coxsackie virus type A), agranulocytic ulcers in aplastic anaemia usually drug induced or leukaemic, erythema multiforme and Stevens–Johnson syndrome, Behçet's syndrome, and under dental plates (often monilia).

Behçet's disease

A disease of unknown aetiology characterised by a relapsing iritis associated with crops of oral (100%) and genital (75%) ulceration. It is twice as common in males and the peak age of onset is in the twenties. There may also be a migrating superficial thrombophlebitis (25%) which may occasionally present with deep vein thrombosis (and occasionally pulmonary involvement), arthralgia of large joints (60%), erythema nodosum (65%) and neurological complications (10%). The diagnosis is chiefly clinical though the erythrocyte sedimentation rate (ESR) is usually over 50 mm/h and there is a neutrophilia. It is treated with anti-inflammatory drugs (steroidal and non-steroidal) and with anticoagulants when indicated. Cytotoxic drugs (azathioprine or cyclophosphamide), colchicine and thalidomide have been used in the more severe cases.

BULLOUS LESIONS

Drugs may produce bullous eruptions. There are four other primary bullous skin disorders which are well regconised. All are rare.

Dermatitis herpetiformis

All patients have a gluten-sensitive enteropathy, though in 50% it is subclinical. The skin of the limbs and trunk is affected. In 80% histocompatibility locus antigen (HLA) B8 is present. Subepidermal immunoglobulin A (IgA) is usually present.

Clinical presentation

Symmetrical clusters of urticarial lesions on the occiput, interscapular and gluteal regions and extensor aspects of the elbows and knees. Vesicles follow and only rarely become bullous as skin trauma is provoked by the intolerable itching. There are seldom lesions in the mouth and there is no fever.

Prognosis and management

The disease starts acutely and may remit spontaneously, but tends to become chronic. Secondary bacterial infection is common. Dapsone is the drug of choice for the skin lesion.

Pemphigus vulgaris

Clinical presentation

A rare disease of middle age, some of the characteristics of which are explained by the very superficial site of the lesion: there is splitting in the epidermis above the basal layer. Degeneration of the cells of the epidermis (acantholysis) is seen on skin biopsy. IgG is present on the intercellular substance. Clinically it presents with widespread erosions and relatively few bullae (because they rupture so easily) spread over the limbs and trunk. Most (90%) patients have lesions in the mouth and these may be the only lesions at first. The surrounding skin is normal. The superficial skin layer can be moved over the deeper layers (Nikolsky's sign) and tends to disintegrate allowing secondary infection. Lesions appear at sites of pressure and trauma and are then extremely painful. There is fever and severe constitutional disturbance. It may be precipitated by drugs, e.g. penicillamine.

Complications and management

Secondary bacterial infection is common and septicaemia may result. Protein loss from weeping skin may occur in widespread disease. Prednisolone (initially 60–100 mg, later reduced) may be required to control the eruptions. The prognosis is poor without treatment, but it can be no more than inconvenient in mild, treated cases.

Pemphigoid

A disease of the elderly in which the lesion is at the basement membrane between the dermis and epidermis—deeper in the skin than in pemphigus. IgG is deposited in the basement membrane zone. Acantholysis is not seen on histology. Clinically it presents after prodromal itch for a few weeks, with the sudden onset of bullae on the limbs and, to a lesser extent, on the trunk. The large, tense subepidermal bullae have less tendency to break than in pemphigus but can be provoked by trauma. Nikolsky's sign is negative. The surrounding skin shows erythematous patches. Mucosal ulceration is rare (10%). Secondary infection is common, and the patients are not usually ill.

Management

Steroids (prednisolone 40–60 mg daily) are required to control the eruption and may be required in low dose for years.

Erythema multiforme

Clinical presentation

A generalised disease that may present in well people or sometimes with prodromal symptoms of fever, sore throat, headache, arthralgia and gastroenteritis. These are followed by a pleomorphic erythematous eruption which may become bullous. The forearms and legs are commonly affected first and the rash may spread centripetally to involve the entire body. The buccal mucosa may be involved. Target lesions—concentric rings of differing shades of erythema— are characteristic but late. The disease remits spontaneously in 5–6 weeks but may recur.

'Stevens–Johnson syndrome' is a severe form of erythema multiforme characterised by systemic illness with lesions in the mouth, conjunctiva, anal and genital regions.

Aetiology
The disease sometimes follows drug therapy (sulphonamides, penicillin, salicylates and barbiturates) and herpes simplex infection. The aetiology often remains unknown.

Management
Withdraw drugs.

Local treatment with mild potency steroids for pruritus.

Stevens–Johnson syndrome may require steroids to suppress the eruption but infection must be identified and specifically treated.

Skin pigmentation
This is usually racial or due to sun tanning. Other causes include pregnancy and the oral contraceptive (chloasma), Addison's disease, Nelson's syndrome (post-adrenalectomy), haemochromatosis, cirrhosis, uraemia, heavy metal and chronic arsenic poisoning. In neurofibromatosis the patches are of varying size, discrete and associated with subcutaneous neurofibromata. In Peutz–Jeghers syndrome there are small discrete patches around the mouth and multiple small intestinal polyps. Other dermatological causes include the post-inflammatory changes which follow a number of dermatoses. Remember cosmetic preparations intended to simulate suntan. The café au lait pigmentation of bacterial endocarditis is now rarely seen because patients are treated early.

Haematology

ANAEMIA

The symptoms given by all anaemias are much the same though the rate of onset of anaemia, age of the patient and symptoms from other aspects of an underlying disease process may alter the presenting symptomatology. These are tiredness, physical fatigue and dyspnoea: with angina, heart failure and confusion in older people.

Classification (pages 91–5)

1 *Deficiency*
- Iron (including sideroblastic anaemia)
- B_{12}
- Folic acid

2 *Haemolysis*

Abnormal red cells (intrinsic disorders):
- *Membrane disorder*: hereditary spherocytosis; hereditary elliptocytosis
- *Haemoglobinopathy*: sickle cell anaemia; thalassaemia
- *Enzyme deficiency*: G6PD; pyruvate kinase

Normal red cells (extrinsic disorders):
- *Immune*: newborn, autoimmune (especially systemic lupus erythematosus); lymphomas (especially chronic lymphocytic leukaemia and Hodgkin's disease); cold haemoglobinuria, drug-induced (methyldopa, mefenamic acid)
- *Non-immune:*
  (a) *Mechanical haemolytic anaemias*: disseminated intravascular coagulation, thrombotic thrombocytopenic purpura, haemolytic uraemic syndrome, prosthetic heart valves and march haemoglobinuria
  (b) *Infections*: malaria, clostridium perfringens, viral infections
  (c) *Paroxysmal nocturnal haemoglobinuria*
  (d) *Drugs*: e.g. oxidative damage, Dapsone, salazopyrine

3 *Marrow failure*
- *aplasia*
- *suppression*: idiopathic or secondary to infiltration, drugs, infections or other disorders such as uraemia, hypothyroidism and chronic disease
- *dyserythropoeisis*: myelodysplastic syndrome

Iron deficiency anaemia

Diagnosis

The peripheral blood count shows hypochromia (mean corpuscular haemoglobin—MCH <27 pg) and microcytosis (mean corpuscular volume

MCV< 80 fl), possibly with poikilocytosis (variation in shape) and anisocytosis (variation in size). The serum iron is low and the transferrin (or total iron binding capacity—TIBC) raised—with a low saturation. Serum ferritin reflects the state of the iron stores and is therefore low. There is a reduction in stainable iron in the marrow. The cause of the iron deficiency must be identified and corrected. In premenopausal women, excess menstrual loss is often the cause, though this should not be accepted uncritically because other important causes may be present as well. Slow gastrointestinal loss is a common cause, with peptic ulceration, gastric carcinoma and carcinoma of the descending colon commonest of the causes which usually give symptoms. Carcinoma of the ascending colon or caecum frequently produces no symptoms and its possible presence must be considered positively in all cases of iron deficiency anaemia. (Other causes of hypochromic, microcytic anaemia include thalassaemia, and anaemia secondary to chronic disease where serum iron and TIBC are usually reduced and ferritin normal or even raised (since it is an acute phase protein)). The bone marrow shows adequate iron in macrophages but reduced amounts in developing erythroblasts. Collagen disease such as rheumatoid arthritis, and renal failure are two of the commoner causes.) *Examination* will include assessment of pallor (very imprecise) glossitis, angular stomatitis, koilonychia, rectal examination. Also investigate for carcinoma of colon if there is a change of bowel habit.

Management

Ferrous sulphate, 200 mg bd before food is usually all that is required. The reticulocyte count rises first and then the haemoglobin (at about 1 g per week) but iron should be continued for another 3 months to replenish the stores.

B$_{12}$ and folic acid deficiency

Vitamin B$_{12}$ is present in liver, and small amounts also in milk and dairy products, and requires intrinsic factor for absorption. Folic acid is found in green vegetables and liver.

B$_{12}$ deficiency

This is usually cause by lack of intrinsic factor: B$_{12}$ deficiency due to the presence of parietal cell and intrinsic factor antibodies is the most common cause in the UK. Rare causes of B$_{12}$ deficiency include gastrectomy, intestinal blind loops (in which bacteria multiply using up B$_{12}$), a vegan diet, Crohn's disease involving the absorbing surface in the terminal ileum, other causes of malabsorption and *Diphyllobothrium latum*—a Finnish tape worm which consumes B$_{12}$.

Folate deficiency

1 *Dietary deficiency.* In the UK this is most commonly seen in chronic alcoholics, the poor and the elderly who get no green vegetables. In the tropics it is often seen in association with multiple deficiencies and with gut infection and infestation.

2 *Malabsorption* (page 270).

3 *Increased requirement.* Haemolysis (increased red cell formation) requires

folate more than B_{12}; pregnancy and infancy.

4   Therapy with phenytoin interferes with folate metabolism.

Pernicious anaemia

This is due to the inability to produce intrinsic factor leading to deficient B_{12} absorption. Stores of B_{12} last 3–4 years. Achlorhydria is invariably present. It is associated with other organ-specific autoimmune disorders (page 168).

Clinical features

Pernicious anaemia occurs in the middle-aged and elderly and is more common in women. Exhaustion and lethargy are the commonest presenting complaints though the anaemia may be noticed incidentally. Classically, the skin has a pale lemon tint, the hair is snow white and the sclera may be slightly jaundiced due to mild haemolysis which is a typical feature. Cardiac failure is common if the anaemia is marked. The tongue may be tender, smooth and red due to atrophy of the mucosa. Peripheral neuropathy may be the presenting feature with pain, soreness or numbness of the feet on walking. Later, features of subacute combined degeneration of the cord may develop (page 148). The spleen is sometimes palpable. There is an increased incidence of gastric carcinoma.

Diagnosis

The haemoglobin may be very low, i.e. 3–4 g or less. The blood film shows oral macrocytes usually with anisocytosis and poikilocytosis, and the MCV is usually >100 fl. The total white blood cell (WBC) count may fall due to reduced numbers of both lymphocytes and neutrophils. Some neutrophils may show hypersegmentation of the nuclei (>5 lobes). There may also be a moderate fall in the platelet count. Reticulocytes are generally not increased until treatment is started. Giant metamyelocytes and megaloblasts are present in the marrow which is hypercellular, evidence that anaemia is in part due to suppression of cell release. Serum bilirubin is raised, haptoglobins reduced, and urobilinogen is present in the urine as a result of reduced red cell survival and ineffective erythropoiesis. Antibodies to parietal cells are present in >90% of patients and to intrinsic factor in approximately 55%. Not all individuals who have parietal cell antibodies have pernicious anaemia.

Treatment

Vitamin B_{12} as hydroxocobalamin 1 mg (1000 µg) is given twice in the first week, then weekly until the blood count is normal and then every 3 months for life.

The response of the marrow to therapy is very rapid with an early reticulocyte response maximal on the 4–6th day. The haemoglobin follows this and rises about 1 g/dl every 1–2 weeks. The WBC and platelets will be normal in about 7 days.

The rapid production of cells with therapy may reveal an associated deficiency of, and demand for, iron, potassium or folic acid and supplements should be given where necessary.

Neurological features of B_{12} deficiency usually improve to some degree: sensory abnormalities more completely than motor, and peripheral neuropathy more than myelopathy. However, neurological features may remain static and occasionally even deteriorate.

NB If folic acid is given alone to patients with pernicious anaemia the neurological features may become worse.

Blood transfusion contains enough B_{12} to correct the marrow and to make interpretation of serum B_{12} levels difficult. It may precipitate heart failure and death—some authorities believe that transfusion *must never* be given to patients with pernicious anaemia. A poor response to B_{12} therapy suggests that the diagnosis is wrong.

Haemolytic anaemia (table 26)

Haemolysisis is characterised by jaundice with a raised unconjugated serum bilirubin, increased urobilinogen in urine and stools, decreased haptoglobins, and reticulocytosis. The blood film may show polychromasia, spherocytes, crenated and fragmented red cells. There may be features of:

- Rapid red cell destruction—increased plasma haemoglobin, methaemalbuminaemia, decreased haptoglobins, haemoglobinuria and haemosiderinuria.
- Excess red cell formation—reticulocytosis and erythroid hyperplasia and increased folate requirements.

Table 26.   Classification of haemolytic anaemias.

Intrinsic red cell disorders	Extrinsic red cell disorders
Membrane disorder *Hereditary spherocytosis; hereditary elliptocytosis	**Immune** *Isoimmune* Mismatched transfusion, haemolytic disease of the new *Autoimmune* (i) Warm antibodies —Idiopathic —Secondary (CLL, SLE, lymphoma, carcinoma, (
Enzyme deficiency *G6PD; pyruvate kinase	
Haemoglobinopathy Sickle cell anaemia; thalassaemia	(ii) Cold—agglutinins —Idiopathic —Secondary (Mycoplasma, glandular fever, lymph —Lysis
	Non-immune March haemoglobinuria; postcardiotomy; microangiopathic haemolytic anaemia (thrombotic thrombocytopenic purpura); paroxysmal nocturnal haemoglobulinuria (page 361)

*Denotes most frequent

Hereditary spherocytosis

An autosomal dominant disorder which causes increased osmotic fragility and produces spherocytes in the peripheral blood. Patients present with intermittent jaundice which may be confused with Gilbert's syndrome or recurrent hepatitis. Gallstones, leg ulcers, splenomegaly and haemolytic or aplastic crises during intercurrent infections may occur.

Splenectomy relieves the symptoms but does not cure the underlying defect.

Hereditary elliptocytosis

This is also inherited as an autosomal dominant and produces elliptical RBCs, variable degrees of haemolysis and rarely splenomegaly.

Glucose-6-phosphate dehydrogenase (G6PD) deficiency

A disease found in Africa, the Mediterranean, the Middle and Far East. Inheritance is sex-linked on the X chromosome (i.e. affected males always show clinical manifestations but females will have variable degrees of haemolysis). Because of the phenomenon of random inactivation of the X chromosome, females will have two populations of red blood cells (RBCs), one normal and one G6PD-deficient: the susceptibilty to haemolysis will be greater, the greater the size of the deficient population. In the UK, acute haemolytic episodes are usually drug-induced (sulphonamides, primaquine) or occur during acute infections. Other features are neonatal jaundice and favism.

The diagnosis is confirmed by reduced or absent enzyme activity in the red cells.

Haemoglobinopathies

Adult haemoglobin (HbA) is 95% of haemoglobin in adults and possesses two α and two β chains ($\alpha_2\beta_2$).

Fetal haemoglobin (HbF) is <0.5% of haemoglobin in adults and possesses two α and two γ chains ($\alpha_2\gamma_2$).

Sickle cell haemoglobin (HbS) possesses two α and two abnormal β chains

Haemoglobin A_2(HbA$_2$) is <3% of haemoglobin in adults and possesses two α and two δ chains ($\alpha_2\delta_2$)

Sickle cell disease

A disease found in Africa, the Middle East, Mediterranean and India, transmitted as an autosomal dominant. Sickle cell trait occurs in heterozygotes (HbA–HbS) whose haemoglobin contains characteristically 60% HbA and 40% HbS. Patients with the trait are usually symptom-free except when the oxygen tension is very low, e.g. altitude and anoxic anaesthesia. The outlook is excellent. The prevalence of the gene is probably because the S haemoglobin protects against the serious and occasionally lethal effects of falciparum malaria.

Sickle cell anaemia occurs in homozygotes (HbS–HbS) and the abnormal haemoglobin renders the RBCs susceptible to very small reductions in oxygen tension leading to the sickling phenomenon and abnormal sequestration with thrombosis in small arterioles with subsequent infarction which may affect any part of the body.

Clinical features

Anaemia occurs within the first months of life as levels of HbF fall. Acute haemolytic crises begin after 6 months causing bone infarcts which are common, and children may present with pain and swelling in the fingers and toes (dactylitis). Infarcts may cause abdominal pain, haematuria or cerebrovascular accidents. Splenic infarction is common and by the age of 1 most children are functionally asplenic. Repeated renal infarction causes tubular damage and failure to concentrate urine compounding sickle cell crises.

Prognosis

The disease carries a high infant and child mortality from thrombosis to a vital organ or infection, with pneumococcus the most common as a result of hyposplenism. Children who survive beyond 4–5 years continue to have chronic ill health with anaemia, haemolytic and thrombotic crises, leg ulcers and infections (which may precipitate crises), and rarely survive beyond 35–40 years. Folate supplements are required throughout life. Pneumococcal vaccine should be given and penicillin prescribed to reduce mortality from *Pneumococcus*.

Thalassaemia

Thalassaemia is found in the Middle and Far East and the Mediterranean, and is due to deficient α or β chain synthesis.

The deficiency is genetically determined and results in α thalassaemia or β thalassaemia. In the latter, γ chains continue to be produced in excess into adult life and excess fetal haemoglobin (HbF) is present.

Beta thalassaemia minor trait (heterozygote)

This often produces no symptoms or a mild microcytic hypochromic anaemia which may be confused with iron deficiency. It is diagnosed by finding a raised HbA_2 level generally (4–7%). HbF levels may also be slightly raised (1–3%).

Beta thalassaemia major (homozygote)

Both parents possess the trait. Patients are relatively normal at birth (little β chain anyway) but develop severe anaemia later with failure to thrive and are prone to infection. The anaemia is hypochromic and the film contains target cells (Mexican hat cells) and stippling. Erythroid hyperplasia occurs in the marrow and chain precipitation appears as inclusion bodies on supravital staining.

Infants who survive develop hepatosplenomegaly, bossing of the skull, brittle and overgrown long bones, gallstones and leg ulcers.

Treatment consists of transfusion to maintain the Hb at 10 g/dl but this, combined with increased iron absorption results in iron overload. Desferrioxamine is given to reduce haemosiderosis (page 258) with folic acid replacement, and splenectomy may be indicated if hypersplenism supervenes. Bone marrow transplantation has been used successfully.

Paroxysmal nocturnal haemoglobinuria

A rare disorder in which a clone of red cells is more sensitive to lysis by plasma complement, particularly in an acid environment. The clinical features occur in the over-30s who develop paroxysmal haemolysis (with anaemia, macrocytosis, reticulocytosis, haemoglobinuria and haemosiderinuria). There is a tendency to intravascular thrombosis. Patients may become pancytopenic because the membrane abnormality also affects the other cell lines.

Ham's acid lysis test is positive and the red cell acetylcholinesterase reduced.

Anaemia secondary to chronic disease (ASCD)

There is an anaemia down to about 10 g/dl, usually normocytic (though sometimes slightly microcytic), associated in particular with chronic infection, malignant disease, chronic renal failure and the collagen diseases. The serum iron is characteristically reduced, and so is the transferrin ('iron binding capacity')—unlike the findings in iron deficiency anaemia. The marrow iron stores are increased, but the iron is not incorporated fully into red cell precursors. The ESR is usually raised (and also ferritin and other acute phase proteins). Haematinics have no significant effect. ASCD can be complicated by true iron deficiency anaemia, for instance when rheumatoid arthritis is treated with NSAIDs, or collagen disease with steroids, because blood loss may occur from gastric erosions or an ulcer.

Marrow aplasia

Patients present with anaemia and/or spontaneous bleeding due to lack of platelets and/or infection due to lack of polymorphonuclear granulocytes. A peripheral blood film reveals a pancytopenia though one cell line may be affected more than the others. A bone marrow aspiration is performed. If it is difficult to aspirate (possible myelofibrosis or malignancy), a trephine biopsy may be necessary to obtain a diagnostic specimen of marrow. The drugs which most commonly cause marrow suppression include phenylbutazone (now only on hospital prescription), indomethacin, chloramphenicol, and cytotoxic drugs. 50% are idiopathic. Remember ionising radiation.

Some marrow suppression is associated with uraemia, rheumatoid arthritis and hypothyroidism.

Myelodysplastic syndrome (MDS) refers to peripheral cytopenia with cellular marrow. It presents mostly as a serendipitous finding on a routine peripheral blood film, usually as macrocytosis (with normal B_{12}, folates, liver and thyroid function tests, and γ-GT). Less commonly, it may present as a refractory anaemia, pancytopenia, neutropenia, or thrombocytopenia. Marrow examination shows a dysmyelopoietic picture with excess blasts—with normal or increased cellularity.

There are six major subgroups with decreasingly satisfactory prognoses:
- Refractory anaemia with sideroblasts (RAS)—with >15% ringed sideroblasts, but none in the periphery
- Refractory anaemia (RA). Less than 5% blasts in a dyserythropoietic marrow, but no blasts in the peripheral blood

- Refractory anaemia with excess blasts (RAEB)—amounting to 5–20% nucleated marrow cells
- Refractory anaemia in transformation (RAEB-t)—with 20–30% sideroblasts or >5% in the periphery or of Auer's rods in the blast cells regardless of the marrow blast count
- Chronic myelomonocytic leukaemia (CMML)—with a peripheral monocyte count $>1 \times 10^9$ and monocytic precursors in the marrow. Philadelphia chromosome negative
- Acute myeloblastic leukaemia (AML)

Treatment

Haematinics have usually been tried and found to be ineffective. Blood transfusion is necessary and has to be repeated regularly.

Prognosis depends on the occasional transformation to blasts and is then that of the leukaemia, with bone marrow failure.

Complications

Anaemia (requiring the transfusion of about 1 unit of blood per week), infection, haemorrhage and blast transformation.

LEUKAEMIAS

Acute lymphatic leukaemia (ALL)

Clinical features

A severe disorder occurring at any age but more common in children and adolescents who present with features of:
- Marrow infiltration, with anaemia (exhaustion, lethargy and pallor), thrombocytopenia (purpura and spontaneous bleeding) and granulocytopenia (infection, e.g. sore throat)
- Lymphatic tissue infiltration, with lymphadenopathy and hepatosplenomegaly
- Infiltration into other tissues such as nervous tissue

Diagnosis

The WBC count may be very high or normal and the platelets usually reduced. Lymphoblasts may or may not be present in the peripheral blood but are always present in the bone marrow.

Management

Specific therapy is aimed at including remission by combinations of cytotoxic agents and irradiation of the CNS (leukaemia is often present in the CNS when the patient presents). Many drugs are currently under trial. Weekly vincristine with daily prednisolone with asparaginase, daunorubicin or doxorubicin is the regime most commonly used and is combined with cranial irradiation and intrathecal methotrexate after the blast cells have disappeared. Remission, as judged by absence of blast cells in the marrow, is usual, and a 5-year survival of 80% can be expected in children. Children who survive this long and remain in complete remission throughout are probably 'cured'. The prognosis of adults is much worse. Maintenance therapy is with cytotoxic agents such as 6-mercaptopurine or methotrexate. Bone marrow transplantation remains an experimental procedure though the results are improving rapidly. Opportunistic infection occasionally with unusual organisms such as TB, *Pseudomonas, Clostridium difficile, Pneumocystis carinii, Monilia, Aspergillus, Cryptococcus* or cytomegalovirus remains a constant danger and must be treated urgently and energetically. Live vaccines should be avoided.

NB Leukaemic patients are treated best in units with specialist experience who are also in the best position to evaluate different drug regimens, to treat the complications of cytotoxic drugs and the uncommon secondary infections which they may promote, and who have optimum experience with marrow transplantation.

Chronic lymphatic leukaemia (CLL)

Clinical features

A disease of the over-50s in which there may be no clinical symptoms or signs, CLL being detected on investigation for other reasons, e.g. preoperative blood count. About 60% of patients have features of anaemia, fever and intercurrent infection. Examination may show pallor, lymphadenopathy and splenomegaly and, rarely, pleural or pericardial effusions, and infiltration of skin or salivary glands. There is an increased incidence of epithelial malignancies, e.g. gut, bronchus.

Diagnosis

Investigation shows anaemia (which may be partially haemolytic and Coombs' positive), granulocytopenia and thrombocytopenia, and a raised peripheral lymphocyte count of more than 5×10^9/litre or a marrow with more than 40% lymphocytes.

Management

Patients who are free of symptoms, signs and other haematological abnormality do not require treatment. If symptoms occur, chlorambucil (0.2 mg/kg daily or 6–10 mg daily for 2 weeks every month) combined if necessary with radiotherapy to reduce the size of large masses of glands. Prednisolone may be used especially if haemolysis is present. Intercurrent infection is a potentially serious complication, especially during drug therapy with immunosuppressive agents. It is less frequent than in acute lymphoblastic leukaemia (ALL) or acute myeloid leukaemia (AML). Symptom-free patients may remain healthy for 15–20 years. The overall 5-year survival is 50%.

Acute myeloid leukaemia (AML)

Clinical features

An extremely serious disease affecting all ages but less common in childhood. Patients present with features of:

Infection: sore throat, 'influenza', septicaemia.

Leukaemic infiltration: anaemia, thrombocytopenia (bleeding gums), granulocytopenia (infection typically with ulceration of the throat) and skin rash.

The diagnosis is made on finding myeloblast cells in the peripheral blood or the marrow.

Management

Untreated the patients rarely survive more than a few months. Even with intensive therapy the outlook is only about 1–2 years. Currently, cytosine arabinoside, 6-thioguanine and daunorubicin may be expected to give an initial remission of 75%. Of these, the 5-year survival is 35–40%. Anaemia and intercurrent infection as in ALL partly secondary to leukaemia and also drug-induced are serious complications. Improved survival figures are partly due to better supportive care with newer antibiotics and platelet and granulocyte infusions. Marrow transplantation after marrow ablation by radiotherapy has been successfully achieved.

Chronic myeloid leukaemia (CML)

Clinical features

This usually present in the 30–50s with an insidious onset of anaemia, leading to weight loss and fever. Marrow infiltration may cause bone pain, thrombocytopenia (with bleeding), and granulocytopenia (with intercurrent infection). The spleen and sometimes the liver are greatly enlarged and abdominal pain may result from splenic infarcts.

Investigation

The WBC count may be very high (e.g. 500×10^9/litre). The marrow possesses large numbers of myeloid precursors and mature granulocytes—as compared with AML where the cells are myeloblasts.

The Philadelphia chromosome is seen as a specific small abnormal chromosome (a No. 22 with the long arms translocated to No. 9) and is present in virtually all cases and is diagnostic.

Management

Busulphan (Myleran) is the drug of first choice. After a time (median 2–3 years), blastic transformation occurs to ALL or AML. This is almost always highly resistant to therapy. Marrow transplantation offers the only hope of cure. Infection, often with opportunistic organisms (page 363), must be treated energetically but is uncommon.

MULTIPLE MYELOMATOSIS

This is one of the paraproteinaemias. It occurs usually after the age of 50 years. It is a malignant disorder of plasma cells in the bone marrow which produce an excessive amount of an immunoglobulin, usually IgG (but also IgA or IgM) and often including light chains from this molecule (present as Bence–Jones

protein). The clinical features are due to:
- the abnormal protein: greatly raised ESR, renal failure, infections
- bone involvement: bone pain, fractures, hypercalcaemia
- marrow replacement: normocytic anaemia, leucopenia, thrombocytopenia—
infection especially zoster during treatment

Diagnosis

Diagnosis depends on the presence of at least two of the three major criteria: (a) The bone marrow aspirate is often diagnostic with an excess (>30%) of plasma cells, (b) Plasma protein electrophoresis will usually show a myeloma band in the gamma region, with immunosuppression, and immunoelectrophoresis of plasma and urine will characterise the type and degree of immunoglobulin abnormality present, and (c) Bone X-rays may show typical multiple osteolytic areas. Occasionally, a 'benign paraproteinaemia', virtually always IgG, may occur with <30 g/litre and without any of the other diagnostic features of myeloma. It is rarely significant but should always be followed up because myeloma may develop. Even when there are bone lesions, the alkaline phosphotase is classically normal.

Treatment

Therapy with combinations of melphalan (or cyclophosphamide), prednisolone, doxorubicin, BCNU, or vincristine are used, with radiotherapy to bone lesions. Infections are especially common during therapy with immunosuppressive agents and they must be investigated and treated urgently. A high fluid intake may protect the kidneys.

HODGKIN'S DISEASE

Clinical features

The usual presentation is painless enlargement of a group of rubbery superficial lymph nodes, commonly in the cervical chain. The disease may spread to involve the remainder of the reticuloendothelial system including the liver and spleen. There may be systemic symptoms of anaemia (which usually is normochromic, noromocytic but sometimes haemolytic), fever, anorexia, weight loss, night sweats, and pruritus. The diagnosis is made on lymph node biopsy.

Staging

The choice of therapy in Hodgkin's disease depends upon the clinical staging. In terms of prognosis it is important to know whether the disease has spread beyond the clinically observed regions, and in some centres laparotomy with liver biopsy is performed. A CT scan above and below the diaphragm can avoid the need for laparotomy:

I   A single region (usually one side of the neck).

II   Two regions involved on the same side of the diaphragm.

III Disease above and below diaphragm but limited to the reticuloendothelial system (nodes, spleen) excluding the liver.

IV Widespread disease involving bone marrow, liver, and lung.

Subclasses of each stage indicate the absence—class A—or presence—class B—of systemic symptoms of weight loss (>10% in 6 months), fever (>38°C), or night sweats.

Treatment

Stages IA and IIA are treated by radiotherapy. Chemotherapy is given to all others. About 80% of patients so treated survive 5 years and 60% of the original number are 'disease free'. The presence of symptoms worsens the prognosis, and the absence or deficiency of lymphocytes in the histological section indicates a very poor outlook, whereas the outlook is very good if lymphocytes are the predominant cell type.

NON-HODGKIN'S LYMPHOMA

A heterogeneous group of lymphomas which occurs most frequently between 50 and 80 years. It may present as Hodgkin's disease but tends to be more widespread in the body and the mediastinum is less frequently involved. The commonest presentation is lymphadenopathy but other tissues are commonly (25%) the site of presentation i.e. skin, gut, marrow, testis and CNS. Diagnosis is based on lymph node biopsy, and classification depends partly on whether the lymphocytes are T-cell or B-cell derived. There may or may not be destruction of normal architecture and Dorothy Reed-Sternberg cells are absent. Staging is similar to Hodgkin's disease, though histology is more important for prognosis in non-Hodgkin's lymphoma. Treatment is with radiotherapy and chemotherapy but the outlook is worse than with Hodgkin's disease.

INFECTIOUS MONONUCLEOSIS

Glandular fever. A common disease of the young with an excellent prognosis, usually transmitted by saliva and mouth to mouth contact ('the kissing disease') and associated with the Epstein–Barr virus, the agent which is associated with Burkitt's lymphoma.

Clinical presentation

An influenzal-type illness with malaise, fever, muscle and joint aches and sore throat. Examination reveals a dirty tonsillar exudate and palatal petechiae with generalised lymphadenopathy and splenomegaly. A macular–papular rash is common, and more frequent if ampicillin is given for the sore throat. Mesenteric adenitis with appendicitis may occur.

Investigation

The disease is confirmed by a leucocytosis with 60–80% of atypical mononuclear cells (large cells with granular nuclei and blue foamy cytoplasm—glandular fever cells), and a positive 'monospot' or raised Epstein–Barr virus antibodies. Thrombocytopenia and abnormal liver function tests are common but virtually never severe.

Complications

Tonsillar swelling may be very severe and even prevent swallowing of saliva. Lethargy may last for up to 6 months.

Differential diagnosis

The disease may be confused with:
- Acute tonsillitis
- Infections which produce a similar rash, e.g. measles, rubella, secondary syphilis
- Infections which produce similar malaise and lymphadenopathy, e.g. toxoplasmosis, brucellosis and tuberculosis
- Diseases associated with immunosuppression (page 384) such as lymphomas and leukaemias especially when treated; patients with transplants on steroids, azathioprine, and cyclosporin; acquired immune deficiency syndrome (AIDS)—where persistent lymphadenopathy, Kaposi's sarcoma and opportunistic infection particularly with pneumocystis pneumonia are common features
- Drug hypersensivity
- Acute appendicitis
- Acute leukaemia on finding lymphocytosis with atypical cells in a patient with splenomegaly and thrombocytopenia
- Hodgkin's disease

NB   Diphtheria should not be forgotten.

Treatment

Usually rest, aspirin gargles, anaesthetic lozenges and ice-cream for the sore throat are sufficient. If the tonsillar enlargement is great and swallowing very difficult (anginose glandular fever—usually with severe general symptoms) a short course of steroids (prednisolone 40 mg daily reducing by 10 mg daily and stopping after 4 days) rapidly reduces the symptoms.

POSTVIRAL SYNDROME

It is well-recognised after glandular fever, but also follows infection with influenza, *Mycoplasma (pneumoniae)*, *Streptococcus* (sore throat) and other common infections. The usual common feature is exhaustion on minimal exertion sometimes with myalgia occurring in a previously fit person without a history of clear depression or anxiety syndromes. There are no helpful physical signs. Patients often become depressed and may be considered to be malingering. There is no diagnostic test (enterovirus in stool or in muscle on electron microscopy are unproven). Routine tests including WBC, ESR, C-reactive protein (CRP), thyroid function tests (TFTs), chest X-ray (CXR) are normal. The differential diagnosis includes primary depression, hypothyroidism, Addison's disease and possibly underlying lymphoma. The prognosis is usually excellent though the exhaustion can persist for many months and even years. A very small number never recover and remain severely disabled.

Drug overdoses

Self-administered drug poisoning accounts for 10% of all acute medical admissions to hospital. Accidental poisoning is common in children and drugs are best kept in 'child-proof' containers out of their reach. In adults the common drugs taken are: the tricyclic antidepressants (e.g. amitriptyline, nortriptyline protriptyline), the benzodiazepines (e.g. diazepam, nitrazepam, chlordiazep oxide), household substances (e.g. bleach, detergents), paracetamol, coprox amol and aspirin. Barbiturates are now less commonly abused. The weedkiller paraquat and insecticides (e.g. organophosphates) are occasionally taken accidentally. Carbon monoxide poisoning from domestic gas no longer occurs in areas where North Sea gas is used and carbon monoxide poisoning is usually now due to incomplete combustion from blocked flues and car exhausts.

Clinical presentation (table 27, pages 370–371)
Most patients who take overdoses are still conscious when seen and will usually state which tablets they have taken and/or bring the bottle. If unconscious, the other causes of coma must be considered even if a bottle is found in the pockets (see page 123). It is well worth searching for a diabetic (to exclude hypoglycaemia) or steroid card, or a hospital outpatient card. Relatives or friends may know whether the patient is currently under treatment. Patients often take more than one drug and very often alcohol in addition.

Management
1 Maintain the airways and ventilation.
2 Remove the drug with emetics if fully conscious or by gastric lavage with tracheal intubation if not (except with corrosives), and diuresis or dialysis if indicated (table 28, page 373).
3 General care of the unconscious patient—nursing, physiotherapy, fluid balance, maintenance of renal function and treatment of shock.
4 Psychiatric assessment.
5 Poisons centres.

Ventilation
After ensuring that the airway is clear the patient should be admitted to hospital. It may be necessary to insert an endotracheal tube and give oxygen. Artificial ventilation is rarely necessary but spontaneous ventilation should be assessed regularly and the decision to ventilate decided on the basis of a falling minute ventilation (e.g. <4 litres/min)

NB Severe respiratory depression from morphine or dextropropoxyphene is reversed with naloxone.

Remove poison from stomach and blood

The object is to remove drugs before they are absorbed. Gastric lavage is used in most centres. Forced vomiting is less efficient in removing tablets though more commonly used in paediatric practice and should only be performed in the conscious. It is very important to explain what is happening to the patient and friends and relatives because the procedure is frightening and unpleasant.

The head of the bed should be lowered and, in unconscious patients, the trachea intubated and the cuff inflated to prevent inhalation.
Specimens should be saved from gastric lavage for identification, and blood levels of likely poisons determined if these may be useful guides to determining the need for intensive therapy, e.g. forced alkaline diuresis.

Alkaline diuresis and dialysis. The alkalinity is more important than the quantity of urine and a normal urine output is adequate for effect (1.5–2 litre/24 h) though it seems reasonable to load the circulation at the onset if the cardiovascular system is stable and can cope. Salicylates in severe overdose may be removed by alkaline diuresis, and also by peritoneal dialysis or haemodialysis: amitriptyline, diazepam, nitrazepam and paracetamol cannot. The decision to use these techniques depends upon the patient's general condition, particularly if this is deteriorating. It is useful to know the initial blood level of salicylate because an initially high level in a deteriorating patient is an indication for diuresis or dialysis. Contraindications are renal failure, shock and heart failure. The value of these techniques for other specific poisons may be obtained by contacting specialist poisons centres.

In paracetamol overdose, the use of oral methionine or intravenous N-acetylcysteine is determined by (a) the initial blood level; and (b) the time after ingestion using standard charts that are available for reference (usually pinned to casualty department notice boards).

Care of the unconscious patient and shock

Expert nursing is essential and aimed at care of the airway and prevention of chest infection and bed sores. Fluid intake and output, and assessment of renal function may be critical, particularly if the patient is hypotensive. This is commonly seen with barbiturate and phenothiazine poisoning. Most young patients will maintain good renal function at a systolic blood pressure of 80 mmHg and sometimes less. In the elderly or if there is doubt about renal perfusion, monitor the central venous pressure to detect hypovolaemia (maintain at 2–5 cm of water) and continously monitor the urine output.

Chest infections due to inhalation or recumbency should be treated energetically with physiotherapy and antibiotics.

Psychiatric assessment

When the patient has recovered a careful assessment is required with the object of aiding the acute problem and preventing further attempts. About 10% of patients who take overdoses seriously intend suicide and 10–20% take a further overdose. It is useful to interview family and friends about the immediate

Table 27.   Clinical features of common drug overdose

Drug	Clinical features	Notes
Aspirin	Hyperventilation, visual disturbance, tinnitus, nausea, vomiting, acidosis	May be well on admission and later very ill Bicarbonate IV for severe acidosis
Barbiturates	Drowsiness and coma, hypotension, hypoventilation, red wheals on pressure points of limbs, wide dilated pupils, absent reflexes	Most patients require supportive therapy only. Ventilation rarely required
Digoxin	N&V arrhythmias	Common if potassium levels are reduced (diuretic therapy)
Benzodiazepines	Drowsiness to coma	Rarely fatal and very rarely requires ventilation (potentiated by alcohol)
Phenothiazines (e.g. chlorpromazine)	Hypotension, hypothermia, arrhythmias and dystonic movements; respiratory and cerebral depression	May require: 1. Diazepam for fits 2. Anti-arrhythmics 3. Orphenadrine for dystonia
β-blockers	Bradycardia and shock	Glucagon for severe reduced blood pressure 10 mg i.v. infusion 3 mg/h
Lithium	Nausea, vomiting, muscle tremor, rigidity and twitching with or without nystagmus and dystharia Apathy proceeding to coma	
Tricyclic antidepressants	Dry mouth, convulsions, arrhythmias, fits, respiratory depression, coma, dilated pupils	1. Diazepam for hyperexcitability 2. Physostigmine to block anticholinergic effects
Paracetamol	Hepatotoxicity is usually apparent at 48 h (LFTs prothrombin time)	Monitor liver function for up to 2 weeks if initially abnormal
Paraquat	Respiratory failure 10–14 days later	Oral Fuller's Earth, followed by oral MgSO$_4$
Morphine and heroin	Hypoventilation, perspiration, pin-point pupils	Injection marks
Iron	Nausea and vomiting, agitation, liver damage	Usually seen in children Chelate gastric iron with desferrioxamine solution for gastric lavage. Chelate absorbed iron with desferrioxamine i.m.
Methanol and ethylene glycol	Blurred vision, acidosis	Gastric lavage with 3% HCO$_3$ and give ethanol to block methanol–acetaldehyde

background and their willingness to help in care after discharge. The patient may admit to planning a future suicidal attempt and a lack of plans for the future may be evidence of depression. The patient should be asked about:

• previous depression and suicide attempts

Diuresis or dialysis	Specific antidotes

Alkaline diuresis successful
Start if initial blood level over
   2.8 mmol/litre (500 mg./litre) or
   if condition deteriorates
	Nil

Rarely required	Nil
Not indicated	Fab digoxin-specific antibody fragments
No value	Flumazenil
No value	Nil
No value	Prenalterol

Forced diuresis or haemodialysis if
   concentration is 5 mmol/litre
   acutely
	Nil

No value	Nil
	N-acetylcysteine i.v. Methionine p.o.
Haemodialysis early (about 6 h) if more than minimal quantities	
No value	Naloxone 0.01–0.02 mg/kg i.v. repeated as necessary
No value	Desferrioxamine
With heavier intoxication	Ethanol

- personal instability with a history of many jobs and different personal relationships
- evidence of schizophrenic personality and schizophrenic thoughts
- family history of depression, schizophrenia, alcohol abuse

- social history, especially living alone

NB   (a) Both aspirin poisoning and hypoglycaemia produce sweating; (b) both aspirin poisoning and diabetic ketoacidosis produce confusion, hyperventilation and glycosuria; (c) most patients with drug overdose rarely require more than active supportive therapy; and (d) keep drugs away from children.

Specialist centres

Advice about poisons, dangerous blood levels and the optimum treatment may be obtained at all times from specialist poisons centres.

Centre	Telephone number(s)
London	071 407 7600 or 071 635 9191
Edinburgh	031 229 2477 or 031 228 6907
Dublin	0001 379964 or 0001 379966
Cardiff	0222 709901
Leeds	0532 430715 or 0532 432799
Manchester	061 740 2254
Newcastle	091 232 5131 or 091 232 1525 (working hours only)
Belfast	0232 231947 or 0232 240503 (working hours only)

Imported diseases and infections

Within the community virus infections of the upper respiratory and gastrointestinal tract are the most common, followed by common virus infections usually of children such as measles, german measles, chickenpox and mumps, and the venereal diseases. Infections seen more frequently in hospitals usually relate easily to a single body system and are dealt with there. (Pneumonia page 291, carditis page 176, gastroenteritis page 52, hepatitis page 249, pyelonephritis page 242, and meningitis page 138, and see table 16, pages 140–141).

Less frequent, but in diagnostic and management terms more difficult, are the imported diseases, septicaemia, pyrexia of unknown origin and infections of the immune-suppressed (see pages 378 and 384). The common infections, likely organisms and antibiotics of choice are shown in table 29 (pages 374–375).

IMPORTED DISEASES

The common diseases of travellers (table 28) returning to temperate climates are malaria, acute gastroenteritis including typhoid and worm infestation. Diarrhoea in returning travellers requires investigation for worms and parasites (especially *Giardia* and *Amoeba*) but usually no organism is found and the symptoms settle spontaneously or with simple therapy. Other diseases common in the tropics but rarely seen in returning travellers include infectious hepatitis, tuberculosis, schistosomiasis, hydatid disease, poliomyelitis, tetanus, cholera, leprosy and trypanosomiasis.

Table 28. Diseases of the returning traveller

Common	Malaria
	Typhoid
	Diarrhoea (page 52) often viral as pathogens rarely found but consider:
	Giardia lamblia and worms
	Amoebic colitis ⎫ which must be distinguished from
	Salmonella and ⎬ ulcerative colitis and Crohn's disease
	Shigella infection ⎭
	Tropical sprue (page 273)
	Infectious hepatitis
Rare	TB—usually not acute and more likely in Asian immigrants
	Amoebic liver abscess
	Hydatid liver cyst
Exceedingly rare	Rabies
	Cholera
	Exotic viruses—Lassa fever
	Marburg
	Ebola

Table 29. Common infections and antibiotics of first choice

Infection	Likely organism	Antibacterial of choice (adult doses whilst awaiting microbiolo⟨
(a) ENT		
Sore throat	Viral	Nil
	Haemolytic streptococcus (*Streptococcus pyogenes*)	Pencillin V oral 250 mg qds (i.m. × 1 or 2 doses initially if severe) or erythromycin 250 mg qds if allergic to penicillin
Sinusitis	*Strep. pneumoniae* (pneumococcus) *Haemophilus influenzae*	Amoxycillin 250–500 mg tds, cotrimoxazole 2 bd or trimethoprim 200 mg bd
Otitis media	As above plus haemolytic streptococcus *H. influenzae* in under fives	Amoxycillin under 5 years old: 20 mg/kg/24 h
Acute epiglottitis	*H. influenzae*	Maintain airway plus cefotaxime or chloramphenicol
Urinary tract		
Acute cystitis	*E. coli* (85%)	Trimethoprim 200 mg bd or cotrimoxazole 2 bd
Acute pyelonephritis	*Proteus vulgaris* (5%)	

NB   Recurrent infection or 'odd' organisms, e.g. *Klebsiella, Pseudomonas*, suggest an underlying abnormalit⟨ such as stone or tumour and further investigation is required. It is rarely possible to clear infection if there is a⟨ indwelling catheter (only treat if systemically ill). It is best to remove it if possible, and if not try instilling a⟨ antiseptic, e.g. chlorhexidine 0.2%. Antibiotic use encourages the development of resistant organisms.
NB   Persistent bacteriuria is difficult to eradicate but patients can be kept relatively symptom free with regular dail⟨ ampicillin 500 mg or nitrofurantoin 100 mg *nocte* or cotrimoxazole 1 tablet *nocte*.

(b) Bone and soft tissue		
Cellulitis	Haemolytic streptococcus *Staph. aureus*	Cloxacillin 500 mg qds, flucloxacillin 250–500 mg qds⟨ orally (by injection initially if
Drip sites	*Staph. aureus*	severe) for 7–10 days
Erysipelas	Haemolytic streptococcus	Penicillin (by injection initially for 24–48 h)
Osteomyelitis	*Staph. aureus* *H. influenzae* in under fives	Flucloxacillin or cloxacillin by injection plus amoxycillin in under fives

NB   Treatment of osteomyelitis may be started by injection for 5–7 days depending upon response and may need⟨ to continue for about 6 weeks.

(c) Gastrointestinal infections		
Acute gastroenteritis	Viral	Nil
	Campylobacter	Erythromycin 250–500 mg qds for 7 days
Dysentry	Bacillary (*Shigella* species)	Ciprofloxacin (or chloramphenicol or ampicillin or cotrimoxazole) If septicaemic doses as for typhoid
	Amoebic-entamoeba histolytica	Metronidazole 800 mg 8-hourly for 5 days
Typhoid	*Salmonella typhi*	If septicaemic ciprofloxacin 200 mg bd i.v. for 24 hours, then 500 mg bd to complete 10–14 days. (Chloramphenicol, ampicillin or cotrimoxazole are alternatives.)

Table 29. (Continued)

Infection	Likely organism	Antibacterial of choice (adult doses whilst awaiting microbiology)
Salmonella food poisoning	*Salmonella* species (>1000)	Nil (usually) unless septicaemic
Pseudomembranous colitis	*Clostridium difficile*	Metronidazole 400 tds or Vancomycin 500 mg qds orally for 7 days
Acute cholangitis	*E. coli*	Penicillin plus gentamicin or cefotaxime (one-third of biliary coliform resistant to ampicillin/amoxycillin)

NB Patients with mild gastroenteritis without systemic illness or suspected systemic infection and who are excreting *Shigella* or *Salmonella* (including *S. typhi*) do not require antibiotics. The major problem is usually dehydration which may lead to deep venous thrombosis and pulmonary embolism in adults. Children need fluid and electrolyte replacement. Dioralyte sachets or electrosol tablets (which contain no dextrose) dissolved in water are satisfactory except in severe depletion.

(d)   Chest infections

In hospital practice Gram-stain of sputum may identify the organism

Acute bronchitis	Viral	Nil
Acute on chronic bronchitis	Bacterial	Amoxycillin 250–500 mg qds
	(*H. influenzae*)	Cotrimoxazole 2 bd
	(*Strep. pneumoniae*)	Trimethoprin 200 g bd
Bronchopneumonia (off the streets)	*Strep. pneumoniae* *Mycoplasma pneumoniae* *Legionella pneumoniae* (rare *H. influenzae* 5% psittacosis)	Erythromycin 500 mg–1g qds
If very unwell or immuno-suppressed consider		
	Coliforms *Klebsiella* Staphylococci during flu epidemics	Erythromycin plus third generation cephalosporin (cefotaxime, cefoxitime)
	Pneumocystis in AIDS	Pentamidine by inhalation Septrin by mouth or i.v.
Meningitis (adult)—most are viral (90%)		
Viral		
Herpes simplex		Acyclovir
Bacterial		
Pneumococcal Meningococcal	*Strep. pneumoniae* } N. meningitidis	Penicillin by injection in large doses 12/20 g/24 h for 5–10 days
Haemophilus (more common in children)	*H. influenzae*	Cefotaxime 4–8 g daily (adult) (Chloramphenicol by injection 1 g 6–8 hourly in adults 50–100 mg/kg/24 h in hourly doses (children) is an alternative)

MALARIA

A disease of the subtropics and where the anopheline mosquito is found. Transmission is via the mosquito which carries infected blood from infected to uninfected man. The mosquito lives chiefly between latitude 15° north and south and not more than 5000 feet above sea level.

Clinical features

The patient presents with fever and rigors usually within 4 weeks of returning from or travelling through a malarial zone. Occasionally symptoms may not develop for 12 months or more. The patient has usually failed to take antimalarials regularly, not slept under mosquito nets or failed to continue prophylaxis for 6 weeks after returning. The fever may be tertian (a 3-day pattern with fever peaking every other day *(Plasmodium vivax* and *P. ovale)*, quartan (a 4-day pattern with fever peaking every third day), or subtertian (a non-specific febrile pattern: *P. falciparum)*. Diagnosis depends upon clinical awareness and then seeing the parasite in a blood film. The species of parasite may be differentiated by an experienced observer. In England, *P. falciparum* and *P. vivax* are most frequently seen in travellers from Africa and Asia. Malignant tertian malaria refers to *P. falciparum* which very occasionally produces high levels of parasitaemia (only *P. falciparum* gives RBC parasitaemia of >1–2%), serious complications of cerebral malaria or acute haemolysis and renal failure (blackwater fever).

Prophylaxis

Prophylaxis is by a combination of: (a) mosquito control, (b) sleeping under mosquito nets, and (c) specific prevention with proguanil (Paludrine) 200 mg daily, with chloroquine 300 mg twice weekly. For regions known to have chloroquine-resistant malaria, Malaprim (pyrimethamine with dapsone) or Fansidar (pyrimethamine with sulphadoxine) have been used, but now only under expert guidance because of serious and potentially lethal side-effects. Prophylaxis should be continued for 6 weeks after returning home.

NB   Before advising travellers, check whether they are entering a malarial zone, and seek advice from the nearest centre for tropical diseases about the current recommended prophylaxis because drug resistance, particularly of *P. falciparum* malaria is continually changing.

Treatment

Acute attacks

Patients with malaria should be given oral quinine. Intravenous quinine is potentially dangerous because it may produce cardiac asystole but is used in those who are vomiting or too ill to take oral therapy. Exchange transfusion may be required in very ill patients with high parasitaemia—consider levels above 10%. Some require full intensive care including treatment of cerebral oedema, renal and liver failure, and shock. Hypoglycaemia from a combination of liver failure and quinine-induced insulin secretion is easily overlooked; and pulmonary oedema from fluid overload is common in those treated for shock.

After treatment of the acute attack, falciparum malaria is cleared with Fansidar or tetracycline, and vivax with primaquine (check the glucose-6-phosphate dehydrogenase status first).

TYPHOID

Clinical features

Symptoms begin with malaise, headache, dry cough and vague abdominal pain, up to 21 days after returning from a typhoid area. Travellers to any area with poor sanitation are at risk and typhoid occasionally occurs in non-travellers. In the first week fever is marked with cough and constipation which are typical features. In the second week, the fever persists, the abdomen distends, diarrhoea may or may not occur and rose spots develop as crops of pale pink macules on the sides of the abdomen. Delirium and death (10%) may occur in the third week in untreated cases.

NB Symptoms of dry cough, constipation and fever should be sufficient to alert the clinician, particularly in returning holiday-makers.

Investigation

Leucopenia and neutropenia may or may not be present. Blood culture is mandatory if typhoid is suspected and culture of urine and stool should also be performed.

Treatment

Salmonella typhi responds to ciprofloxacin chloramphenicol, ampicillin or cotrimoxazole (Septrin). Ciprofloxacin is the drug of first choice.

NB (a) It is unnecessary to give antibiotics to patients who are clinically well, but from whom S. typhi is grown from the stools. If these patients are given antibiotics, they are more likely to become chronic excretors of resistant S. typhi (antibiotic-induced resistance), (b) typhoid must be reported to the public health authorities, and (c) excretors of S. typhi are not allowed to work in the food industry.

DYSENTERY

Bacillary dysentery

Bacillary dysentery is caused by the genus Shigella. Sonne is the most common and occurs in outbreaks in children's homes, and shiga produces the most serious clinical form of the disease including septicaemia.

It is transmitted by faecal contamination of food and water and 2–4 days after ingestion produces acute diarrhoea sometimes accompanied by abdominal colic, vomiting and tenesmus. If severe, there is rectal blood, mucus and pus.

Asymptomatic carriage can occur.

The disease is prevented by good sanitation and clean water supplies and good personal hygiene.

Infected patients should be isolated and rehydrated. Antibiotics (ampicillin, cotrimoxazole, ciprofloxacin or chloramphenicol) are required if the patient is septicaemic.

The public health service must be informed and patients and close contacts should not handle food until the stool cultures are negative.

Shigella dysentery can be confused with salmonella food poisoning, amoebic and ulcerative colitis (pages 52, 266).

Amoebic dysentery

An infection of the colon by the protozoon *Entamoeba histolytica*. In the acute dysenteric form, the illness begins suddenly with fever, abdominal pain, nausea, vomiting and diarrhoea containing mucus and blood. More commonly, amoebic colitis presents less acutely with intermittent diarrhoea with or without abdominal pain, mucus and blood.

The major complications are hepatic abscesses and pericolic amoebomas which can be confused with colonic carcinoma. The diagnosis is made by finding trophozoites or cysts in fresh faeces, rectal mucus or rectal biopsy and supported by a positive complement fixation test.

Metronidazole is the treatment of choice for all invasive forms of amoebiasis, but abscesses may have to be drained if they do not resolve on drug therapy. Diloxanide is used to eradicate chronic amoebic cysts.

Cyst excretors should not handle food, and the contacts screened. Acute amoebiasis can be confused with bacillary dysentery, salmonella food poisoning, and ulcerative colitis, and chronic infection with *giardia lamblia*, tropical sprue, ulcerative colitis and diverticular disease (page 275).

GIARDIASIS

Giardia lamblia is a flagellate protozoon which infects the small intestinal wall but not the blood. Viable cysts are ingested with contaminated food and may be excreted asymptomatically, or produce diarrhoea and steatorrhea.

The diagnosis is confirmed by the presence of trophozoites or cysts in stools or duodenal aspirates.

Tinidazole or metronidazole are the drugs of choice.

PYREXIA OF UNKNOWN ORIGIN (PUO)

There are many definitions of PUO. In practice, the difficulty arises when the cause is unidentified after the clear clinical possibilities have been excluded, and a basic set of tests performed. It is usually a hospital problem. A broad-spectrum antibiotic has usually been given. The causes are listed in Table 30 (page 380).

Special points in the history

- Exposure to infection (meals away from home, febrile illness in household contacts, unpasturised milk or cheese, undercooked eggs and poultry)
- Occupation, especially if a doctor or nurse (factitious fever). Farmer,

veterinary surgeon, sewer worker, forester, (for brucella, leptospira, anthrax, cat-bite fever, Lyme disease)
- Drug history, e.g antibiotics, methyldopa, hydralazine, phenytoin, including non-prescribed preparations
- Travel (malaria, amoebiasis), and sexual history
- Pets, including dogs, cats and birds

Special points in examination
NB Repeat regularly, e.g. on alternate days if the fever persists
- *Cardiovascular*. Murmurs, especially if changing, suggest infective endocarditis. Tender temporal arteries. Dressler's syndrome.
- *Respiratory*. Crackles (crepitations or rales) for early pneumonia (e.g. Legionnaire's). Sinuses. Consider recurrent pulmonary thromboembolic disease
- *Abdomen*. Palpable liver, gall bladder or spleen (with or without tenderness).
- *Musculoskeletal*. Muscle stiffness and tenderness of collagen diseases, e.g. polymyalgia rheumatica
- *Skin rashes* (drugs, rose spots of typhoid). Splinter haemorrhages, Osler's nodes.
- *Lymphatic*. Glands (all group)
- *Check all orifices*: mouth (teeth for apical abscesses, ears, perineum (anus and genito-urinary tract)

Basic screening tests already performed (check)
Most will need to be repeated until a diagnosis has been achieved.
- *Haemoglobin*. If anaemia is present and considerable, it is usually relevant. If iron deficient and there is no overt blood loss, exclude gut malignancy
- *White blood cell (WBC) count*. Neutrophilia is associated with pyogenic infection and neoplasia, and neutropenia with viral infection. Lymphocytosis may suggest tubercle. Leukaemia and infectious mononucleosis are usually associated with abnormal peripheral counts and cell types (remember direct tests for infectious mononucleosis. Eosinophilia may suggest parasites or polyarteritis nodosa
- *Erythrocyte sedimentation rate*. If over 100 mm/h, check for myeloma, polymyalgia rheumatica, and secondaries from carcinoma in bone or liver (also see page 95)
- *Mid-stream urine*. Haematuria, possibly microscopic, occurs with bacterial endocarditis, renal carcinoma, polyarteritis nodosa and leptospirosis. WBCs in infection. Early morning urine for acid-fast bacillus (AFB). **NB** Glycosuria suggests infection somewhere
- *Chest X-ray*. Carcinoma (primary or secondary) in lungs, and bone metastases. Miliary shadowing in miliary TB and sarcoid. Hilar nodes in TB, lymphoma, sarcoid and carcinoma
- Sputum for micrcoorganisms including AFB
- Liver function tests (LFTs) for secondary or primary malignancy, abscess, biliary disease, hepatitis (page 47)
- Infectious mononucleosis screening test e.g. Monospot
- Blood culture ($\times 3$)

Further tests commonly required as determined by clinical leads

- Agglutination/ELISA tests for Salmonellae, Brucella and Coxiella
- Viral, mycoplasma and HIV antibody titres immediately and 2 weeks later
- ASO titre and rheumatoid factors
- Autoimmune screen (etc)
- Sonar and/or CT scan of abdomen for liver abscesses, and for secondaries, for renal tumours and abscesses, and for splenic enlargement, and of the pelvis for pelvic lesions
- Echocardiography for vegetations
- Computerised tomography scanning of chest and abdomen for lymphadenopathy

Table 30. Mnemonic list (IMAGINE)

Infections	*Bacterial.* Bacilliary endocarditis and septicaemia (including 'culture-negative') *Collections of pus Subphrenic Intrahepatic Perirenal Pelvic Pleura Bone (osteomyelitis) *Viral/rickettsial* (including hepatitis B) *Protozoal* Malaria, amoeba, spirochaetes *Specific* TB* (all sites), typhoid, brucella, Lyme disease (*Borrelia burgdorferi*)
Malignancy	Kidney and liver (primary and secondary) Pancreas, micrometasases, lymphoma* (Hodgkin's and non-Hodgkin's), leukaemia
Autoimmune diseases	*Systemic lupus erythematosus, polyarteritis nodosa Chronic active hepatitis Rheumatoid disease, Still's disease (including adult Still's disease page 173)
Granulomata	Sarcoid Crohn's disease
Iatrogenic	Drug fever
Nurses—and doctors and all paramedicals	Factitious fever
Etcetera	Consult exhaustive lists in big books, but remember that the cause is more often a rare manifestation of a common disease than a common manifestation of a rare disease

*Denotes a more likely cause of PUO—all are treatable and all are potentially curable.

Invasive procedures as indicated
- Temporal artery biopsy
- Liver needle biopsy (TB, granulomata, neoplasm)
- Muscle biopsy
- Laparoscopy and laparotomy are seldom necessary since the advent of modern scanning

Go back again and again to take a new history, to re-examine the relevant areas, and to repeat selected investigations, especially those which might have been performed 'too early' i.e. before they could have become abnormal.

OTHER IMPORTED PATHOGENS: NEMATODES, SCHISTOSOMES

The worms listed in table 31 are found world-wide and not uncommonly in travellers who live rough or enter areas of poor sanitation.

Table 31. Worms commonly found in areas of poor sanitation

Worm	Major clinical features	Treatment
Threadworm (*Enterobius vermicularis*)	Anal itch Worm on stool	Piperazine Thiabendazole (treat all household members to prevent reinfection)
Roundworm (*Ascaris lumbricoides*)	Worm on stool	Piperazine
Hookworm (*Necator americanus; Ancylostoma duodenale*)	Nil. If severe infection, iron-deficient anaemia; malnutrition in children. Eggs or worms in stools	Bephenium (Alcopar) Pyrantel Tetrachloroethylene
Schistosoma 1. *S. mansoni* (spur on side) 2. *S. haematobium* (spur on tail)	Fever and eosinophilia Initially diarrhoea Haematuria	Oxamniquine Metriphonate Praziquantel (for both)

SEPTICAEMIA (bacteriaemia)

Traditionally this is classified as Gram positive, Gram negative or unknown. In practice bacteriaemia occurs most often postoperatively. Less commonly patients are admitted from home with suspected bacteriaemia often without an obvious source or site of infection (see table 32).

Post-operative bacteriaemia

The clinical features are of fever, often swinging and with rigors, and later hypotension and oliguria. The major differential diagnosis of postoperative shock is pulmonary embolism.

Management

General measures include good nursing care and fluid and electrolyte balance, and in severe cases intensive therapy including treatment of shock and renal failure.

Table 32.   Septicaemia: guidelines to therapy

(a)   *Postoperative*
1   Drain pus.
2   Expert supportive or intensive care:
  (a)   Fluids
  (b)   Electrolytes
  (c)   Urine output and renal failure
  (d)   Shock
  (e)   DIC
3   Treat infection with antibiotics.

Operation site	Likely organism	Antibiotics of choice ('Blind therapy' while awaiting cultures)
Gastrointestinal	Coliforms and anaerobes	Gentamicin, metronidazole plus ampicillin (ampicillin plus gentamicin for *Strep. faecalis*)
Hepatobiliary	Coliforms and *Strep. faecalis*	Gentamicin plus ampicillin
Urinary	Coliforms	Ampicillin and gentamicin or cefotaxime
Gynaecoclogical	Staphylococci (skin) and anaerobes (vagina)	Flucloxacillin and metronidazole (augmentin for minor infection)
Cardiothoracic/CNS	Staphylococci (skin)	Flucloxacillin

(b)   *Off the streets* (differential diagnosis influenza, or malaria in travellers)
1   Observe for site of infection:
  • Throat
  • Leg ulcer
  • Wound
  • History of urinary or chest infection
  • Rash—drugs, virus, staphylococcus/streptococcus
  • Hidden infection—ENT and teeth, pelvis, liver, kidney
2   Urgent investigation:
  • WBC
  • CXR
  • Urine examination and culture
  • Blood cultures (± stool)
  • Ultrasound of liver and kidney for abscesses
3   Management:
  • Drain pus if present
  • General expert supportive or intensive care
  • Antibiotic therapy:

Table 32. (Continued)

Site of infection	Likely organism	Antibiotics of choice
Skin	Staphylococci, (± toxic shock syndrome) β-haemolytic Strep.	Flucloxacillin
Gynaecological (vaginitis, abortion)	E. coli anaerobes, Strep. faecalis, Clostridia, Staph., Strep. (coliforms and Strep. faecilis)	Penicillin and gentamicin and metronidazole (anaerobes)
Nil obvious	Probably Staph. or Strep.	Flucloxacillin
	Abscess:	
	Liver (Strep. milleri	Drain plus penicillin
	Amoebae)	Drain plus metronidazole
	Biliary (E. coli and Strep. faecalis)	Gentamicin plus ampicillin
	Renal (E. coli and Strep. faecalis)	Gentamicin plus ampicillin

NB *Shocked patients:*
- Monitor right atrial pressure (+ 8–10 cm H_2O) and maintain circulating volume.
- Monitor left atrial pressure (pulmonary artery flow catheter)
- Inotropes (dopamine, dobutamine)
- Monitor urine output and renal function—dialysis may be required.
- Treat DIC.

NB *Antibiotic choice:*
- Always seek expert microbiological advice as choice and dosage alters with changing character of organisms
- Use i.v. therapy initially to guarantee adequate blood levels

Special measures. A wound abscess is often the site of infection and obvious pus must be drained. This may result in a rapid fall in temperature and obviate the need for antibiotics.

The choice of antibiotic depends upon the organism grown from the wound or blood. If the patient's condition demands that treatment must be started before microbiological cultures are available, the site type of operation allows a best guess at the likely organism. The choice of antibiotic depends in turn upon the likely organism and local knowledge of antibiotic sensitivities (see table 29, pages 374–375).

The key management points are:

1 Drain pus.
2 Antibiotics (see table 29 for appropriate choice).
3 Expert nursing care.
4 Fluid balance and monitor renal function.

If the patient is shocked:

5 Treat hypovolaemia with plasma or equivalent.
6 Give expert intensive care monitoring:
   (a) renal function and fluid balance
   (b) right atrial pressure
   (c) left atrial pressure (pulmonary artery flow catheter).
7 Inotropes—dopamine to increase pumping efficiency for hypotension and

increased renal blood flow. Dopamine will also cause arteriole relaxation to reduce afterload if systemic vascular resistance is high.

8 Treat disseminated intravascular coagulation (DIC) by replacing deficient blood factors as measured. The presence of DIC indicates a poor prognosis, and the best means of treatment remains uncertain. Endotoxin triggers both extrinsic and intrinsic coagulation systems leading to consumption of coagulation factors and in turn to the widespread bleeding of DIC. Preventing the triggering mechanism (e.g. with tumour necrosis factor monoclonal antibodies) may form the basis of future treatment.

NB Steroids are not of proven value in septicaemic shock unless there is associated adrenal damage (short synacthen test).

INFECTIONS IN THE IMMUNOCOMPROMISED

Immune suppression is seen most often in patients with leukaemia, lymphoma, myeloma and following transplantation and results from a combination of the disease and/or the drugs used to treat them. The picture is of recurrent infections often with organisms which otherwise rarely cause infection (see pneumonia page 291, myeloma page 364 and leukaemia page 362). Mortality is high and investigation and treatment must not be delayed.

• AIDS is the other important cause (page 384).

• Rarely increased susceptibility to pneumococcal septicaemia may follow splenectomy and is most common in young children. It can be prevented by immunization.

• The very rare susceptibility to staphycoccal septicaemia following chicken pox is probably the result of impaired neutrophil function.

Investigation

Initially the most useful urgent tests are the WBC for lymphocytosis, or neutrophilia, urine for protein and microscopy and a chest X-ray as signs of consolidation may be sparse and easily missed despite obvious radiological abnormalities. Blood cultures should be set up at the same time. If the site of infection remains obscure, ultrasound or radioactive scan of the liver may reveal an abscess—rare but treatable. Renal and biliary abscesses are much less common.

General and specific measures of management are the same as for septicaemia. Antibiotic therapy is often required before the results of blood cultures and sensitivities are known, and choice is guided by knowing the likely organism(s).

AIDS (acquired immune deficiency syndrome)

This follows infection with the human immune deficiency virus (HIV). This disorder of T-cell mediated immunity is most common in homosexuals with many partners, and drug addicts who inject the agent. It has occurred in haemophiliacs given infected cryoprecipitate and has been transmitted during childbirth similarly to hepatitis B. Diagnosis of infection is confirmed by detection of antibodies to HIV. Blood specimens should be handled in the same way as those from cases suspected of hepatitis B infection. Patients present with fever, weight loss, fatigue and generalised persistent lymphadenopathy. There is a greatly increased risk of Kaposi's sarcoma of the skin and other uncommon lymphomas. Opportunistic infections become common. Infection with *Pneumocystis pneumoniae* is the most common, but tuberculosis and virus infections particularly cytomegalovirus; herpes simplex and herpes zoster occur as do fungal infections with *Aspergillus, Cryptococcus,* and *Monilia.* Diffuse toxoplasmosis, particularly cerebral, also occurs. Chronic persistent diarrhoea is a debilitating complication often caused by infection with *Cryptosporidium.*

Communicable Diseases Centre (CDC) Atlanta classification

Group I   Acute seroconversion illness
Group II   Asymptomatic infection
Group III   Persistent generalised lymphadenopathy
Group IV   AIDS related complex (ARC) and AIDS subgroup

(a)   ARC (constitutional disease)
(b)   Neurological disease
(c)   Opportunistic infection
(d)   Secondary cancers
(e)   Other conditions

The mortality of AIDS is over 50% and the underlying condition appears to be incurable. Treatment is with azidothymidine (AZT) which prolongs life and occasionally gives greatly improved general health, gancyclovir, and Foscarnet (see table 33). Pneumocystisis responds to cotrimoxazole and recurrence is prevented by regular inhalations of pentamidine.

Drugs used in AIDS

The likely opportunistic infections and therapy of choice are shown in table 33. Of these gancyclovir, Foscarnet in addition to zidovudine have a special role in the treatment of AIDS and its complications.

Table 33.   Common treatable opportunistic infection of AIDS and the therapy of choice

Common treatable opportunistic infections	Therapy of choice	Prophylaxis
Pneumocystis carinii pneumonia	Pentamidine by inhalation or Septrin	Pentamidine or Septrin
Toxoplasmic encephalitis	Pyrimethamine + Sulphadiazine	Nil
Cryptococcal meningitis	Amphotericin B + 5-flucytosine or Fluconazole	Fluconazole
Cytomegalovirus	Gancyclovir or Foscarnet	Gancyclovir or Foscarnet
Herpes simplex and zoster	Acylovir	
Mycobacterial TB	Standard TB therapy	

Gancyclovir. This analogue of thymidine is used to treat acute cytomegalovirus infection, and is currently being tried prophylactically to prevent recurrence. Gancyclovir, a prodrug, is converted to gancyclovir triphosphate within the cells, and this inhibits viral DNA polymerase. Leucopenia and thrombocytopenia are important side effects.

Foscarnet (trisodium phosphonoformate) is an alternative to gancyclovir though not yet as well tested. It acts to inhibit both human herpes virus and DNA polymerase, and also retrovirus reverse transcriptase.

AZT (azidothymidine) is used to treat patients with AIDS and those with complications prior to developing the full blown disease. It appears to increase both life quality and expectancy. It is converted in the cell to zidovudine triphosphate which acts to inhibit viral reverse transcriptase. The major adverse effects are anaemia, neutropenia and leucopenia, which are most common if the T-helper cell count is low. Nausea, myalgia and insomnia are common.

Recommended reading

Membership candidates and senior students with sufficient time should look at the recommended journals and the *Drugs and Therapeutics Bulletin* regularly. Robinson and Stott remains an excellent manual of emergency treatment. Roitt, and Zilva and Pannall are the best introductions to Immunology and Clinical Biochemistry respectively. When exhaustion and boredom make further formal study impossible, selected articles from the two annuals, *Symposium on Advanced Medicine* and *Advances in Internal Medicine*, will come as light relief and may even add a hint of interest. All other titles are reference books which we have found useful from time to time. They are expensive and should be held in all medical lending libraries. If, as is often the case, a reference book fails to answer your specific question, we suggest that you do as we do; ask a Senior Registrar.

Journals
Leading articles and annotations in the *Lancet, British Medical Journal* and *New England Journal of Medicine*.
Quarterly Journal of Medicine.
Hospital Update.
Medicine–monthly add-on series.
British Journal of Hospital Medicine.

General texts
Braunwald, E. et al. eds. (1987) *Harrison's Principles of Internal Medicine*, 11th edn. McGraw-Hill, New York.

Comprehensive textbooks
Wyngaarden J.B. & Smith L.H. eds (1988) *Cecil's Textbook of Medicine*, 18th edn. W.B. Saunders, Philadelphia.
Weatherall D.J., Ledingham J.G.G. & Warrell D.A. eds (1987) *Oxford Textbook of Medicine, 2nd edn*. Oxford University Press, Oxford.

Special texts
Robinson R.O. & Stott R. (1987) *Medical Emergencies*, 5th edn. Heinemann, London.
Advances in Internal Medicine (annually). Year Book Medical Publications, Chicago.
Symposium on Advanced Medicine (annually). Pitman, London.

Specialist texts

Chest disease
Seaton A. Seaton D. & Leitch A.G. (1989) *Crofton and Douglas's*

Respiratory Diseases (4th edn). Blackwell Scientific Publications, Oxford.

Cardiology

Braunwald E.: (1988) *Heart Disease—A Textbook of Cardiovascular Medicine,* 3rd edn. W. B. Saunders, Philadelphia.

Julian D. G. (1989) *Disease of the Heart.* Baillière-Tindall, London.

Hurst, J. W. (1986) *The Heart,* 6th edn. McGraw-Hill, New York.

Schamroth L. (1990) *An Introduction to Electrocardiography,* 7th edn Blackwell Scientific Publications, Oxford.

Endocrinology

Hall R. & Besser M. (1989) *Fundamentals of Clinical Endocrinology,* 4th edn. Pitman, London.

Diabetes

Tattersall R. B. Gale A.M. (1989) *Diabetes. Clinical Management.* Churchill Livingstone, Edinburgh.

Kidney Disease

Strauss M.B. & Welt L.G. (1979) *Diseases of the Kidney,*   3rd edn. Williams and Wilkins, Baltimore.

Sweny P., Farrington, K. & Moorhead, J. F. (1989) *The Kidney and its Disorders.* Blackwell Scientific Publications, Oxford.

Gastroenterology and liver disease

Sherlock S. (1989) *Diseases of the Liver and Biliary System,* 8th edn. Blackwell Scientific Publications, Oxford.

Sleisenger M.H. & Fordtran J.S. (1988) *Gastrointestinal Disease,* 4th edn. W.B. Saunders, Philadelphia.

Haematology

Firkin, F. Chestermann, C. Penington D. & Rush B. (1989) *de Gruchy's Clinical Haematology in Medical Practice.* 5th edn. Blackwell Scientific Publications, Oxford.

Hoffbrand A.V. & Pettit J.E. (1984) *Essential Haematology,* 2nd edn. Blackwell Scientific Publications, Oxford.

Immunology

Roitt I.M. (1988) *Essential Immunology,* 6th edn. Blackwell Scientific Publications, Oxford.

Dermatology

Hunter J.A.A., Savin J.A. & Dahl M.V. (1989) *Clinical Dermatology.* Blackwell Scientific Publications, Oxford.

Marks R. (1984) *Practical Problems in Dermatology.* VCH Publishers, Cambridge.

Rook, A.,Wilkinson D.S.,Ebling F.J.G., Champion H. & Burton J.L. (1986) *Textbook of Dermatology,* 4th edn. Blackwell Scientific Publications, Oxford.

Neurology

Adams R.D. & Victor M. (1977) *Principles of Neurology.* McGraw-Hill, New York.

Bickerstaff E.R. & Spillane J.A. (1989) *Neurological Examination in Clinical Practice*, 5th edn. Blackwell Scientific Publications, Oxford.

Patten, J.P. (1983) *Neurological Differential Diagnosis: an Illustrated Approach.* Harold Stark Ltd, London.

Psychiatry

Gelder M. *et al.* (1983) *Oxford Textbook of Psychiatry.* Oxford University Press, Oxford.

Rees W.L. (1982) *A Short Textbook of Psychiatry*, 3rd edn. Hodder & Stoughton, London.

Rose N. ed (1988) *Essential Psychiatry.* Blackwell Scientific Publications, Oxford.

Rheumatology

Mason M. & Currey H.L.F. (1986) *Introduction to Clinical Rheumatology*, 3rd edn. Pitman, London.

Radiology

Armstrong P. & Wastie M.L. (1987) *Diagnostic Imaging*, 2nd edn. Blackwell Scientific Publications, Oxford.

Dixon A.K. (1983) *Body CT.* Churchill Livingstone, Edinburgh.

Infectious diseases

Hoeprick P.D. & Jordan M.C. (1989) *Infectious Diseases*, 4th edn. J. B. Lippincott, Philadelphia.

Mandell, G.L. *et al.* eds (1989) *Principles and Practice of Infectious Diseases*, 3rd edn. Churchill Livingstone, Edinburgh.

Pharmacology and therapeutics

British National Formulary, current issue. British Medical Association and The Pharmaceutical Press, London.

Gilman A.G., Goodman L.S. & Gilman A. eds (1980) *The Pharmacological Basis of Therapeutics*, 7th edn. Collier-Macmillan, London.

Martindale's Extra Pharmacopoeia (1982) 28th edn. Pharmaceutical Press, London.

Drugs and Therapeutics Bulletin.

Statistics

Bland M. (1987) *An Introduction to Medical Statistics.* Oxford University Press, Oxford.

Clinical biochemistry

Zilva J.F. & Pannall P.R. (1984) *Clinical Chemistry in Diagnosis and Treatment*, 4th edn. Lloyd-Luke, London.

SI units conversion table

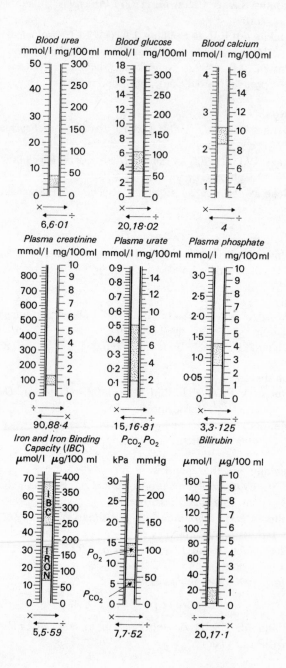

Figures in italics give the exact conversion factor, those in roman give a rough approximation. Shaded areas indicate norms.

Index